OVERVI

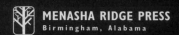

MENASHA RIDGE PRESS
Birmingham, Alabama

60 HIKES WITHIN 60 MILES

SAN FRANCISCO

INCLUDING **NORTH BAY**,
EAST BAY, PENINSULA,
and **SOUTH BAY**

THIRD EDITION

JANE HUBER

60 HIKES WITHIN 60 MILES: SAN FRANCISCO

Copyright © 2013 Jane Huber
All rights reserved
Printed in the United States of America
Published by Menasha Ridge Press
Distributed by Publishers Group West
Third edition, second printing 2014
ISBN-13: 978-0-89732-508-0; eISBN 978-0-89732-509-7

Cataloging-in-Publication Data is available from the Library of Congress.

Editor: Ritchey Halphen
Cover design and cartography: Scott McGrew
Text design: Steveco International
Cover and interior photos: Jane Huber except where noted on-page
Proofreader: Julie Hall Bosché
Indexer: Ann Cassar / Cassar Technical Services

MENASHA RIDGE PRESS
P.O. Box 43673
Birmingham, Alabama 35243
menasharidge.com

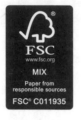 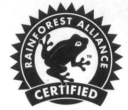

DISCLAIMER

This book is meant only as a guide to select trails in the San Francisco area and does not guarantee hiker safety—you hike at your own risk. Neither Menasha Ridge Press nor Jane Huber is liable for property loss or damage, personal injury, or death that may result from accessing or hiking the trails described in this guide. Be especially cautious when walking in potentially hazardous terrains with, for example, steep inclines or drop-offs. Do not attempt to explore terrain that may be beyond your abilities. Please read carefully the introduction to this book, as well as safety information from other sources. Familiarize yourself with current weather reports and maps of the area you plan to visit (in addition to the maps provided in this guidebook). Be cognizant of park regulations, and always follow them. While every effort has been made to ensure the accuracy of the information in this guidebook, land and road conditions, phone numbers and websites, and other information can change from year to year.

FOR JACK
—J. H.

TABLE OF CONTENTS

ACKNOWLEDGMENTS

THANKS ONCE AGAIN to all the Bay Area Hikers who generously shared trail conditions and observations. Special kudos to Jim Bahn, Raj Hajela, Russell Melick, and Greg Monaghan for their expert fact-checking.

I've been lucky to once again work with Ritchey Halphen—his editing expertise and humor make the publishing process pleasant and easy. Cheers to everyone at Menasha Ridge Press for their support, and a tip of the map to Scott McGrew for his fine cartography.

My husband, Hans Huber, has always been my biggest supporter and continues to help me whenever and however I need him. Our son, Jack, is a determined and tough hiker who warms my heart with his love of nature; it is to him and the children of his generation that this book is dedicated.

—*Jane Huber*

FOREWORD

WELCOME TO MENASHA RIDGE PRESS'S *60 Hikes within 60 Miles,* a series designed to provide hikers with the information they need to find and hike the very best trails surrounding large metropolitan areas.

Our strategy is simple: First, find a hiker who knows the area and loves to hike. Second, ask that person to spend a year researching the most popular and very best trails around. And third, have that person describe each trail in terms of difficulty, scenery, condition, elevation change, and other categories of information that are important to hikers. "Pretend you've just completed a hike and met up with other hikers at the trailhead," we told each author. "Imagine their questions, and be clear in your answers."

An experienced hiker and writer, Jane Huber has selected 60 of the best hikes in and around the San Francisco metropolitan area. From greenways and urban hikes that make use of parklands to flora- and fauna-rich treks along the cliffs and hills in the hinterlands, Jane provides hikers (and walkers) with a great variety of hikes—and all within roughly 60 miles of San Francisco.

You'll get the most from this book if you take a moment to read the Introduction, which explains how to read the trail listings. The "Topographic Maps" section will help you understand how useful topos are on a hike, and will also tell you where to get them. And though this is a where-to rather than a how-to guide, readers who haven't hiked extensively will find the Introduction of particular value.

As much to free the spirit as to free the body, let these hikes elevate you above the urban fray.

All the best,
The Editors at Menasha Ridge Press

ABOUT THE AUTHOR

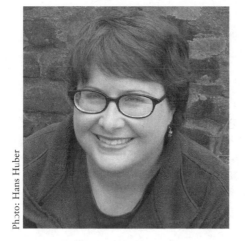

Photo: Hans Huber

JANE HUBER grew up roaming the rural back roads of northern New Jersey. After graduating from Boston University, she moved to New York City to pursue a publishing career. Dazzled by a visit to San Francisco, she soon pulled up stakes and moved west.

Once she got over the shock of driving a stick shift up and down the city's legendarily steep streets, Jane began exploring the Bay Area's parks and open spaces. She created the **Bay Area Hiker** website (**bahiker.com**) in 1999 to share her love of region's natural beauty. A freelance writer and photographer, Jane enjoys volunteering at open-space preserves south of the city in her spare time. She lives with her husband and son in a San Francisco neighborhood populated with hummingbirds and hawks and blessed with views of Mount Tamalpais and Mount Diablo.

PREFACE

I REMEMBER my first Bay Area hike well. On my premier trip to San Francisco, I accompanied two friends on what they promoted as a "walk on the beach." When I showed up with sandals on, they laughed and sent me back for sneakers—this was to be a walk *to* the beach. We drove across the Golden Gate Bridge, then wound uphill through woods on a tiny, curvaceous road. We finally stopped at a parking lot (Mount Tamalpais, Pantoll) and began hiking on Steep Ravine Trail.

I grew up near High Point, the tallest elevation in New Jersey (all of 1,803 feet), and I spent my youth walking along country roads and romping through rural woods. Even when I left New Jersey for six years of city living in Boston and New York, I always walked whenever possible, usually several miles daily. None of this walking had prepared me for Steep Ravine: a descending footpath plummeting through a wooded canyon, where I had to stop and rest (going downhill) because my quads were quivering. I marveled at the foreign scenery—unknown tall trees and lush shrubs—and was suitably impressed by the throngs of happy people on the trail, but in no way did the experience pique my interest in hiking.

I eventually got the nerve to pull up stakes and move to San Francisco, and a few years later a stray impulse triggered an interest in hiking. Once I started, I found I couldn't stop: My passion raged like a fever. I sought out maps and devoured them, studying the contour lines and squiggling trails, awed at the possibilities. I acquired hiking boots, wildflower guides, and sunscreen. I ignored the worried pleas of friends and family who were sure I'd be stalked by psychopaths roaming the trails as I hiked alone. I began learning about the different vegetation and landscapes of the Bay Area: the rolling grassy ridges, steep-sided redwood canyons, and sunbaked hillsides covered with a curious mix of shrubs I would later learn was called chaparral. I'm still exploring today, chasing fragments

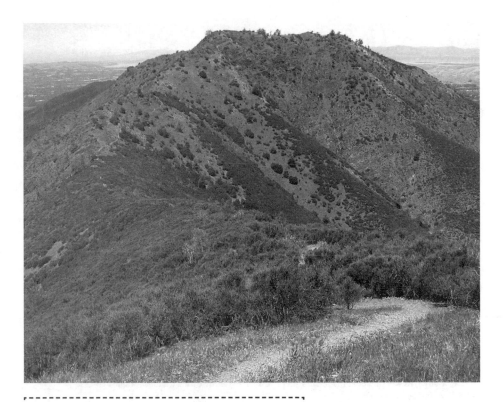

Eagle Peak Trail: an unforgettable adventure at Mount Diablo

of secondhand information about obscure trails, identifying new wildflowers, and learning to tell the difference between painted lady and American lady butterflies.

Consider yourself warned: Hiking in the Bay Area can be intense and addictive. Sure, other areas of California are home to more-esteemed landforms and parks—Yosemite is one of many world-class parks within a day's drive, and backpackers traverse the state on the Pacific Crest Trail. Throughout the Bay Area are many "destination parks," where people from all over the world flock to walk among giant redwoods or whale-watch from a wildflower-dotted coastal bluff. But there are also hundreds of smaller parks unknown to most tourists and even lifelong residents, and short drives (or in some cases bus trips, walks, or bike rides) lead to numerous parks and preserves with stunning views, bountiful wildlife, and quiet trails. These "backyard" preserves are especially beneficial to the residents of the Bay Area's most densely packed cities, San Jose, San Francisco, and Oakland. Local parks provide close-to-home outlets for daily exercise and nature exploration—thousands of people living in the foothills of Mount Tamalpais can literally walk from their front doors for miles, all the way to the top of the mountain if they like. Locals hike parks and open-space preserves bordering the towns of

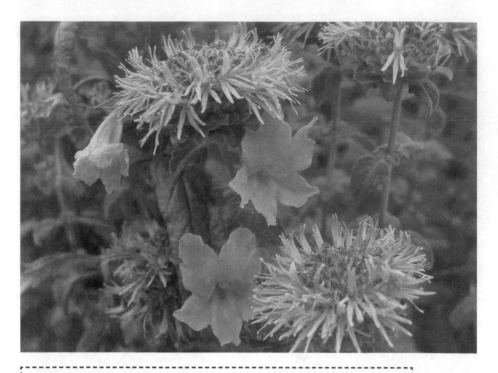

Sticky monkeyflower and coyote mint are just a few of the wildflowers that add fragrance and color to Bay Area trails.

Berkeley, Mill Valley, and Woodside daily, and they take active roles in maintaining the trails. Getting to know your backyard means getting to love your backyard—and we fight for what we love.

This dedication to open space has led many ordinary citizens in rallies to save some of our most cherished Bay Area spots. The campaign to preserve open space began in the era of John Muir, and the list of protected parklands is long and impressive. Battles continue, and development still threatens many special areas. As you make your way over trails throughout the Bay Area, think of what we could have lost and what we've already preserved: old-growth redwoods in Muir Woods saved from logging; Point Reyes National Seashore and the Marin Headlands saved from huge housing complexes; various small parks, including Edgewood, saved from development as golf courses; and many other "common" plots of land preserved to make life a little better for the surrounding community.

What difference does open space make to the Bay Area? It permits residents to depart from the edge of a suburban development onto a path climbing a hillside peppered with wildflowers, where butterflies and damselflies flutter. It beckons hikers off bustling city streets to a park where bobcat prints mark the trail, hawks perch in hundred-year-old oaks, and salmon spawn in clear, cold creeks. It draws nature-lovers from all over the world to redwood canyons so majestic that some find themselves overwhelmed with emotion. These preserved lands will stand long after we're gone, and although the tallest trees will eventually fall, a new generation of saplings will find a protected home in these parks, where manzanitas will put forth sweet-smelling blossoms yearly, mountain lions will roam with stealth and grace, and carpets of wildflowers will bloom whether anyone sees them or not.

Take care of these parks and preserves and treat nature with reverence—you will be handsomely rewarded with lifetime memories. I think of all I've experienced in less than 20 years of hiking Bay Area trails: whales lumbering through the waters off Point Reyes's Chimney Rock; the soft sound of raindrops pattering through woods at Castle Rock; a bobcat close enough to pet, transfixed at the edge of a lake at Skyline Ridge; a coyote stepping out of the woods, then vanishing back into the trees on the high slopes of Mount Tam; fresh drifts of snow covering soaring Douglas-firs after an unusual Bay Area winter storm along Skyline Boulevard; dazzling flowers everywhere, so many incredible springtime displays that I often felt giddy from the splendor.

We never made it all the way to the beach that fateful day, but I've been back to Steep Ravine since. I now know the plants that line the trail and the creatures that roam the woods, and I sometimes utter their names under my breath in passing, as if greeting old friends. My fingers lightly linger on blossoms of trillium, hound's tongue, and violet; trail over the shaggy bark on redwoods and Douglas-fir; and caress the smooth trunks of aromatic bay. I watch the silent flutter of a buckeye butterfly and the slow, languid crawl of a banana slug. Unseen mammals who creep about at night have left their calling cards, and I look for coyote scat at the trail junctions and raccoon footprints in mud along the creek.

The hike through Steep Ravine to Stinson Beach, combined with a return ascent through Douglas-fir woods and the high grassy ridges of Mount Tam, is one of the hikes I've included in this book. It's an incredible trek that highlights the best of Bay Area hiking—easy access from San Francisco, a variety of vegetation, and a sense of peacefulness weaving through a wild landscape.

Whether you hike for exercise, for nature study, or in companionship with others, San Francisco Bay Area trails are incredibly diverse and beautiful. I hope you'll delight in discovering these parks and preserves.

60 HIKES BY CATEGORY

HIKE CATEGORIES		
★ < 3 miles	★ > 6 miles	✓ kid-friendly
★ 3–6 miles	★ configuration	✓ dogs allowed
DIFFICULTY		
ıll = easy	ıll = moderate	ıll = strenuous
CONFIGURATION		
B = balloon / F8 = figure eight	L = loop	OB = out-and-back / S = spiral

REGION Hike Number/Hike Name	page	< 3 miles	3–6 miles	> 6 miles	configuration	kid-friendly	dogs allowed
NORTH BAY							
1 Angel Island State Park	16		ıll		B	✓	
2 Annadel State Park	20			ıll*	F8		
3 China Camp State Park	25		ıll		L		
4 Jack London State Historic Park	30		ıll		OB		
5 Marin Headlands	34	ıll			B	✓	
6 Mt. Burdell Open Space Preserve	39	ıll			B		✓
7 Mt. Tamalpais: Cataract Falls–Potrero Meadows Loop	44		ıll*		L		
8 Mt. Tamalpais: Matt Davis–Steep Ravine Loop	49		ıll		L		
9 Mt. Tamalpais: Mountain Home–Muir Woods Loop	54		ıll		L	✓	
10 Mt. Tamalpais: Phoenix Lake	59		ıll		B		✓
11 Point Reyes National Seashore: Bear Valley to Arch Rock	64			ıll	OB	✓	

Mixed difficulty (e.g., mostly easy with moderate sections)

REGION Hike Number/Hike Name	page	< 3 miles	3-6 miles	> 6 miles	configuration	kid-friendly	dogs allowed
NORTH BAY *(continued)*							
12 Point Reyes National Seashore: Estero to Drakes Bay	68			▮▮▮	OB	✓	
13 Point Reyes National Seashore: Tomales Point	72			▮▮▮	OB	✓	
14 Ring Mountain Open Space Preserve	76	▮▮▮			B	✓	✓
15 Robert Louis Stevenson State Park	80			▮▮▮	OB		
16 Samuel P. Taylor State Park	84			▮▮▮	B	✓	
17 Skyline Wilderness Park	89		▮▮▮		B		
18 Sugarloaf Ridge State Park	94			▮▮▮	L	✓	
19 Tomales Bay State Park	100	▮▮▮			L	✓	
EAST BAY							
20 Anthony Chabot Regional Park	106		▮▮▮		L		✓
21 Black Diamond Mines Regional Preserve	110		▮▮▮*		L	✓	✓
22 Briones Regional Park	115		▮▮▮		B	✓	✓
23 Coyote Hills Regional Park	119		▮▮▮		L	✓	
24 Huckleberry Botanic Regional Preserve	124	▮▮▮			L	✓	
25 Las Trampas Regional Wilderness	128		▮▮▮		L		✓
26 Los Vaqueros Watershed	132		▮▮▮		B	✓	
27 Mission Peak Regional Preserve	136			▮▮▮	OB		✓
28 Morgan Territory Regional Preserve	139		▮▮▮		L		✓
29 Mt. Diablo State Park: Donner Canyon Waterfall Loop	142		▮▮▮		B		
30 Mt. Diablo State Park: Mary Bowerman Trail	146	▮▮▮			L	✓	
31 Mt. Diablo State Park: Mitchell Canyon–Eagle Peak Loop	150			▮▮▮	L		
32 Redwood Regional Park	155		▮▮▮		L	✓	✓
33 Round Valley Regional Preserve	158		▮▮▮		L	✓	
34 Sunol Regional Wilderness	162		▮▮▮		L		✓
35 Tilden Regional Park	168		▮▮▮		OB	✓	✓

REGION Hike Number/Hike Name	page	< 3 miles	3–6 miles	> 6 miles	configuration	kid-friendly	dogs allowed
PENINSULA AND SOUTH BAY							
36 Almaden Quicksilver County Park	174			▪	B		✓
37 Año Nuevo State Park	178		▪		B	✓	
38 Big Basin Redwoods State Park: Waterfall Loop	182			▪	L		
Castle Rock State Park	187		▪		F8	✓	
Edgewood County Park and Natural Preserve	192		▪		B	✓	
Henry Cowell Redwoods State Park	196		▪		F8	✓	
42 Henry W. Coe State Park	200		▪		L		
43 Joseph D. Grant County Park	204			▪	B		
44 Montara Mountain	209			▪	B	✓	
45 Monte Bello Open Space Preserve	214			▪	L	✓	
46 Portola Redwoods State Park	219			▪	L		
47 Pulgas Ridge Open Space Preserve	224	▪			L	✓	✓
48 Purisima Creek Redwoods Open Space Preserve	228			▪	L		
49 Rancho San Antonio Open Space Preserve	232			▪*	F8	✓	
50 Russian Ridge Open Space Preserve	237		▪		B	✓	
51 San Bruno Mountain State and County Park	241		▪		L	✓	
52 Sierra Azul Open Space Preserve	245		▪		OB	✓	
53 Skyline Ridge Open Space Preserve	249		▪		L	✓	
54 Sweeney Ridge	254		▪*		OB	✓	✓
55 Uvas Canyon County Park	258		▪		B	✓	✓
56 Windy Hill Open Space Preserve	263			▪	L		
CITY OF SAN FRANCISCO							
57 Golden Gate Park: Stow Lake	270	▪			S	✓	✓
58 Lands End	274	▪			OB	✓	✓
59 Mt. Davidson	278	▪			B	✓	✓
60 The Presidio: Batteries to Bluffs Trail	283	▪			OB	✓	

Mixed difficulty

HIKE CATEGORIES

✓ public transit	✓ wildlife	✓ wildflowers	✓ redwoods
✓ good for runners	✓ scenic views	✓ waterfalls	

REGION / Hike Number/Hike Name	page	public transit	wildlife	wildflowers	redwoods	good for runners	scenic views	waterfalls
NORTH BAY								
1 Angel Island State Park	16	✓		✓			✓	
2 Annadel State Park	20		✓	✓				
3 China Camp State Park	25			✓		✓		
4 Jack London State Historic Park	30			✓				
5 Marin Headlands	34	✓					✓	✓
6 Mt. Burdell Open Space Preserve	39			✓				
7 Mt. Tamalpais: Cataract Falls–Potrero Meadows Loop	44			✓	✓			✓
8 Mt. Tamalpais: Matt Davis–Steep Ravine Loop	49	✓		✓	✓		✓	✓
9 Mt. Tamalpais: Mountain Home–Muir Woods Loop	54	✓			✓			✓
10 Mt. Tamalpais: Phoenix Lake	59			✓		✓		
11 Point Reyes National Seashore: Bear Valley to Arch Rock	64	✓					✓	
12 Point Reyes National Seashore: Estero to Drakes Bay	68						✓	
13 Point Reyes National Seashore: Tomales Point	72		✓	✓			✓	
14 Ring Mountain Open Space Preserve	76			✓			✓	
15 Robert Louis Stevenson State Park	80						✓	

REGION Hike Number/Hike Name	page	public transit	wildlife	wildflowers	redwoods	good for runners	scenic views	waterfalls
NORTH BAY *(continued)*								
Samuel P. Taylor State Park	84			✓			✓	✓
7 Skyline Wilderness Park	89			✓				
8 Sugarloaf Ridge State Park	94			✓			✓	
9 Tomales Bay State Park	100						✓	
EAST BAY								
Anthony Chabot Regional Park	106			✓				
Black Diamond Mines Regional Preserve	110			✓				
2 Briones Regional Park	115			✓		✓		
3 Coyote Hills Regional Park	119					✓	✓	
4 Huckleberry Botanic Regional Preserve	124			✓				
25 Las Trampas Regional Wilderness	128			✓		✓	✓	
26 Los Vaqueros Watershed	132	✓		✓			✓	
Mission Peak Regional Preserve	136	✓					✓	
8 Morgan Territory Regional Preserve	139			✓				
Mt. Diablo State Park: Donner Canyon Waterfall Loop	142			✓			✓	✓
Mt. Diablo State Park: Mary Bowerman Trail	146						✓	
31 Mt. Diablo State Park: Mitchell Canyon–Eagle Peak Loop	150			✓			✓	
2 Redwood Regional Park	155				✓			
3 Round Valley Regional Preserve	158		✓					
34 Sunol Regional Wilderness	162			✓			✓	
5 Tilden Regional Park	168					✓		
PENINSULA AND SOUTH BAY								
36 Almaden Quicksilver County Park	174			✓				
37 Año Nuevo State Park	178		✓					
38 Big Basin Redwoods State Park: Waterfall Loop	182				✓			✓
39 Castle Rock State Park	187			✓			✓	✓

REGION Hike Number/Hike Name	page	public transit	wildlife	wildflowers	redwoods	good for runners	scenic views	waterfalls
PENINSULA AND SOUTH BAY *(continued)*								
40 Edgewood County Park and Natural Preserve	192		✓			✓		
41 Henry Cowell Redwoods State Park	196				✓			
42 Henry W. Coe State Park	200		✓				✓	
43 Joseph D. Grant County Park	204		✓				✓	
44 Montara Mountain	209	✓					✓	✓
45 Monte Bello Open Space Preserve	214		✓				✓	
46 Portola Redwoods State Park	219				✓			✓
47 Pulgas Ridge Open Space Preserve	224		✓			✓		
48 Purisima Creek Redwoods Open Space Preserve	228				✓			
49 Rancho San Antonio Open Space Preserve	232	✓	✓			✓		
50 Russian Ridge Open Space Preserve	237		✓			✓	✓	
51 San Bruno Mountain State and County Park	241		✓				✓	
52 Sierra Azul Open Space Preserve	245		✓			✓	✓	
53 Skyline Ridge Open Space Preserve	249		✓			✓	✓	
54 Sweeney Ridge	254		✓				✓	
55 Uvas Canyon County Park	258				✓			✓
56 Windy Hill Open Space Preserve	263		✓				✓	
CITY OF SAN FRANCISCO								
57 Golden Gate Park: Stow Lake	270	✓				✓		
58 Lands End	274	✓					✓	✓
59 Mt. Davidson	278	✓					✓	
60 The Presidio: Batteries to Bluffs Trail	283	✓		✓			✓	✓

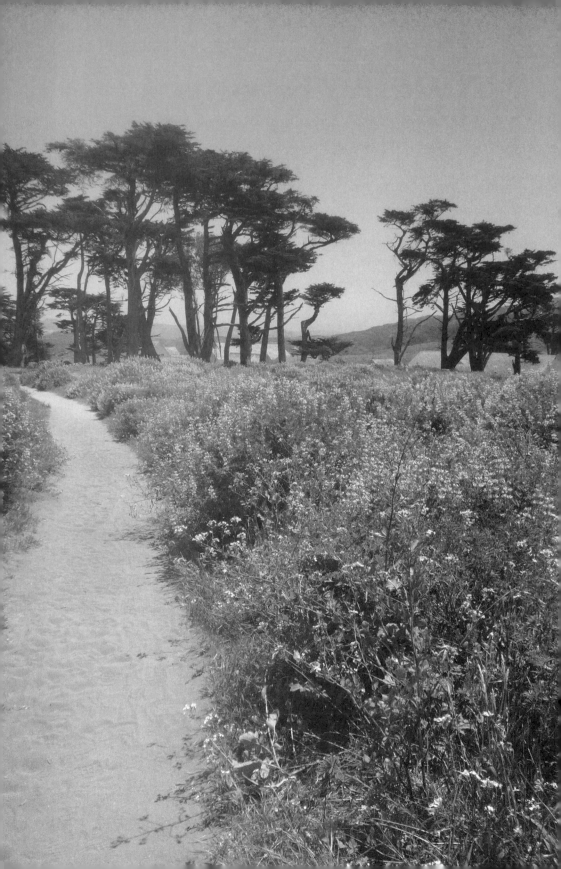

INTRODUCTION

WELCOME TO *60 Hikes within 60 Miles: San Francisco.* If you're new to hiking or even if you're a seasoned trailsmith, take a few minutes to read the following pages. They explain how this book is organized and how to use it.

HOW TO USE THIS GUIDEBOOK

OVERVIEW MAP, MAP KEY, AND MAP LEGEND

The overview map on the inside front cover shows the primary trailheads for all 60 hikes. The numbers on the overview map pair with the key on the facing page. A legend explaining the map symbols used throughout the book appears on the inside back cover.

REGIONAL MAPS

The book is divided into regions, and prefacing each regional section is an overview map. The regional maps provide more detail than the overview map, bringing you closer to the hikes.

TRAIL MAPS

In addition to the overview map on the inside cover, a detailed map of each hike's route appears with its profile. On each of these maps, symbols indicate the trailhead, the complete route, significant features, facilities, and topographic landmarks such as creeks, overlooks, and peaks.

To produce the highly accurate maps in this book, I used a handheld GPS unit to gather data while hiking each route, then sent that data to Menasha Ridge Press's expert cartographers. Be aware, though, that your GPS device is no substitute for sound, sensible navigation that takes into account the conditions that you observe while hiking.

« Towering cypresses at Tomales Point

Further, despite the high quality of the maps in this guidebook, I strongly recommend that you always carry an additional map, such as the ones noted in "Maps" in each hike's Key At-a-Glance Information.

ELEVATION PROFILES

Each hike contains a detailed elevation profile that corresponds directly to the trail map. This graphical element provides a quick look at the trail from the side, enabling you to visualize how the trail rises and falls. On the diagram's vertical axis, or height scale, the number of feet indicated between each tick mark lets you visualize the climb. To avoid making flat hikes look steep and steep hikes appear flat, varying height scales provide an accurate image of each hike's climbing challenge. Elevation profiles for loop hikes show total distance; those for out-and-back hikes show only one-way distance.

GPS INFORMATION

As noted in "Trail Maps," on the previous page, I used a handheld GPS unit to obtain geographic data and sent the information to the cartographers at Menasha Ridge. Provided for each hike profile, the GPS coordinates—the intersection of latitude (north) and longitude (west)—will orient you from the trailhead. In some cases, you can park within viewing distance of a trailhead. Other hiking routes require a short walk to the trailhead from a parking area. As a complementary aid to navigation, I've also provided street addresses where appropriate.

The latitude–longitude grid system is likely quite familiar to you, but here's a refresher, pertinent to visualizing the coordinates:

Imaginary lines of latitude—called *parallels* and approximately 69 miles apart from each other—run horizontally around the globe. The equator is established to be 0°, and each parallel is indicated by degrees from the equator: up to 90°N at the North Pole, and down to 90°S at the South Pole.

Imaginary lines of longitude—called *meridians*—run perpendicular to lines of latitude and are likewise indicated by degrees. Starting from 0° at the Prime Meridian in Greenwich, England, they continue to the east and west until they meet 180° later at the International Date Line in the Pacific Ocean. At the equator, longitude lines also are approximately 69 miles apart, but that distance narrows as the meridians converge toward the North and South Poles.

In this book, latitude and longitude are expressed in degree–decimal minute format. For example, the coordinates for Hike 1, Angel Island State Park (page 16), are as follows: **N37° 52.128' W122° 26.070'**. To convert GPS coordinates given in degrees, minutes, and seconds to degrees and decimal minutes, divide the seconds by 60. For more on GPS technology, visit **usgs.gov**.

HIKE PROFILES

Each hike contains seven key items: an In Brief description of the trail, a Key At-a-Glance Information box, directions to the trail, GPS coordinates, a trail map, an elevation profile, and a trail description. Many hikes also include notes on things to see and do nearby.

IN BRIEF

A "taste of the trail." Think of this section as a snapshot focused on the historical landmarks, beautiful vistas, and other sights you may encounter on the hike.

KEY AT-A-GLANCE INFORMATION

This gives you a quick idea of the statistics and specifics of each hike:

LENGTH How long the trail is from start to finish. There may be options to shorten or extend the hikes, but the mileage corresponds to the described hike. Use the Description as a guide to customizing the hike for your ability or time constraints.

CONFIGURATION A description of what the trail might look like from overhead. Trails can be loops, out-and-backs (trails on which one enters and leaves along the same path), figure eights, or balloons. Sometimes the descriptions might surprise you.

DIFFICULTY The degree of effort an average hiker should expect on a given hike. For simplicity, the trails are rated as *easy, moderate,* or *strenuous.*

SCENERY A short summary of the hike's attractions and what to expect in terms of plant life, wildlife, natural wonders, and historic features.

EXPOSURE A quick check of how much sun you can expect on your shoulders during the hike.

TRAFFIC Indicates how busy the trail might be on an average day. Trail traffic, of course, varies from day to day and season to season.

TRAIL SURFACE Indicates whether the path is paved, rocky, gravel, dirt, board-walk, or a mixture of elements.

HIKING TIME How long it took me to hike the trail. I like to dawdle, and I can easily fritter away time watching butterflies or admiring wildflowers. On average, I cover 2 miles an hour (more mileage hiking downhill, less on steady ascents, particularly during hot weather). If you're an experienced hiker in great shape, you'll finish the hikes with time to spare, but if you're a beginner or you like to stop and smell the manzanitas, allow for a little extra.

SEASON Tells you when the trail is best experienced, to accommodate extremes in weather and/or ensure the best nature-viewing. Except where specific hours are noted, all hikes are accessible daily, sunrise–sunset.

ACCESS A listing of any required fees or permits.

MAPS Which supplementary map is the best or easiest (in my opinion) for a particular hike, and where to get it.

FACILITIES Restrooms, phones, water, and other niceties available at the trailhead or nearby.

SPECIAL COMMENTS Provides you with those little extra details that don't fit into any of the above categories. These may include insider information or special considerations about the trail, access, warnings, or ideas for enhancing your hiking experience.

CONTACTS Listed here are phone numbers and/or websites for checking trail conditions and gleaning other basic information.

DRIVING DISTANCE How far the hike is by car from a starting point given in the Directions—for example, the Golden Gate Bridge toll plaza.

DIRECTIONS

These will help you locate each trailhead. California numbers its freeway exits; when pertinent, exit numbers are included.

GPS INFORMATION

Trailhead coordinates and/or street addresses can be used in addition to the Directions if you enter the data into your GPS unit before you set out. See page 2 for more information.

DESCRIPTION

The heart of each hike, summarizing the trail's essence and highlighting any special traits the hike has to offer. The route is clearly outlined, including any landmarks, side trips, and possible alternate routes along the way. Ultimately, the Description will help you choose which hikes are best for you.

NEARBY ACTIVITIES

Not every hike has this listing, but for hikes that do, look here for information about appealing attractions in the vicinity of the trail.

WEATHER

Bay Area weather is mild, with a Mediterranean-like climate that generally ranges from the 40s to the 80s, inviting year-round hikes. Microclimates throughout the Bay Area span a wide range of temperatures and conditions, particularly in summer and winter. On a typical summer day, the weather may be clear and warm along the Sonoma coast, scorchingly hot and dry inland around Mount Diablo, and completely fogbound in San Francisco. During the rainy season, generally November–March, coastal mountains are inundated with rainfall, and the Bay Area's highest peaks are occasionally dusted with snow. City residents may go for a week without even switching on the heater. Locals learn to avoid getting caught out in weather shifts by carrying layers wherever they go, and this is a practical solution for hikers as well. Stuff a lightweight fleece jacket, one of those anoraks that compress down to nearly nothing, and a hat into your backpack, and you're generally prepared for light rain and cool snaps. Beware of fog, which commonly collects on high ridges near the coast, mostly in summer; it often blows in very quickly and can make for a nasty hike, as it completely obscures landmarks and trail junctions. A safe policy is to descend as soon as you see the fog headed your way.

Because heavy storms almost always damage trails, particularly in forested canyon parks, you should check weather conditions before you head out in winter and early spring. Trails get substantially less use in winter, but I adore hiking through forests in light rain (Castle Rock State Park in the fog is particularly enchanting). In summer, unless you prefer hot, dry heat, avoid exposed destinations in Alameda, Contra Costa, Napa, Santa Clara, and Sonoma Counties, where temperatures can soar to nearly 100 degrees. Summer is a good time to visit forested parks, particularly near the coast. Spring and autumn are the most easygoing seasons, although some parks close during high fire danger (red-flag days), until the rains begin in late fall.

MEAN TEMPERATURES BY MONTH: SAN FRANCISCO AREA						
	JAN	FEB	MAR	APR	MAY	JUN
HIGH	46°F	50°F	59°F	71°F	78°F	85°F
LOW	23°F	25°F	31°F	39°F	48°F	56°F
	JUL	AUG	SEP	OCT	NOV	DEC
HIGH	88°F	86°F	81°F	71°F	61°F	50°F
LOW	60°F	59°F	52°F	41°F	34°F	25°F

WATER

How much is enough? Well, one simple physiological fact should convince you to err on the side of excess when deciding how much water to pack: a hiker walking steadily in 90° heat needs about 10 quarts of fluid per day—that's 2.5 gallons. A good rule of thumb is to hydrate before your hike, carry (and drink) 6 ounces of water for every mile you plan to hike, and hydrate again after the hike. For most people, the pleasures of hiking make carrying water a relatively minor price to pay to remain safe and healthy, so pack more water than you anticipate needing, even for short hikes.

If you find yourself tempted to drink "found water," proceed with extreme caution. Many ponds and lakes you'll encounter are fairly stagnant, and the water tastes terrible. Drinking such water presents inherent risks for thirsty trekkers. Giardia parasites contaminate many water sources and cause the intestinal ailment giardiasis, which can last for weeks after onset. For more information, visit the Centers for Disease Control and Prevention website: **cdc.gov/parasites/giardia.**

Effective treatment is essential before you use any water source you've found along the trail. Boiling water for 2–3 minutes is always a safe measure for camping, but day hikers can consider iodine tablets, approved chemical mixes, filtration units rated for giardia, and ultraviolet filtration. Some of these methods (for example, filtration with an added carbon filter) remove bad tastes typical in stagnant water, while others add their own taste. Even if you've brought your own water, consider bringing along a means of water purification in case you've underestimated your consumption needs.

CLOTHING

Weather, unexpected trail conditions, fatigue, extended hiking duration, and wrong turns can individually or collectively turn a great outing into a very uncomfortable one at best. Some helpful guidelines:

- **Choose silk, wool, or moisture-wicking synthetics for maximum comfort in all of your hiking attire—from hats to socks and in between. Cotton is fine if the weather remains dry and stable, but you won't be happy if that fabric gets wet.**

- **Always wear a hat, or at least tuck one into your day pack or hitch it to your belt. Hats offer all-weather sun and wind protection as well as warmth if it turns cold.**

- **Be ready to layer up or down as the day progresses and the mercury rises or falls. Today's outdoor wear makes layering easy, with such designs as jackets that convert to vests and zip-off or button-up legs.**

- **Mosquitoes, poison oak, and thorny bushes found along many trails can generate short-term discomfort and long-term agony. A lightweight pair of pants and a long-sleeved shirt can go a long way toward protecting you from these pests.**

- **Wear hiking boots or sturdy hiking sandals with toe protection. Flip-flopping along a paved urban greenway is one thing, but you should never hike a trail in open sandals or casual sneakers. Your bones and arches need support, and your skin needs protection.**

- **Pair that footwear with good socks. If you prefer not to sheathe your feet when wearing hiking sandals, tuck the socks into your day pack—you may need them if temperatures plummet or if you hit rocky turf and pebbles begin to irritate your feet.**

- **Don't leave rainwear behind, even if the day dawns clear and sunny. Tuck into your day pack, or tie around your waist, a jacket that's breathable and either water-resistant or waterproof. Investigate different choices at your local outdoors retailer. If you're a frequent hiker, ideally you'll have more than one rainwear weight, material, and style in your closet to protect you in all seasons in your regional climate and hiking microclimates.**

THE TEN ESSENTIALS

One of the first rules of hiking is to be prepared for anything. The simplest way to be prepared is to carry the "Ten Essentials." In addition to carrying the items listed below, you need to know how to use them, especially navigational aids. Always consider worst-case scenarios such as getting lost, hiking back in the dark, broken gear (for example, a broken hip strap on your pack or a water filter that gets plugged), twisting an ankle, or a brutal thunderstorm. These items don't cost a lot of money, don't take up much room in a pack, and don't weigh much—but they might just save your life.

Extra food: trail mix, granola bars, or other high-energy snacks.

Extra clothes: raingear, a change of socks, and, depending on the season, a warm hat and gloves.

Flashlight or headlamp with extra bulb and batteries.

Insect repellent. For some areas and seasons, this is vital.

Maps and a high-quality compass. Don't leave home without them, even if you know the terrain well from previous hikes. As previously noted, bring maps in addition to those in this guidebook, and consult them before you hike. If you're GPS-savvy, bring that device, too, but don't rely on it as your sole navigational tool—battery life is limited, after all—and be sure to check its accuracy against that of your maps and compass.

Pocketknife and/or multitool.

Sun protection: sunglasses, lip balm, sunscreen (check the expiration date), and sun hat.

Water. Again, bring more than you think you'll drink. Depending on your destination, you may want to bring a container and iodine or a filter for purifying water in case you run out.

Whistle. It could become your best friend in an emergency.

Windproof matches and/or a lighter, as well as a fire starter.

FIRST-AID KIT

In addition to the preceding items, the ones that follow may seem daunting to carry along for a day hike. But any paramedic will tell you that the products listed here are just the basics. The reality of hiking is that you can be out for a week of backpacking and acquire only a mosquito bite . . . or you can hike for an hour, slip, and suffer a cut or broken bone. Fortunately, the items listed pack into a very small space. Convenient prepackaged kits are available at your pharmacy or online.

Ace bandages or Spenco joint wraps

Adhesive bandages

Antibiotic ointment (such as Neosporin)

Aspirin, acetaminophen (Tylenol), or ibuprofen (Advil)

Athletic tape

Blister kit (such as Moleskin or Spenco 2nd Skin)

Butterfly-closure bandages

Diphenhydramine (Benadryl), in case of allergic reactions

Epinephrine in a prefilled syringe (EpiPen), typically available by prescription only, for people known to have severe allergic reactions to hiking mishaps such as bee stings

Gauze (one roll and a half-dozen 4-by-4-inch pads)

Hydrogen peroxide or iodine

HIKING WITH CHILDREN

No one is too young for a hike in the outdoors. Be mindful, though. Flat, short, and shaded trails are best with an infant. Toddlers who haven't quite mastered walking can still tag along, riding on an adult's back in a child carrier. Use common sense to judge a youngster's capacity to hike a particular trail, and be ready for the child to tire quickly and need to be carried.

When packing for the hike, remember the child's needs as well as your own. Make sure children are adequately clothed for the weather, have proper shoes, and are protected from the sun with sunscreen. Kids dehydrate quickly, so make sure you have plenty of fluids for everyone. Hikes suitable for children are noted in the 60 Hikes by Category chart on pages xiv–xvi.

Finally, when hiking with kids, remember that the trip will be a compromise. A child's energy and enthusiasm alternate between bursts of speed and long stops to examine snails, sticks, dirt, and other attractions.

GENERAL SAFETY

While many hikers hit the trail full of enthusiasm and energy, others may find themselves feeling apprehensive about possible outdoor hazards. Although potentially dangerous situations can occur anywhere, your hike can be as safe and enjoyable as you had hoped, as long as you use sound judgment and prepare yourself before hitting the trail. Here are a few tips to make your trip safer and easier:

- **Hike with a buddy. Not only is there safety in numbers, but a hiking companion can help you if you twist an ankle on the trail or if you get lost, can assist in carrying food and water, and can be a partner in discovery. A buddy is good to bring along not only to infrequently traveled or remote areas but also to urban areas.**

- **If you're hiking alone, leave your hiking itinerary with someone you trust, and let him or her know when you return.**

- **Don't count on a mobile phone for your safety. Reception may be spotty or nonexistent on the trail, even on an urban walk—especially one embraced by towering trees.**

- **Always carry food and water, even on short hikes. Food will give you energy and sustain you in an emergency until help arrives. Bring more water than you think you'll need—we can't emphasize this enough. Hydrate throughout your hike and at regular intervals; don't wait until you feel thirsty. Treat water from a stream or other source before drinking it.**

- **Ask questions. Public-land employees are on hand to help. It's a lot easier to solicit advice before a problem occurs, and it will help you avoid a mishap away from civilization when it's too late to amend an error.**

- **Stay on designated trails. Most hikers get lost when they leave the path. Even on the most clearly marked trails, you usually reach a point where you have to stop and consider the direction in which to head. If you become** disoriented, don't panic. As soon as you think you may be off-track, stop, assess your current direction, and then retrace your steps back to the point where you went awry. Using a map, compass, and this book—and keeping in mind what you've passed thus far—reorient yourself and trust your judgment about which way to continue. If you become absolutely unsure of how to continue, return to your vehicle the way you came in. Should you become completely lost and have no idea how to return to the trailhead, remaining in place along the trail and waiting for help is most often the best option for adults and always the best option for children.

- Always carry a whistle. It may become a lifesaver if you get lost or hurt.

- Be especially careful when crossing streams. Whether you're fording the stream or crossing on a log, make every step count. If you have any doubt about maintaining your balance on a foot log, go ahead and ford the stream instead. When fording a stream, use a trekking pole or stout stick for balance and *face upstream as you cross.* If a stream seems too deep to ford, turn back. Whatever is on the other side isn't worth risking your life for.

- Be careful at overlooks. While these areas may provide spectacular views, they are potentially hazardous. Stay back from the edge of outcrops, and be absolutely sure of your footing.

- Standing dead trees and storm-damaged living trees pose a hazard to hikers and tent campers. These trees may have loose or broken limbs that could fall at any time. When choosing a spot to rest, camp, or snack, *look up.*

- Know the symptoms of heat exhaustion, or hyperthermia. Light-headedness and loss of energy are the first two indicators. If you feel these symptoms coming on, find some shade, drink your water, remove as many layers of clothing as practical, and stay put until you cool down. Marching through heat exhaustion leads to heatstroke—which can be deadly. If you should be sweating and you're not, that's the signature warning sign. If you or a companion reaches this point, your hike is over: Do whatever you can to cool down, and seek medical help immediately.

- Likewise, know the symptoms of subnormal body temperature, or hypothermia. Shivering and forgetfulness are the two most common indicators of this stealthy killer. Hypothermia can occur at any elevation, even in the summer—especially if you're wearing lightweight cotton clothing. If symptoms develop, get to shelter, hot liquids, and dry clothes ASAP.

- Most importantly, take along your brain. A cool, calculating mind is the single most important asset on the trail. Think before you act. Watch your step. Plan ahead. Avoiding accidents before they happen is the best way to ensure a rewarding and relaxing hike.

PLANT AND ANIMAL HAZARDS

Hikers should be aware of the concerns on the following pages regarding plant life and wildlife:

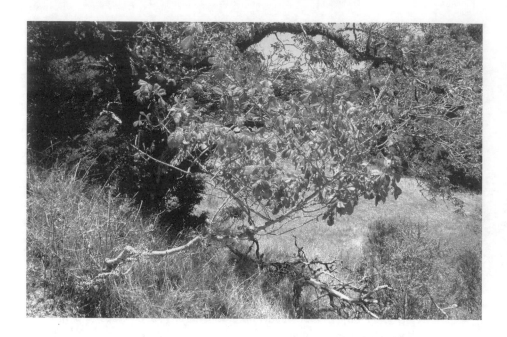

POISON OAK This deciduous plant *(above)* grows as a sparse ground cover, vine, or shrub; regardless of its form, poison oak always has three leaflets. It's easiest to spot in summer and early autumn, when the leaves flush bright-red. Beware of unknown bare-branched shrubs and vines in winter—the entire plant can cause a rash, no matter what the season.

Urushiol, the oil in the sap of the plant, is responsible for the rash. Reactions may start almost immediately or not appear until a week after exposure. Raised lines and/or blisters will appear, accompanied by a terrible itch. Try to refrain from scratching, though, because bacteria under your fingernails can cause an infection. Wash and dry the affected area thoroughly, applying calamine lotion to help dry out the rash. If the itching or blistering is severe, seek medical attention.

Most people come into contact with poison oak while bushwhacking or traveling off-trail, so stay on established trails whenever possible. If you do knowingly touch the plant, you must remove the oil within 15–20 minutes to avoid a reaction. Rinsing off the oil with cool water—hot water spreads it—is impractical on the trail, but some commercial products such as Tecnu are effective in removing urushiol from your skin. To keep from spreading the misery to someone else, wash not only any exposed parts of your body but also any oil-contaminated clothes, hiking gear, and pets.

SNAKES The most common snakes you'll encounter along Bay Area trails are non-poisonous gopher and garter snakes. The only venomous snakes in the Bay Area are rattlesnakes, but sightings of these pit vipers are generally infrequent, occurring most commonly in dry, rocky, or exposed zones during the warmest months of the year. The standard advice for hiking in rattlesnake territory is as follows:

- **Don't put your hands or feet where you can't see them—at the top of a rock outcrop, for example, or in tall grass or a log pile.**
- **Be extra-cautious in hot weather, when snakes are more active.**
- **Scan the trail continuously as you hike.**
- **Keep kids from running ahead on the trail. Bites to children are more severe than those to adults.**

Should you encounter a rattlesnake, its body language will reveal its mood. A coiled rattler is primed for a strike, while a relaxed rattler is more sanguine (although snakes have been reported to lunge). If the snake is within striking distance, stand motionless and wait for it to calm down and move on. Taking small, slow steps backward is another smart strategy. If you're out of immediate range, you can either skirt the snake or wait for it to move. Some people believe tapping the ground with a stick—from a safe distance, rather than in the snake's face—will encourage the snake to move on.

Gopher snakes resemble rattlesnakes; both species have a similar cream, tan, and brown pattern. The easiest way to tell them apart—again, of course, from a safe distance—is by head shape: A gopher snake *(below right)* has no distinction from its "neck" to its head, while a rattler *(below left)* has a diamond-shaped head. Both, by the way, make noises to warn off predators, rattlesnakes by shaking their rattles and gopher snakes by vibrating their tails against the ground.

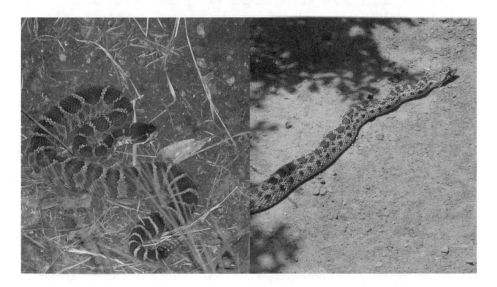

TICKS These arachnids like to hang out in the brush that grows along trails. July is the peak month for ticks in the Bay Area, but you should be tick-aware throughout the spring, summer, and fall. The ticks that alight onto you while hiking will be very small, sometimes so tiny that you won't be able to spot them. All ticks need to attach for several hours before they can transmit disease.

A few precautions: Use insect repellent that contains DEET. Wear light-colored clothing, which will make it easy for you to spot ticks before they migrate to your skin. When your hike is done, inspect your hair, the back of your neck, your armpits, and your socks. During your posthike shower, take a moment to do a more complete body check. To remove a tick that is already embedded, use tweezers made especially for this purpose. Treat the bite with disinfectant solution.

TOPOGRAPHIC MAPS

The maps in this book have been produced with great care and, used with the hike text, will direct you to the trail and help you stay on-course. However, you'll find superior detail and valuable information in the U.S. Geological Survey's 7.5-minute-series topographic maps. At **MyTopo.com**, for example, you can view and print USGS topos of the entire United States free of charge. Online services such as **Trails.com** charge annual fees for additional features such as shaded relief, which makes the topography stand out more. If you expect to print out many topo maps each year, it might be worth paying for such extras. The downside to USGS maps is that most are outdated, having been created 20–30 years ago; nevertheless, they provide excellent topographic detail.

A fabulous alternative to topo maps is **Google Earth** (**earth.google.com**), which allows you to zoom into a hiking area and view it from overhead via satellite imagery. In addition, note that Bay Area land-management agencies provide free trail maps at their websites.

If you're new to hiking, you might be wondering, "What's a topo map?" In short, it indicates not only linear distance but elevation as well, using contour lines. These lines spread across the map like dozens of intricate spiderwebs. Each line represents a particular elevation, and at the base of each topo a contour's interval designation is given. If, for example, the contour interval is 20 feet, then the distance between each contour line is 20 feet. Follow five contour lines up on the same map, and the elevation has increased by 100 feet.

In addition to the sources listed previously and in Appendix B, you'll find topos at major universities and some public libraries, as well as online at **nationalmap.gov** and **store.usgs.gov**.

A NOTE ABOUT WHEELCHAIR ACCESS

In a select few cases, I've noted sections of trail that are wheelchair-accessible. While some other hikes in this book are technically accessible, meaning they contain no impediments such as stairs, they involve considerable changes in elevation that would likely challenge even those with exceptional maneuvering abilities.

TRAIL ETIQUETTE

Whether you're hiking in a city, county, state, or national park, always remember that great care and resources (from nature as well as from your tax dollars) have gone into creating these spaces. Treat the trail, wildlife, and fellow hikers with respect.

Here are a few general principles to keep in mind while you're on the trail:

- *Hike on open trails only.* Respect trail and road closures (ask if you're not sure), avoid possible trespassing on private land, and obtain all permits and authorization as required. Also, leave gates as you found them or as marked.

- *Be sensitive to the ground beneath you.* This also means staying on the existing trail and not blazing any new trails. Pack out what you pack in. Leave No Trace ethics make hiking and camping more fun for others (see lnt.org for more information).

- *Never spook animals.* An unannounced approach, a sudden movement, or a loud noise can startle them. A surprised snake or skunk can be dangerous to you, others, and itself. Give animals extra room and time to adjust to your presence.

- *Plan ahead.* Know your equipment, your ability, and the area in which you are hiking—and prepare accordingly. Be self-sufficient at all times; carry necessary supplies for changes in weather or other conditions. A well-executed trip is a satisfaction to you and to others.

- *Be courteous to other hikers, bikers, and equestrians* you encounter on the trails. Hikers and bikers should yield to equestrians, bikers should yield to hikers, and, whenever safe, everyone should yield to uphill hikers, bikers, or equestrians.

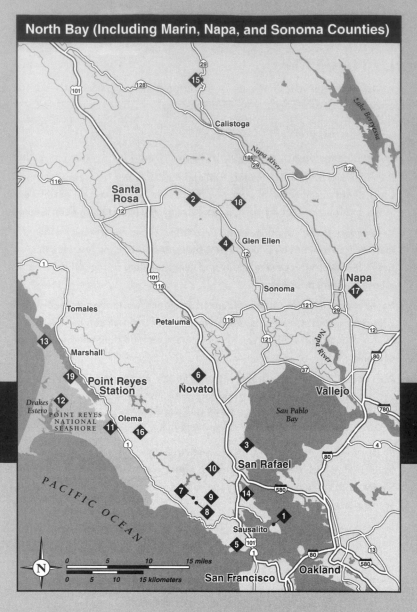

North Bay (Including Marin, Napa, and Sonoma Counties)

NORTH BAY
(INCLUDING MARIN, SONOMA, AND NAPA COUNTIES)

1 ANGEL ISLAND STATE PARK

KEY AT-A-GLANCE INFORMATION

LENGTH: 5 miles

CONFIGURATION: Balloon

DIFFICULTY: Easy

SCENERY: Coast-live-oak and California bay woods, grassland, chaparral, 360-degree views of the Bay Area from the top of Mount Livermore

EXPOSURE: Mix of sun and shade, with full sun at the top

TRAFFIC: Moderate—busy in summer, lighter in the off-season

TRAIL SURFACE: Dirt trails

HIKING TIME: 3 hours

SEASON: Year-round, 8 a.m.–sunset, but ferry service is limited during the off-season, generally September–May. Good any time of year.

ACCESS: Blue and Gold Fleet's $17 round-trip ferry ticket ($9.50 for children ages 6–12) includes park admission.

MAPS: Available at the park's visitor center and at the ferry landing; download it free at tinyurl.com/angel islandspmap.

FACILITIES: Toilets and drinking water at the trailhead

SPECIAL COMMENTS: Contact Blue and Gold Fleet, 415-773-1188 or blueandgoldfleet.com, for a ferry schedule. No dogs allowed on the island.

CONTACTS: 415-435-5390, tinyurl .com/angelislandstatepark

DRIVING DISTANCE: Not applicable

GPS INFORMATION

N37° 52.128' W122° 26.070'

IN BRIEF

Angel Island is a perfect day trip, where the journey to the trailhead rivals the hike for sheer relaxation and beauty. Because you can reach Angel Island only by boat, sit back and enjoy the ferry ride, then climb to the top of the island and back, with incredible 360-degree views nearly the entire trip. Just keep an eye on the clock to make sure you catch that last ferry.

DESCRIPTION

San Francisco Bay's largest island, rising out of the water between Marin and San Francisco, has served as a cattle ranch, military base, quarantine station, immigration facility, prisoner-of-war detention center, and Nike missile site. When the federal government abandoned the island in the late 1940s, it became part of the state-park system, though missile sites operated until 1962. Years of restoration, the elimination of planted nonnative vegetation, and the passage of time have allowed coast-live-oak woods

----

Directions ————————→

Angel Island is accessible by boat only. If you start a journey to Angel Island from a location served by BART or Muni trains, it makes perfect sense to take public transportation to the ferry landing at San Francisco's Pier 41. Take BART or Muni to the Embarcadero station, come above ground and transfer to the F Line (on the Embarcadero across from the Ferry Building), and proceed west to the Fisherman's Wharf stop. Ferries to Angel Island also depart from Tiburon and Alameda. If you want to drive to the ferry, the easiest and most direct route to Fisherman's Wharf from the Bay Bridge is via the Embarcadero. From the Golden Gate Bridge, take Lombard Street to Van Ness Avenue to North Point Street, then park in one of the parking garages at Fisherman's Wharf.

Angel Island State Park

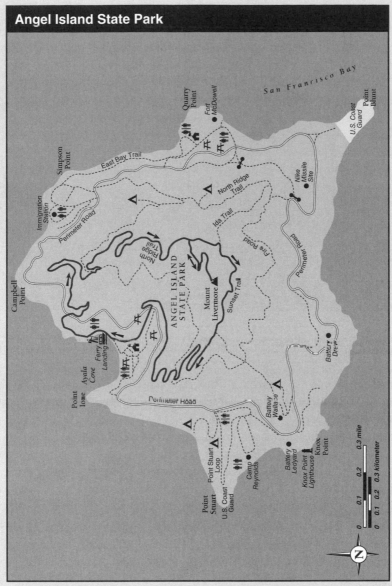

San Francisco Bay

Quarry Point

Fort McDowell

Point Blunt

U.S. Coast Guard

Simpson Point

East Bay Trail

North Ridge Trail

Nike Missile Site

Immigration Station

Perimeter Road

Ida Trail

North Ridge Trail

Fire Road

Perimeter Road

Campbell Point

ANGEL ISLAND STATE PARK

Mount Livermore

Sunset Trail

Battery Drew

Point Ione

Ayala Cove

Ferry Landing

Perimeter Road

Battery Wallace

Point Stuart Loop

Battery Ledyard

Knox Point Lighthouse

Knox Point

Camp Reynolds

Point Stuart

U.S. Coast Guard

0.3 mile

0.2

0.1

0.3 kilometer

0.2

0.1

0

N

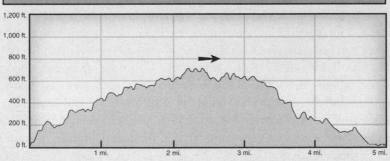

1,200 ft.

1,000 ft.

800 ft.

600 ft.

400 ft.

200 ft.

0 ft.

1 mi.   2 mi.   3 mi.   4 mi.   5 mi.

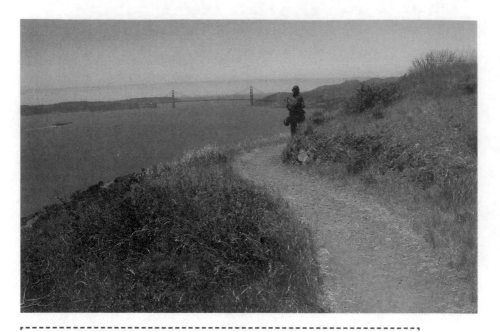

Angel Island's Sunset Trail affords 360-degree views of Bay Area landmarks including the Golden Gate Bridge.

and grassland to make a comeback. Park staff have returned the island's highest peak, Mount Livermore, to its original state by restoring acres of dirt pushed off the summit by the military.

Angel Island offers two main hikes: a nearly level 5-mile circuit around the island on a fire road, and this loop, a combination of Northridge and Sunset Trails, with a short out-and-back spur to the summit. The park is busy during tourist season, but once when I visited with a friend in early summer, we disembarked from a nearly full ferry, then watched as the crowds made a beeline for the visitor center. On the trails, we crossed paths with only a dozen other hikers—trails are even quieter in winter, when clear days promise long views, and early spring, when the wildflower displays are legendary.

Begin from the ferry landing on Northridge Trail, which sets off to the left (north) of the restrooms. As it leaves the shoreline area, this path climbs through pine, toyon, and coast live oak, ascends some long, steep stairs past a few picnic tables, then reaches a cluster of eucalyptus and paved Perimeter Road at 0.1 mile. Continue on the far side of the pavement on Northridge Trail, entering a more natural area where clarkia and Indian pink bloom in early summer. The narrow path winds uphill through shaded woods of California bay and hazelnut. When Northridge Trail emerges from the woods on the northernmost flank of the island, enjoy views north across Raccoon Strait to the Tiburon peninsula. Wind through a patch of manzanita charred by fire, where new shrubs are quickly reinvigorating the hillsides. At 0.9 mile, turn left onto a fire road for a few feet, then veer right, continuing on Northridge Trail.

After one last foray through chaparral, the path, still ascending easily, takes a long tour through quiet woods of coast live oak, where you might also see madrone, gooseberry, huge thickets of hazelnut, and poison oak. Northridge Trail levels out as it reaches a grassy plateau dotted with coyote brush; here, iris and paintbrush bloom in spring, and coyote mint, venus thistle, and buckwheat flower in summer. There are good views, too—west to Mount Tamalpais, and uphill to Mount Livermore's summit. Under a few pines at 1.8 miles, Northridge Trail ends at a T-junction. Turn right, following the sign to Mount Livermore.

At an easygoing rate, the trail climbs past coast live oak into grassland. You'll likely see butterflies, including California sister and a variety of swallowtails fluttering about in summer, along with fast-moving swifts and more-languid vultures and hawks riding the thermal currents. After two bends in the trail, the path makes a final push to the summit, climbing through grassy slopes dotted with young coyote brush, reintroduced after the restoration of the peak. At 2.1 miles, you'll reach the top of Mount Livermore, where views are simply incredible and, even in summer's haze, include the Golden Gate Bridge stretching from San Francisco's Presidio to Marin's rolling Headlands; Alcatraz Island; Mount Tamalpais; the downtown San Francisco skyline; Mount Diablo; Treasure Island; and the Bay Bridge. Descend back to the previous junction, then continue right on Sunset Trail.

As you drop down onto the island's south slope, unobstructed views extend downhill to Point Blunt, an active Coast Guard station. This area is still scarred from development and restoration efforts, which have left some burned pines and a sense of disarray. Sunset Trail crosses an old, closed road and begins to angle across a hillside, heading west. Bushes of sticky monkeyflower, coyote brush, poison oak, and sagebrush frame awesome views of the world's most famous span, its signature "international orange" paint scheme so pretty against a clear blue sky. Sunset Trail descends a ridge, offering splendid views of Sausalito, Belvedere Island, the Marin Headlands, and Mount Tam, then veers right into coast-live-oak woods.

At one last little sunny viewpoint, a bench invites a lingering break, and the trail then begins a campaign of switchbacks. Some shortcuts are worn into the hillside here, but please stay on the trail, which is well graded. Poison oak and Italian thistle crowd the trail in places in summer. At 3.5 miles, veer right on a fire road for a few feet, then turn left, back onto Sunset Trail. Switchbacks continue, mostly through California bay and coast-live-oak woods. Just past a water tank and a cluster of picnic tables, the trail bends left, runs along the road, then ends at 4.6 miles. Cross the road near a paved route descending to group picnic areas, then veer right, following the sign to the dock area.

This wide trail starts out paved but soon shifts to dirt. As you descend toward the visitor center, you might notice several nonnative plants, including pride of Madeira, a shrub with big purple flower spikes, and broom, a wispy bush that bears yellow, sweet-smelling, pealike blossoms. The trail turns sharply left, then ends at the side of the visitor center, where a grassy picnic area fronts the shoreline at Ayala Cove. Turn right and walk on a paved road the remaining distance back to the ferry landing.

2 ANNADEL STATE PARK

KEY AT-A-GLANCE INFORMATION

LENGTH: 6.2 miles

CONFIGURATION: Figure-eight

DIFFICULTY: Easy–moderate

SCENERY: Woods, grassland, oaks, and lake

EXPOSURE: First and last section shaded, the rest mostly full sun

TRAFFIC: Medium weekdays, heavy weekends

TRAIL SURFACE: Rocky dirt fire roads and trails

HIKING TIME: 3 hours

SEASON: Year-round, 8 a.m.–sunset; Channel Drive entrance gate open 9 a.m.–6 p.m. Spring is best; it's muddy after rains and hot in summer.

ACCESS: Pay the $6 entrance fee at the ranger station.

MAPS: At the ranger station and tinyurl.com/annadelmap

FACILITIES: Pit toilets at the trailhead

SPECIAL COMMENTS: Dogs are not permitted on park trails. All trails but one are multiuse.

CONTACTS: 707-539-3911, tinyurl .com/annadelsp

DRIVING DISTANCE: 56 miles from the Golden Gate Bridge toll plaza

GPS INFORMATION

N38° 26.669' W122° 36.945'

IN BRIEF

If hikes were marketed like new cars, I'd say that this Annadel loop has the most meadow views per mile. This hike climbs through a forest, loops around a meadow, and skirts the shore of Lake Ilsanjo before returning through woods to the trailhead. Although Annadel is a busy park, heavily used by equestrians and cyclists as well as local walkers and runners, it's worth putting up with the crowds.

DESCRIPTION

Annadel's grassy expanses are at their best in spring, when carpets of flowers bloom at the feet of mature oaks. The park is situated at the north end of the Sonoma Mountains, a long series of rolling hills that run from the eastern outskirts of Santa Rosa to the flats of San Pablo Bay. Like Jack London Historic State Park a few miles to the south (see Hike 4), Annadel has pretty woods and good views, but it also offers lakeside picnic spots, big sweeps of grassland, and oak savanna. Because Annadel is surrounded by residential communities, there are

----

Directions ———————————➤

Leave San Francisco on northbound US 101 and use the Golden Gate Bridge toll plaza as your mileage starting point. Drive about 50 miles north on US 101, then take Exit 488B on CA 12. Drive east toward Sonoma/Napa 1.5 miles, then turn left onto CA 12 East/Farmers Lane. After 0.7 mile, turn right onto Montgomery Drive. Drive east 3 miles, then turn right onto Channel Drive. After less than 0.1 mile, continue straight where the road makes a sharp turn right toward Spring Lake. Drive into the park, stop and pay the entrance fee at the ranger station, then continue to the parking lot at the end of the road.

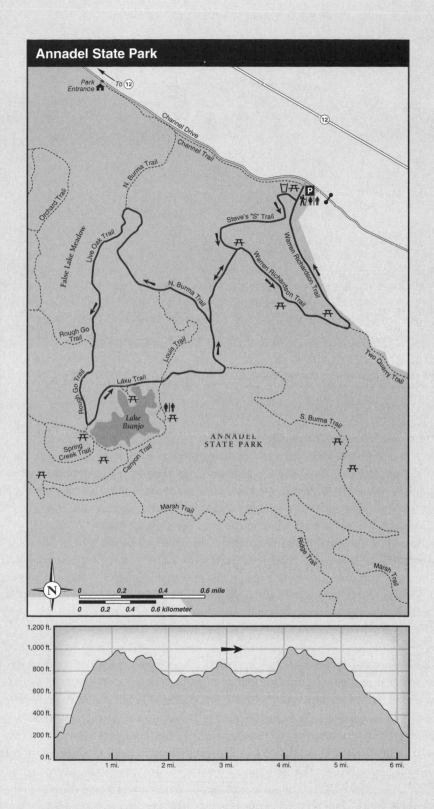

Annadel State Park

Park Entrance ⌂ To 12

Channel Drive

Channel Trail

N. Burma Trail

Orchard Trail

False Lake Meadow

Live Oak Trail

N. Burma Trail

Rough Go Trail

Rough Go Trail

Louis Trail

Lake Trail

Lake Ilsanjo

Spring Creek Trail

Canyon Trail

Steve's "S" Trail

Warren Richardson Trail

Warren Richardson Trail

Two Quarry Trail

ANNADEL STATE PARK

S. Burma Trail

Marsh Trail

Ridge Trail

Marsh Trail

N

| 0 | 0.2 | 0.4 | 0.6 mile |
| 0 | 0.2 0.4 | 0.6 kilometer |

1,200 ft.
1,000 ft.
800 ft.
600 ft.
400 ft.
200 ft.
0 ft.

1 mi.   2 mi.   3 mi.   4 mi.   5 mi.   6 mi.

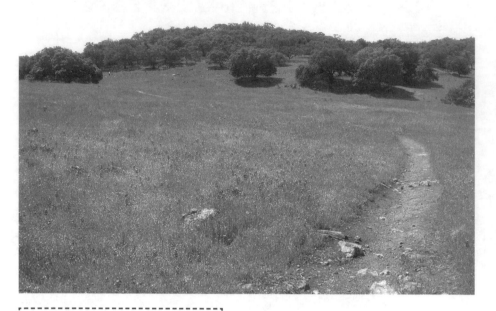

Old oaks and grassland line Live Oak Trail.

quite a few trailheads, many paths and trails, and lots of loop opportunities. In the past few years park staff have cracked down on shortcuts and old, erosive routes, and the number of official trails is now much smaller—you'll still find faint paths and bike cuts, but all the legitimate routes are signed and appear on the map. As you hike you'll surely notice rocks and boulders all over the place, evidence of the cobblestone quarrying that took place in the area before the 1920s.

Begin from the middle of the parking lot, uphill on W. Richardson Trail. After about 200 feet on the fire road, turn right onto Steve's "S" Trail. The park's sole hiking-only path begins a mostly easy climb through an open forest of California bay, Douglas-fir, coast live oak, and black oak. You might see woodland star and iris in spring. Views are obscured by the forest, and noise from the surrounding neighborhoods is steady, but the hubbub fades as the trail progresses uphill. Look for shiny black shards of obsidian on the trail—American Indian tribes used the rock for arrow points and spearheads. In some spots, there's so much obsidian directly on the trail that you might initially mistake it for broken glass. As the trail makes its way across the wooded flanks of the hillside, boulders loom in the shadows, beneath Douglas-fir and California bay. Steve's "S" Trail crosses a little creek, then bends sharply left. On one spring hike I saw a deer moving through the woods out of the corner of my eye and heard turkeys yodeling in the distance. At the 1-mile mark, the trail ends near a picnic table, at a junction with W. Richardson Trail. Turn right.

The fire road ascends slightly, leaving the forest for a grassy savanna where deciduous black and Oregon oaks mingle with evergreen coast live oak and manzanitas. Spring wildflowers include Linanthus, lupines, blue-eyed grass, pop-corn flower, goldfields, blue-dicks, and hound's tongue. At 1.3 miles, turn right onto North Burma Trail.

The setting, with oaks sprinkled through grassland, is incredibly scenic and invites daydreams, but be sure to stay alert for mountain bikes on this narrow path. North Burma Trail descends briefly along a sloping hillside, then veers left into a young forest (an old trail to the right, now closed, leads back toward Steve's "S" Trail). Douglas-fir and madrone crowd the rocky, level trail, giving way to manzanita, ceanothus, and poison oak. Among the small boulders strewn about along the trail, look for shooting stars and blue-eyed grass in late winter and a generous amount of golden fairy lanterns in mid-to-late April. At 1.7 miles, the left side of the trail opens up to a descending meadow dotted with oaks, where lupines, popcorn flower, Linanthus, and goldfields were blooming on one mid-spring hike. As the trail proceeds slightly downhill, ceanothus, poison oak, coyote brush, manzanita, and toyon close off views, and Douglas-fir, black oak, and madrone provide occasional shade. At 2.2 miles, North Burma Trail bends left to a junction. Turn left onto Live Oak Trail.

The narrow path runs parallel to False Lake Meadow, a short distance down-hill to the right, mostly screened by an assortment of young Douglas-fir, and coast live, Oregon, and black oak. Because trees line Live Oak Trail at a distance, grassy patches abound where you might see false lupine, blue-eyed grass, lupines, blue-dicks, iris, shooting stars, and Linanthus in spring. Rocks and small boulders are strewn all over the place, and in one spot along the trail you might notice an artistic-looking pile of stones on the right. As the trail travels slightly downslope from a little knoll, you'll pass through a pocket of woods where California bay and buckeye blend into the other trees, then emerge on the western side of a meadow (apparently unnamed although it's one of the park's largest). To the right are unobstructed views down to False Lake Meadow. Expect big patches of lupines along the trail in April, along with some California poppies and blue larkspur. The trail winds past an old, sprawling coast live oak, then ends at 3 miles. Bear left onto Rough Go Trail.

Oaks and manzanita are common along the trail, which descends very gently through rocky grassland. Although Rough Go is heavily trafficked, this is a quiet part of the park, far from the trappings of suburban Santa Rosa. Two rugged Sonoma County peaks, Mounts Hood and St. Helena, loom off in the distance on the left. Just past a bench, Rough Go Trail ends at 3.4 miles. Turn left onto Lake Trail. (If you want to take the long way around the lake, continue past this junc-tion, then turn left at the junction with Spring Creek Trail.)

Lake Ilsanjo is the heart of the park and a regular destination for many visi-tors who enjoy picnicking on the shores of the little reservoir, so you'll likely cross paths with plenty of runners, equestrians, and cyclists in this part of Annadel. This level segment of Lake Trail skirts the northern shoreline at a distance. Even when you can't see it, cries from red-winged blackbirds indicate that the water is close by, off to the right, and the trail is often muddy in all but the driest months of the year. Native bunchgrasses thrive beneath oaks, manzanita, and California bay, in an understory where California buttercups, shooting stars, and iris bloom in spring. At the south edge of the meadow, you might see johnny-tuck and concentrated clusters of Linanthus and goldfields blooming in April. If you're looking for a good spot for lunch, you'll find many picnic tables in the area—try following one of the side paths veering off to the right or left. At 3.9 miles, Lake Trail sweeps right, continuing its loop around the lake. Make a soft left and you're once again on W. Richardson Trail.

This stretch on the fire road starts as an easy climb along a small creek. In spring, red larkspur and yellow buttercups provide a nice contrast to the ferns and creambush beneath Douglas-fir and California bay. South Burma Trail heads right at 4.2 miles—continue left on W. Richardson Trail. You may notice some mature, dead-looking Douglas-firs, most conspicuous in spring and summer, when all the park's trees bear green leaves or needles. Annadel's staff has girdled some Douglas-firs at the transition zones between oak savanna and evergreen forest, an attempt to stop the Douglas-firs from invading the oaks' territory. As these trees die and fall, they will become an important part of the healthy park ecosystem, providing habitat for many wild creatures.

The surface of the fire road may be scored with tracks made by one of the most commonly spotted animals at Annadel, the wild turkey. I've seen turkeys on every Annadel visit, either shuffling through oak woods, searching through the fallen leaves for insects, or tootling down the trails—these big birds make a substantial racket, gobbling back and forth to each other, and although they seem ungainly, they can move surprisingly fast. Wild turkeys can be feisty, too, especially the males (called toms), who keep a close watch on females (hens) during breeding season.

As W. Richardson Trail makes its way north, look left for a last view of the meadow and Lake Ilsanjo. At 4.4 miles, you'll once again reach the junction with North Burma Trail. Stay to the right on the fire road and retrace your steps back to the junction with Steve's "S" Trail at 4.7 miles. Continue right and downhill on W. Richardson Trail.

The fire road begins a moderate descent, through a forest of redwood, Douglas-fir, California bay, and coast live oak. At a hairpin turn about 5.4 miles into the hike, Two Quarry Trail departs on the right, heading into the eastern part of the park. Continue on W. Richardson Trail, which runs at the edge of the woods, presenting nice views of a little egg-shaped hill on the right. A few big-leaf maple trees call attention to themselves in autumn, when they show off their foliage. As the trail descends, traffic and household noise filters through the trees. At 6 miles, you'll return to the junction with Steve's "S" Trail. You can walk the short distance back to the trailhead on the fire road, but I prefer the path on the right, which descends a flight of steps, then ends at the south end of the parking lot.

CHINA CAMP STATE PARK

IN BRIEF

China Camp's rolling, forested hills front San Pablo Bay just minutes from the hustle and bustle of San Rafael. Unlike some other destinations where the trip to the start of your hike seems to take forever, the coffee nestled in your cup holder may still be warm when you pull into the trailhead.

DESCRIPTION

China Camp can feel rather sleepy in autumn and winter, but summer draws loads of visitors for hiking, biking, picnicking, and camping. Miwok Meadows Group Area is a popular (reservations required) day-use site for family gatherings and parties. Back Ranch Meadows Campground hosts 30 walk-in sites strewn throughout pretty woods. The campground is an extremely popular destination in summer, but you can often snag a site at the last minute on an autumn or early-spring weekday; in winter the place is mostly deserted.

Before you start your hike here, take a minute to discuss trail-sharing etiquette with your hiking partners. China Camp is an unusual Bay Area state park, with all but two trails open to hikers, equestrians, and cyclists (most state parks prohibit bikes from narrow trails). You probably won't see many horses, but cycling is popular here, and you'll likely

Directions

Leave San Francisco northbound on US 101 and use the Golden Gate Bridge toll plaza as your mileage starting point. Drive north on US 101 about 15 miles, then take Exit 454, North San Pedro Road. Continue east on North San Pedro Road for 3 miles, then turn right into the park at the campground sign.

KEY AT-A-GLANCE INFORMATION

LENGTH: 7.3 miles

CONFIGURATION: Loop

DIFFICULTY: Moderate

SCENERY: Mixed woods, views

EXPOSURE: Mostly shaded, some full sun

TRAFFIC: Moderate

TRAIL SURFACE: Dirt fire roads and trails

HIKING TIME: 3 hours

SEASON: Daily, 8 a.m.–sunset. Good year-round.

ACCESS: Pay the $5 day-use fee at the entrance kiosk.

MAPS: At entrance kiosk and tinyurl.com/chinacampmap

FACILITIES: Restrooms and drinking water at the campground

SPECIAL COMMENTS: Dogs are not allowed on the trails.
   The park's name dates back to the Chinese shrimp-fishing village that existed here in the 1880s. If you want to learn more about the history of China Camp, visit the Village Area: continue east on North San Pablo Road, past the campground trailhead and ranger station, to the signed China Camp Village Area on the left side of the road.

CONTACTS: 415-456-0761, tinyurl.com/chinacampsp

DRIVING DISTANCE: 18 miles from the Golden Gate Bridge toll plaza

GPS INFORMATION

N38° 0.357' W122° 29.804'

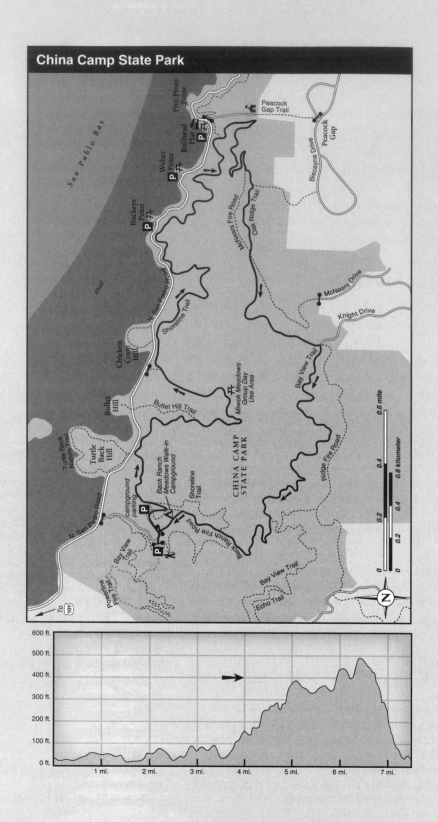

China Camp State Park

Five Pines Point

Peacock Gap Trail

Peacock Gap

Biscayne Drive

Bullhead Flat

P

Weber Point

P

McNears Fire Road

Oak Ridge Trail

Buckeye Point

P

McNears Drive

Knight Drive

N. San Pedro Road

Shoreline Trail

Chicken Coop Hill

Bay View Trail

Bullet Hill

Bullet Hill Trail

Miwok Meadows Group Day Use Area

CHINA CAMP STATE PARK

Turtle Back Nature Trail

Turtle Back Hill

Back Ranch Meadows Walk-in Campground

Shoreline Trail

Ridge Fire Road

Campground parking

P

Back Ranch Fire Road

San pablo Bay

mud

N. San Pedro Road

P

Bay View Trail

Bay View Trail

To 101

Powerline Fire Trail

Echo Trail

N

0.6 mile

0.6 kilometer

0.4

0.4

0.2

0.2

0

0

600 ft.

500 ft.

400 ft.

300 ft.

200 ft.

100 ft.

0 ft.

1 mi.   2 mi.   3 mi.   4 mi.   5 mi.   6 mi.   7 mi.

cross paths with lots of bikes. The protocol for multiuse trails is that bikers yield to hikers and everyone steps aside for horses. However, on China Camp's narrow trails, I find it simpler to step aside for the bikes, particularly when riders are slogging uphill, where momentum is important. In a group, the first hiker who spots a cyclist is advised to call out "Bike!" to the rest of the party, who should then veer onto the right edge of the trail. When hiking with several people, try to remain single-file rather than stretching across the trail. Use special caution near the blind corners on the upper trails at China Camp—down in the flats cyclists expect heavy hiker use, but farther afield they don't seem as prepared for encounters.

Begin from the day-use lot and walk on the paved park road toward the campground. (You can skirt the campground completely via Shoreline Trail, but that option is longer and does not route you past some of the nicest park restrooms in the Bay Area, at the campground.) When we hiked here last, the smell of morning-campfire smoke drifted our way as a wild turkey trotted across the road. When you reach the campground parking lot, pass the restrooms and information signboard, step into the woods, cross a bridge, turn left, pass Campsite 1, then leave the campground area and, after a few steps, meet Shoreline Trail feeding in from the right. The nearly level path runs above a damp area on the left, through grassland dotted with young buckeyes and coyote brush. Deer are common throughout the park, and we saw the first of several here on a summer morning. Without tall trees blocking views, uninterrupted vistas stretch north to the shores of San Pablo Bay and south to the park's tallest hills.

At about the 0.5-mile mark, continue straight on Shoreline Trail, where a path heads left toward Turtle Back Nature Trail. Shoreline Trail runs near North San Pedro Road briefly, then veers right as it skirts a marshy meadow. Look for a pretty buckeye standing alone off to the left, conspicuous in early summer when it's ablaze with clusters of white flowers. Shoreline Trail passes through pockets of California bays and oaks, crosses a creek, then reaches the edge of Miwok Meadows Group Day Use Area. Pass through the parking lot and continue on Shoreline Trail, here a wide dirt road (watch for cars). At a level grade, the trail runs along the edge of sloping woods on the right, where orange sticky monkeyflower blooms in spring and summer.

At 1.5 miles (Miwok Trail used to head uphill here but is now closed), the trail shrinks back to footpath size and once again parallels North San Pedro Road briefly. In early summer, look in the grass along the trail here for yellow mariposa lilies. Shoreline Trail pulls away from the road and heads into woods again, giving hikers an opportunity to spot (or hear) some of the songbirds that call China Camp home. Chickadees are common—listen for their *chick-a-dee-dee-dee* call as they flit through the trees. I've also seen a black phoebe and spotted towhee in this area. With dark-gray heads and backs and white bellies, black phoebes are flycatchers, so look for them perched on tree or shrub branches, while spotted towhees shuffle through the leaf litter on the ground. Spotted towhees are about robin-sized and have rusty bellies. Their black wings are speckled with white, which is most obvious when they

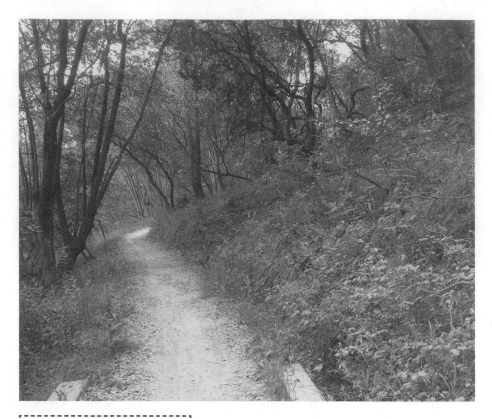

Shaded woods along Shoreline Trail

are in flight. Shoreline Trail winds through patches of grassland and a forest of natives including madrone, coast live and black oak, and California bay. At 3.7 miles, you'll reach a junction with Peacock Gap Trail. Bear right and ascend to a second junction at 3.8 miles, where Peacock Gap Trail continues straight to the park boundary. Bear right, now on Oak Ridge Trail.

The narrow trail weaves uphill through woods dominated by California bays. Switchbacks ease the climb, and soon you'll emerge from the woods at a junction at 4.2 miles. McNears Fire Road heads left and right—continue straight on Oak Ridge Trail. Slightly off the ridgeline, Oak Ridge Trail sweeps across a sloping hillside dotted with oaks and a few manzanita shrubs. Early wildflowers here include milkmaids and shooting stars. Where breaks in the vegetation permit, look off to the left for great views of San Rafael Bay and the Richmond–San Rafael Bridge. Oak Ridge Trail meets McNears Fire Road again at 4.6 miles. The fire road climbs steeply to the left, up a ridge once dominated by nonnative eucalyptus. In 2001 the park removed the trees, so the ridgeline is now bare. Continue straight, still on Oak Ridge Trail. Back in the pretty mixed woods, the trail keeps to a nearly level grade. The shade is welcome on a warm summer day, but in the

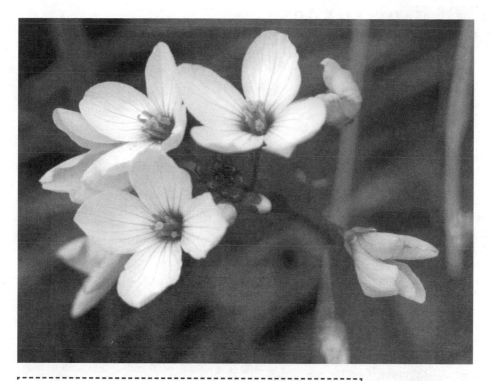

Milkmaids, one of the first flowers to appear in winter woods and grassland

winter expect mud in this section. Oak Ridge Trail ends at 4.9 miles. Continue straight, now on Bay View Trail.

Another singletrack trail, Bay View is one of the park's quietest. Far uphill from the developed area, and without a paved road or trail in sight, the trail provides easy and peaceful strolling under cover of oaks, madrone, and California bay woods. In spring, blue-eyed grass blooms along the trail, and in summer look for California milkwort, a native wildflower with rose-pink petals. Bay View Trail meets Back Ranch Fire Road at 6.4 miles. Bear right.

This steep fire road descends rapidly, switchbacking under power lines. The black oaks mixed through madrone and California bays along the trail shed gorgeous orange leaves here in autumn. After one last steep and slippery patch, Back Ranch Fire Road ends at a junction with Shoreline Trail (the leg left skirts the campground and is an optional route back to the parking lot) at 6.8 miles. Continue straight, and the trail drops into the campground (if you camped here you'd be home now). A spur heads left near the restrooms, but keep going straight to the bridge at 7.1 miles, then turn left and retrace your steps back to the trailhead.

4   JACK LONDON STATE HISTORIC PARK

KEY AT-A-GLANCE INFORMATION

LENGTH: 10.8 miles

CONFIGURATION: Out-and-back with 2 short loops

DIFFICULTY: Moderate, despite the length

SCENERY: Woods, with some grassland

EXPOSURE: Almost completely shaded

TRAFFIC: Moderate around ranch, light on the upper trails

TRAIL SURFACE: Dirt fire roads and trails

HIKING TIME: 6 hours

SEASON: Summer, daily, 9:30 a.m.–5 p.m.; winter, Thursday–Monday, same hours; closed Thanksgiving, December 25, and January 1. Anytime is good, but autumn is perfect.

ACCESS: Pay $10 fee at entrance kiosk.

MAPS: At the entrance kiosk, the park museum, and jacklondonpark.com/jack-london-park-map.html

FACILITIES: Pit toilets and water near the trailhead

SPECIAL COMMENTS: Dogs are permitted on some park trails, but not on every trail in this hike.

CONTACTS: 707-938-5216, jacklondonpark.com

DRIVING DISTANCE: 46 miles from the Golden Gate Bridge toll plaza

GPS INFORMATION

N38° 21.381' W122° 32.692'
2400 London Ranch Rd.
Glen Ellen, CA 95442

IN BRIEF

This out-and-back Bay Area Ridge Trail segment begins on old ranch roads, then ascends on a narrow path through an unspoiled forest of madrones, black oaks, big-leaf maples, buckeyes, redwoods, and California bays. After 5.5 miles you'll reach the end of the trail, and the return segment is downhill (almost) all the way.

DESCRIPTION

Just minutes from the charming wine country village of Glen Ellen, hikers can walk up the forested slopes of Sonoma Mountain, literally following in the footsteps of Jack London, author of *Call of the Wild*. The property, containing London's home and ranch buildings, as well as many surrounding wooded acres, became a state park after London's wife, Charmian, died in 1955. Visitors can tour the "House of Happy Walls," London's grave site, and the remains of Wolf House, London's dream home, which was destroyed by fire before it was ever occupied. For many, that's an

---

Directions ⟶

Leave San Francisco northbound on US 101 and use the Golden Gate Bridge toll plaza as your mileage starting point. Drive about 20 miles north on US 101, then take exit 460A to merge onto CA 37 East toward Napa/Vallejo. After 7.5 miles, turn left (north) onto CA 121. Drive north about 7.5 miles to the junction with CA 116 and continue straight on CA 116. Continue north 1.5 miles, then bear right onto Arnold Drive. Continue north 8.4 miles on Arnold into Glen Ellen, then turn left (west) onto London Ranch Road and drive about 1.2 miles to the park's entrance kiosk. Once past the kiosk, turn right and drive less than 0.1 mile to the parking lot.

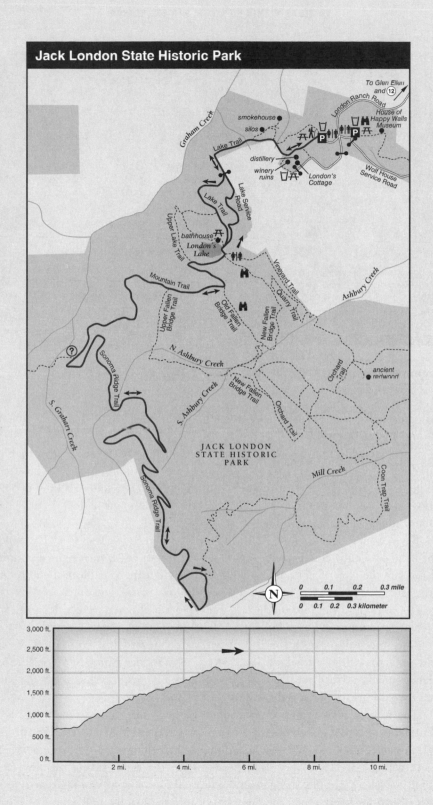

Jack London State Historic Park

To Glen Ellen and (12)

London Ranch Road

House of Happy Walls Museum

Graham Creek

smokehouse
silos

Lake Trail

distillery

winery ruins

London's Cottage

Wolf House Service Road

Lake Trail

Lake Service Road

Upper Lake Trail

bathhouse
London's Lake

Mountain Trail

Vineyard Trail

Ashbury Creek

Upper Fallen Bridge Trail

Old Fallen Bridge Trail

New Fallen Bridge Trail

Quarry Trail

N Ashbury Creek

Orchard Trail

ancient redwood

?

Sonoma Ridge Trail

S Graham Creek

S Ashbury Creek

New Fallen Bridge Trail

Orchard Trail

JACK LONDON STATE HISTORIC PARK

Mill Creek

Coon Trap Trail

Sonoma Ridge Trail

N

| 0 | 0.1 | 0.2 | 0.3 mile |
| 0 | 0.1 | 0.2 | 0.3 kilometer |

3,000 ft.

2,500 ft.

2,000 ft.

1,500 ft.

1,000 ft.

500 ft.

0 ft.

2 mi.   4 mi.   6 mi.   8 mi.   10 mi.

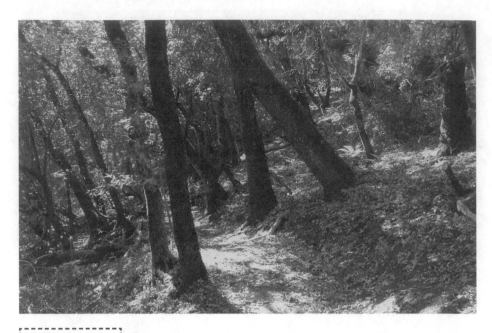

Sonoma Ridge Trail

adequate day trip, but hikers should press on, up the hillsides of Sonoma Mountain and into a gorgeous forest.

This hike adds up to nearly 11 miles, but the trails are so well graded that it's a moderate excursion. The park is a popular stop for summer visitors, but once you get away from the developed areas you might see more squirrels than people. Spring hikes are tempting, but the gentle temperatures and colorful foliage of Indian summer make autumn hikes very enjoyable.

Begin from the parking lot, following the Bay Area Ridge Trail (BART) symbol. When the path ends at a T-junction with a wide gravel road, turn right. London's cottage and the winery ruins are on your left. (If you care to explore them, return to the ranch road when you're done and keep following the signs for BART and the lake.) As you skirt a vineyard on the left, a few more paths on the right depart to the Pig Palace and other old farm buildings. All of these are optional side hikes.

After the trail makes a sharp turn with the vineyard still on the left, a gate stretches across the fire road, also known as Lake Service Road, and you'll reach a signed junction with Lake Trail. At this point you'll have traveled about 0.5 mile from the parking lot. Turn right, still on Lake Trail.

The narrow path begins an easy climb through the woods. On sunny days, light filters down to highlight a few stately redwoods nestled in a forest of madrone, big-leaf maple, black oak, tan oak, and Douglas-fir. Trilliums are very common here in late winter. The Lake Spur Trail heads off to the right, taking the long way around the lake. Continue straight on the Lake Trail as it runs within sight of Lake Service Road for a few paces, then veers back into the woods. At 1 mile, Lake Trail ends at the shore of Bathhouse Lake. Here, turn left, walk a few steps, then turn right onto a fire road also known as Mountain Trail. As the trail swings around the lake, Vineyard Trail departs to the left, with Quarry Trail following in the same direction after a few steps. Continue to the right on Mountain Trail. The ascent begins an easy but steady climb through redwood, California bay, and madrone.

Unless you're visiting on a particularly busy day, the crowds thin with every step past the lake. The fire road reaches a little sloping meadow, known as May's Clearing, at 1.3 miles. Views stretch southeast, as does Fallen Bridge Trail on the left. Keep going uphill on Mountain Trail, browsing through a forest crowded with native Bay Area trees: redwoods, madrones, coast live oaks, big-leaf maples, buckeyes, Douglas-firs, California bays, and Oregon oaks. At 1.6 miles, the other end of Upper Fallen Bridge Trail returns on the left. Keep climbing on Mountain Trail. The trail winds past Pine Tree Meadows, really more of a grassy patch mostly overtaken by the pines. Just when the ascent seems never-ending, the trail dips to cross a creek, then reaches a junction at 2.3 miles. Turn left onto Sonoma Ridge Trail. Beneath a canopy of California bay, the trail gently ascends through a rocky section. Angling up the side of the mountain, you'll enter a more exposed area where oak, toyon, and manzanita mingle with Douglas-fir. The ascent is easy, initially through dense woods of Douglas-fir, California bay, and madrone.

Where the trail crosses Asbury Creek, redwoods are especially prominent and lovely. On the south side of the creek, the landscape shifts a bit, making a long transition to the grassland you'll see at the ridgeline. Buckeye, black oak, big-leaf maple, and manzanita are common, and wherever there are breaks in the forest, you'll get views extending far to the north, east, and south. The most prominent landform is 4,304-foot Mount St. Helena, looming to the north. Switchbacks keep the grade nearly effortless, and the climb passes quickly. Before long you'll find yourself bisecting a grassy slope just under the ridgeline at nearly 2,100 feet.

At 5.3 miles, the trail splits into two legs of a loop. Turn left. After less than 0.1 mile, Coon Trap Trail departs downhill on the left. (Using Coon Trap, I turned this out-and-back hike into a loop on my last visit, but I don't recommend you do the same—the trail is steep and ill-maintained.) Continue to the right, climbing a little, past giant black oaks sprawling through grassland and fences that guard private property on the park boundary to the left. The loop closes at 5.6 miles. Turn left and retrace your steps back to Mountain Trail, then turn right and walk downhill to the junction with Lake Trail at 9.9 miles. This time, stay to the right on Lake Service Road. With plenty of generous curves, the trail sweeps easily downhill through the woods. If you visit after a rainstorm, look for animal footprints in muddy patches. At 10.3 miles, you'll reach the gate and junction with Lake Trail. Continue straight, retracing your steps back to the parking lot.

NEARBY ACTIVITIES

The park museum, Jack London's grave, and the Wolf House ruins sit within the park. Visit **jacklondonpark.com** for more information.

5 MARIN HEADLANDS

KEY AT-A-GLANCE INFORMATION

LENGTH: 5.8 miles

CONFIGURATION: Balloon

DIFFICULTY: Moderate

SCENERY: Coastal scrub, views of the Golden Gate Bridge, the Pacific, the downtown San Francisco skyline, and Mount Tamalpais

EXPOSURE: Full sun

TRAFFIC: Steady year-round; includes mountain bikers and equestrians

TRAIL SURFACE: Fire roads

HIKING TIME: 3 hours

SEASON: Good anytime

ACCESS: Free

MAPS: Obtain the free National Park Service map at the Marin Headlands Visitor Center or tinyurl.com/marin headlandsmap, or buy Tom Harrison Maps' *Southern Marin Trail Map* ($9.95; tomharrisonmaps.com).

FACILITIES: None at trailhead; restrooms and water at visitor center

SPECIAL COMMENTS: Dogs are permitted on some Headlands trails, but not on every trail in this hike (see Nearby Activities for an alternate dog-friendly excursion). Check at the visitor center for specifics.

CONTACTS: 415-331-1540, nps.gov/goga/marin-headlands.htm

DRIVING DISTANCE: 4.4 miles from the Golden Gate Bridge toll plaza

GPS INFORMATION

N37° 49.940' W122° 30.925'

IN BRIEF

The Marin Headlands' softly rolling hills form a picturesque backdrop for travelers driving north across the Golden Gate Bridge, as well as a perfect platform for San Francisco city views that include the world's most beautiful span. You'll begin this hike at the valley floor, climb through coastal scrub along one side of the valley, then crest at the ridgeline and return on the other side of the valley. The entire loop sticks to fire roads and is easy to follow, but expect substantial mountain-bike and equestrian traffic.

DESCRIPTION

The Gerbode Valley trailhead is so close to San Francisco that when traffic conditions

----

Directions ⟶

Leave San Francisco northbound on US 101 and use the Golden Gate Bridge toll plaza as your mileage starting point. Drive 2 miles to the far end of the bridge; then, just past the Vista Point exit, take Exit 442 onto Alexander Avenue. Turn right (east) and drive 0.3 mile toward Sausalito, then turn left onto Bunker Road. Drive 0.1 mile to the mouth of a 0.5-mile one-way tunnel (you may need to wait as long as 5 minutes for your turn). From the other side of the tunnel, continue 1.5 miles more on Bunker Road, then turn right onto a small, unmarked dirt road directly across from the horse stables.

**   The Marin Headlands Visitor Center is open daily, October–March, 9:30 a.m.–4:30 p.m., and Saturday–Monday April–September, same hours. From this hike's trailhead, drive west on Bunker Road about 0.5 mile, and where Bunker curves right, continue straight onto Field Road. After less than 0.1 mile, turn right into the visitor-center parking lot.**

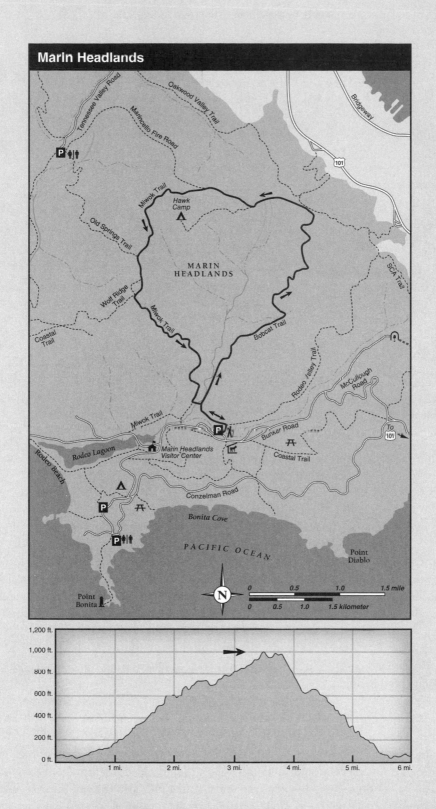

Marin Headlands

Tennessee Valley Road
Oakwood Valley Trail
Marincello Fire Road
Bridgeway
101
Miwok Trail
Hawk Camp
Old Springs Trail
MARIN HEADLANDS
Wolf Ridge Trail
SCA Trail
Miwok Trail
Coastal Trail
Bobcat Trail
Rodeo Valley Trail
McCulough Road
Miwok Trail
P
Bunker Road
To 101
Rodeo Lagoon
Marin Headlands Visitor Center
Coastal Trail
Rodeo Beach
P
Conzelman Road
Bonita Cove
PACIFIC OCEAN
Point Diablo
Point Bonita
N
0   0.5   1.0   1.5 mile
0   0.5   1.0   1.5 kilometer

1,200 ft.
1,000 ft.
800 ft.
600 ft.
400 ft.
200 ft.
0 ft.
1 mi.   2 mi.   3 mi.   4 mi.   5 mi.   6 mi.

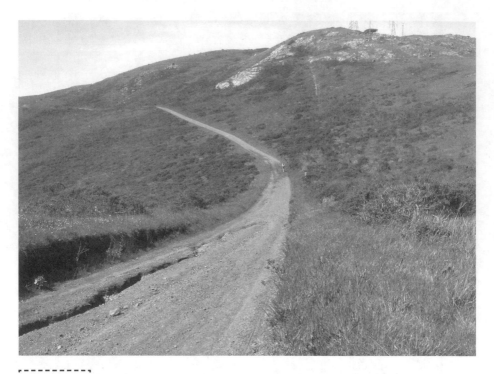

Bobcat Trail

permit a quick escape, you can make the transition from city mouse to country mouse in 15 minutes. Although the Headlands are a stone's throw from the city and US 101, ridges block traffic noise and trails are peaceful. The Headlands are laced with a handful of trails and lots of fire roads, some of them remnants from the land's military past and others part of a development that never happened.

Just north of the Golden Gate, a military installation occupied the area now known as the Marin Headlands until the 1960s. After the bunkers and batteries were shuttered, a developer planned to build a massive housing complex called Marincello. Environmental and community activists squelched the development, and the land eventually became part of the Golden Gate National Recreation Area, managed by the National Park Service. It's high-profile open space, exemplifying what Bay Area preservationists and outdoors enthusiasts cherish: broadly accessible land close to urban areas, with tons of elbow room for animals, wildflowers, and people.

Begin at the signed trailhead, marked by a Bay Area Ridge Trail symbol, immediately crossing a wide footbridge. Keep an eye open for newts in this area during the rainy season. At the far end of the bridge you'll reach a T-junction—turn left onto Rodeo Valley Trail. Grassy hills rise to the right, but the broad fire road keeps to a level grade, running along a damp meadow dotted with coyote brush. At 0.3 mile, Rodeo Valley Trail ends. Bear right onto Bobcat Trail. Ascending gradually, the wide dirt fire road follows the course of a creek on the left, where willow and blackberry thrive and red-winged blackbirds flutter around the fringes of the stream. A stand of tall eucalyptus and a few scattered fruit trees suggest an old settlement in this area. The medicinal eucalyptus aroma mingles with the licorice scent of fennel, which grows with abandon along the trail. As the fire road begins to climb at a more moderate grade, views open up across Gerbode Valley, including glimpses of Miwok Trail. With each step, more of the ocean becomes visible back to the west.

The sides of Bobcat Trail are lined with many native plants. Coyote brush, purple bush lupine, poison oak, lizard's-tail, sticky monkeyflower, coffeeberry, sagebrush, and toyon are common coastal scrub plants, but the fog that is often held in this bowl-shaped valley nourishes some plants, such as creambush, snowberry, and currant, usually found in less exposed locations. Flowers you might see in bloom range from late-winter specialists such as hound's tongue and milkmaids to spring favorites including blue-eyed grass, buttercups, blue-dicks, California poppies, iris, paintbrush, checkerbloom, and fringe cups. In early April, patches of goldfields blaze with color on the highest reaches of the ridge. There are very few trees—just a few clusters of some shrubby coast live oak, cypress, and a particularly squat Douglas-fir.

After a long, steady ascent, the grade eases and huckleberry shrubs appear on the left. Bobcat Trail climbs until it finally levels out at the ridgeline. Fire roads split off to the right at 2.3 miles, with Wolfback Ridge Trail heading back to the south and Rodeo and Alta Trails proceeding north toward a pullout along US 101 and Oakwood Valley Trail. Continue straight on Bobcat. Although this is far from the highest point on the ridgeline, the sweeping views feel well earned. Gerbode Valley slopes down at your feet, and the ocean sparkles to the west. Bobcat Trail passes under some power lines, then takes a dip before rising back to follow the ridge. In spring, California poppies, blue-dicks, checkerbloom, blue-eyed grass, and buttercups blossom through the grass along the trail.

At 2.8 miles, a trail leading to Hawk Camp breaks off to the left. Continue straight on Bobcat, which now makes a final push toward the Headlands' second highest hill. The northern Golden Gate Bridge tower peeks out from between two hills to the south, and then the entire ridge of Mount Tamalpais comes into view to the north. Marincello Fire Road starts a journey to Tennessee Valley at 3.1 miles, on the right. Continue straight on Bobcat Trail. Still climbing through grassland, the trail finally ends at a junction with Miwok Trail and two fire roads that service a Federal Aviation Administration navigational antenna perched at the hilltop. Turn right onto Miwok. The fire road descends, sweeping around the hill while offering grand views to the north of Tennessee Valley and Mount Tam. After a brief ascent, Miwok crests. But before heading downhill, take a moment to appreciate the views south. The Bay and Golden Gate Bridges are visible, as are downtown San Francisco skyscrapers, the Sutro Tower near Twin Peaks, and, farther south, Montara Mountain. If it's not too windy, a little grassy spot off the trail to the left makes a great rest stop. Where Miwok Trail begins a steep descent, the rest of the journey is downhill.

A gopher played peek-a-boo with me along the trail once, popping out of a hole, then diving back down. Although this stretch of trail is closed to cyclists, some riders still brave the harsh descent and massive drainage humps known as water bars, so stay alert for traffic. Reach a junction with Old Spring Trail on the right at 4 miles, but continue straight on Miwok Trail. Trailside vegetation is a bit bland compared to the Bobcat's; you'll see mostly coyote brush, with lots of mule ear sunflowers blooming in summer. This is a good trail for raptor watching, though, particularly in autumn when migratory birds pass through, and year-round you'll probably see vultures soaring overhead. Jagged Wolf Ridge rises off to the right, and the trail drops to reach its namesake trail at 4.3 miles. Stay to the left on Miwok Trail. The descent is relentless, but I always console myself with the thought that at least it's downhill. If you're a bit rusty, your quads will be hollering.

As the trail drops back into Gerbode Valley, the vegetation on the hillside to the right becomes more lush, with ferns, snowberry, poison oak, purple bush lupine, and sagebrush spread across a hillside of coyote brush. Paintbrush, buttercups, and California poppies are the most common "wild" flowers in early spring, but there's also plenty of nonnative Bermuda buttercup, a yellow-blossomed member of the oxalis family related to redwood sorrel. Miwok Trail finally winds its way back to level ground, meeting Bobcat Trail at 5.5 miles. Turn left. The trail crosses over a creek where twinberry, a rather bland shrub most of the year, makes a spectacle of itself in spring, putting forth pairs of orange-red flowers that develop into berries in the summer. After about 300 feet, Bobcat veers left at the start of the Rodeo Valley Trail. Turn right and retrace your steps back to the trailhead.

NEARBY ACTIVITIES

Miwok Trail plays a part in another Headlands loop hike. Continue to the Rodeo Beach trailhead at the end of Bunker Road, and string together Miwok, Wolf Ridge, and Coastal Trails for a 4.3-mile excursion—note that this is one Headlands hike on which dogs are welcome.

MOUNT BURDELL
OPEN SPACE PRESERVE

IN BRIEF

Mount Burdell is a big name for a relatively low Marin County peak. This preserve is backyard wilderness for Novato dog-walkers and runners, and is a great destination for easy-to-moderate hikes like this one—a loop through oaks and grassland to the high flanks of the mountain and the upper reaches of Olompali State Historic Park.

DESCRIPTION

Two parks occupy the slopes of Mount Burdell: Olompali State Historic Park and Mount Burdell Open Space Preserve. The state park, on the east slope, features a small, reconstructed Miwok village and trails that snake uphill through gorgeous oak woods. Unfortunately, traffic noise from US 101 is pervasive in the state park—the open-space preserve is quieter and offers more options for loops through oak savanna, with good wildflower displays in spring.

Begin from roadside parking and veer right, entering the preserve through either a V-shaped stile or a cattle gate. A shortcut path heads to the right, but follow the access path straight, then begin uphill on San Andreas Fire Road. After 300 feet, San Marin Fire Road

- -

Directions

Leave San Francisco northbound on US 101 and use the Golden Gate Bridge toll plaza as your mileage starting point. Drive north 20 miles on US 101 to Novato, and take Exit 463, San Marin Drive/Atherton Avenue. Drive west 2.5 miles on San Marin Drive, then turn right onto San Andreas Drive. Continue uphill 0.5 mile, then park on the right side of road, near the open-space gate.

KEY AT-A-GLANCE INFORMATION

LENGTH: 5.3 miles

CONFIGURATION: Balloon

DIFFICULTY: Moderate

SCENERY: Grassland and oaks

EXPOSURE: Mostly full sun

TRAFFIC: Moderate

TRAIL SURFACE: Rocky dirt trails and fire roads, one paved fire road

HIKING TIME: 2.5 hours

SEASON: Good anytime; nice flowers in late winter and spring.

ACCESS: Free

MAPS: None at the trailhead; download at tinyurl.com/mtburdellmap.

FACILITIES: None

SPECIAL COMMENTS: Dogs are permitted in the preserve but not the state park (one short out-and-back segment of this hike).
Tour the east slope of Burdell Mountain from Olompali State Historic Park, accessed off US 101 (415-892-3383, tinyurl.com/olompalishp).

CONTACTS: 415-473-2816, tinyurl.com/mtburdell

DRIVING DISTANCE: 26.6 miles from the Golden Gate Bridge toll plaza

GPS INFORMATION

N38° 7.809' W122° 36.254'

Mt. Burdell Open Space Preserve

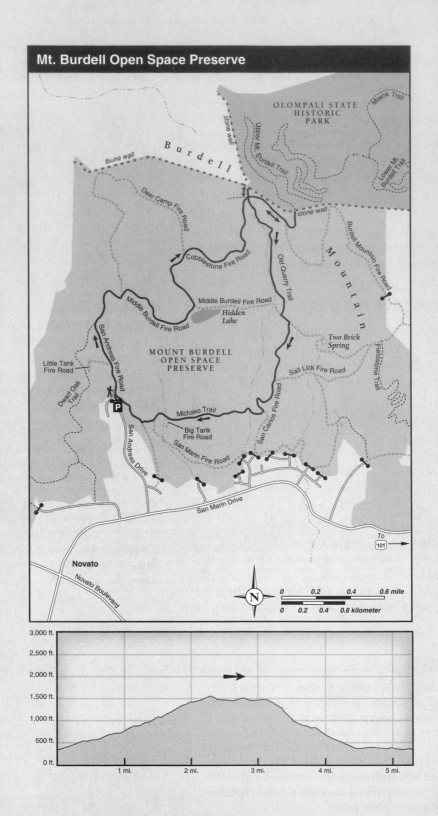

begins on the right near a huge coast live oak. Continue on San Andreas Fire Road, ascending past coast live oak and California bay at a moderate clip. At 0.2 mile, Little Tank Fire Road departs on the left—stick to San Andreas Fire Road and keep climbing. A few black oaks and buckeyes appear; in late winter, look for a good display of Chinese houses on the left side of the trail. San Andreas Fire Road crests at the lip of a bowl-shaped valley at 0.4 mile.

Dwarf Oak Trail heads back downhill on the left—stay to the right on San Andreas Fire Road, ignoring a dead-end fire road heading straight, leading to the park boundary. On one early-April hike, the grass in this valley was completely overtaken by the yellow flowers of blooming johnny-tuck and California butter-cup. Two months later the grassy bowl and oak-dotted slopes ascending out of the valley were a sea of dry, blonde grass. San Andreas Fire Road curves right and ascends again, winding past mature valley oak, California bay, and buckeye, then ends at a fork at 0.7 mile. Deer Camp Fire Road, to the left, is a longer option—for this hike, continue straight, now on Middle Burdell Fire Road.

Blue-dicks and popcorn flower bloom along the trail in early spring, preced-ing a June bonanza of clarkia and elegant brodiaea. Ascending easily, Middle Bur-dell Fire Road is mostly unshaded, although there is one grove of California bay, coast live oak, and buckeye. At 1.1 miles, you'll reach the edge of Hidden Lake, fenced to keep cows (and dogs) out of this sensitive habitat. In dry months the seasonal pond looks like a damp meadow, but in winter it does hold water. Cob-blestone Fire Road begins at 1.2 miles. Turn left.

The fire road initially climbs at an easy-to-moderate grade, but there is one short, rocky, steep stretch. Cobblestones were quarried from the upper slopes of Mount Burdell for San Francisco street construction, and as you progress uphill, the trails and hillsides get increasingly rocky. At 1.5 miles, Deer Camp Fire Road enters from the left—stay to the right on Cobblestone Fire Road. The trail ascends through grassland, with buckeye, California bay, and oaks standing well back on sloping hillsides. In June, look for yellow mariposa lilies blooming along with California poppy, clarkia, and venus thistle. A rough path sweeps off to the right—supposedly a shortcut—but it offers no relief from the climb, so stay to the left. A microwave relay structure is visible to the left, and off to the right one of the old quarries is conspicuous. Cobblestone Fire Road levels out as it approaches the summit area, then ends at a multiple junction at 2.2 miles. A paved fire road heads west (left) to the microwave relay and east to the park boundary. Old Quarry Trail, this hike's return route, departs sharply to the right. Continue straight through the junction, uphill on an unmarked but obvious path.

This little trail ascends through grassland, but beware of a small poison oak shrub crowding the path on the left. The last stretch is very rocky, and the path crests at 2.3 miles at the park boundary, marked by an old stone wall. This rock fence and several others, all built without mortar, were constructed in the late 1800s by Chinese laborers. Return downhill to the paved fire road and turn left.

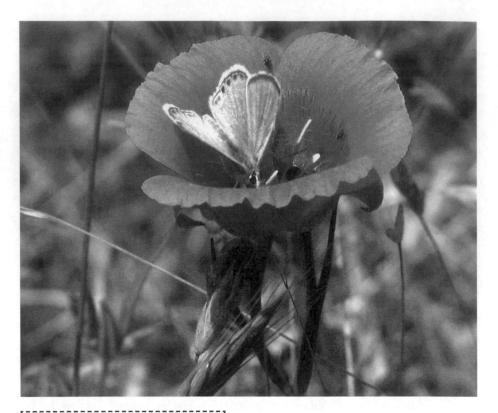

Yellow mariposa lily (and visiting butterfly)

Burdell Mountain Fire Road keeps a level pace as it winds just downslope from the mountain's highest ridge. There's considerable, if distant, noise from US 101, visible downhill to the east. More scenic are views to Big Rock Ridge and Mount Tamalpais to the south. At 2.6 miles, veer left onto an unsigned dirt road that quickly leads to a fence and entry into Olompali State Park. As you enter the state park, a grassy hillside falls steeply to the east, revealing long views of the Petaluma River, upper San Pablo Bay, and the southern tip of the Sonoma Mountains. Two picnic tables here invite a lingering lunch. Follow the trail off to the left through a sparse, grassy forest of California bay to another stone wall crossing the trail at 2.8 miles. If you want to extend this hike, you could continue, winding downhill another 3.5 miles to the next junction. For now, though, retrace your steps back to the junction with Cobblestone Fire Road and Old Quarry Trail at 3.2 miles. Turn left onto Old Quarry Trail.

Descending through grassland, the slight path shifts from easy to steep near a pocket of sagebrush and sticky monkeyflower. Coast live oak, California bay, and buckeye nestle in a little creek bed on the right, as the trail descends into a mostly unshaded canyon. Steep, grassy slopes on the left are scored with animal paths, and you may see deer browsing in this area of the park, where mule ear sunflowers are common in spring. After the steepest section, littered with loose rock, Old Quarry Trail eases up in the middle of a California bay grove, then emerges into grassland. At 3.9 miles, the trail reaches a T-junction with Middle Burdell Fire Road. Turn left.

After about 300 feet of level strolling, turn right onto the continuation of Old Quarry Trail. The descent is steep, but less so than the previous segment, and not nearly as rocky. An expanse of grassland stretches off the sides of the trail, punctuated by oaks and buckeye. Just past a gate and stile, Old Quarry Trail ends at San Carlos Fire Road. Turn right.

The fire road descends easily through coast live oaks, with summer displays of milk thistle. Salt Lick Fire Road sets off to the left at 4.2 miles—stay to the right on San Carlos Fire Road, following an arching curve downhill to the junction with Michako Trail at 4.5 miles. Turn right.

Note the granary tree at this junction—drilled with holes and stuffed with acorns by birds. At a slight descent, Michako Trail passes through another cattle gate, then skips across a small creek. In June large patches of Davy's centaury, a pink flower, bloom in the drying grass, accompanied by sprinkles of elegant brodiaea. The trail forks at another creek crossing—the two legs rejoin shortly. At the 5-mile mark, a fire road crosses the trail, leading left to a water tank. Follow the fire road to the right or continue straight on the trail; the two routes meet at a junction at about 5.1 miles. Veer right, now on San Marin Fire Road.

The green, waxy rock exposed along the trail is serpentine, and this stretch of trail hosts a good display of native flowers in early spring. Nearing the preserve boundary, the trail bends right and descends, then levels out as it approaches the trailhead. Officially, San Marin Fire Road continues to its terminus at San Andreas Fire Road, but a well-worn path shortcuts the route to the left, leading to the entrance gate.

7 MOUNT TAMALPAIS:
CATARACT FALLS–POTRERO MEADOWS LOOP

KEY AT-A-GLANCE INFORMATION

LENGTH: 6.5 miles

CONFIGURATION: Loop

DIFFICULTY: Moderate–strenuous

SCENERY: Grassland, woods, chaparral, and waterfalls

EXPOSURE: Back and forth through shade and sun

TRAFFIC: Moderate on Cataract Trail, otherwise light

TRAIL SURFACE: Dirt fire roads and trails

HIKING TIME: 4 hours (includes lunch break)

SEASON: Good anytime but muddy in winter.

ACCESS: Free at this trailhead

MAPS: None at the trailhead but available online at tinyurl.com/mmwdmaps. I highly recommend Tom Harrison Maps' *Mount Tamalpais* topo ($9.95; tomharrisonmaps.com).

FACILITIES: Pit toilets at the trailhead and at Laurel Dell

SPECIAL COMMENTS: Leashed dogs are welcome on this hike (on Marin Municipal Water District land) but prohibited in the adjacent state park.

CONTACTS: 415-945-1181, marinwater.org

DRIVING DISTANCE: 16 miles from the Golden Gate Bridge toll plaza

GPS INFORMATION

N37° 54.652' W122° 36.765'

IN BRIEF

One of Mount Tamalpais's most compelling assets is its broad variety of possible hikes. You can order up your hike like a San Francisco burrito: hot or mild, small or *grande,* with just rice and beans or the works. This 6.5-mile loop is one of the mountain's wildest, with only two short segments on fire roads and the rest on narrow and rocky hiking-only trails.

DESCRIPTION

Since the first edition of this book, the Marin Municipal Water District has mothballed some of Tam's oldest northside trails by removing their signage and ceasing trail maintenance. Many of these well-worn paths followed too closely to creek beds and were badly eroded and/or steeply routed, but they were scenic and lonely. The hike described here sticks to sanctioned, well-signed trails, but a detailed map of the area is still highly recommended—it's quite easy to get lost on Tam's north slope.

This entire loop is a tour de force of the mountain's magic: you'll experience dense

----

Directions

Leave San Francisco on northbound US 101 and use the Golden Gate Bridge toll plaza as your mileage starting point. Drive about 5.5 miles, then take Exit 445B, CA 1/Mill Valley/Stinson Beach, and drive about 1 mile on Shoreline Highway to the junction with Almonte Boulevard (look for the CA 1 sign). Turn left and drive about 2.5 miles to the junction with Panoramic Highway. Turn right on Panoramic and drive about 5.5 miles to the junction with Pantoll Road. Turn right onto Pantoll and drive another 1.5 miles to the Rock Spring trailhead, at the junction of East and West Ridgecrest Boulevards.

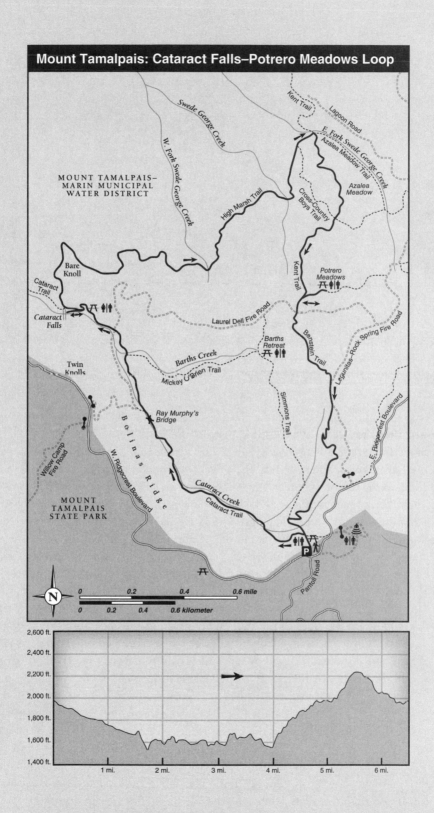

Mount Tamalpais: Cataract Falls–Potrero Meadows Loop

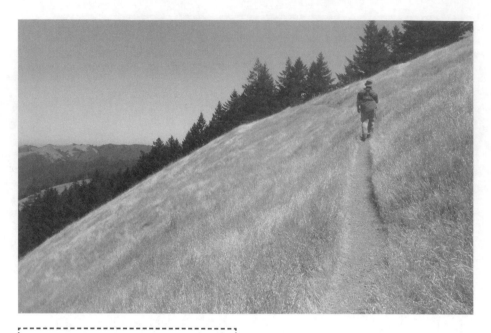

A hiker traverses grassland on High Marsh Trail.

forests, aromatic chaparral, rushing creeks, waterfalls, and flower-dotted meadows. In fact, the hike begins at a meadow, just off the Rock Spring parking lot. Here, Cataract Trail starts a long journey from Tam's high ridges down to the shores of Alpine Lake. Follow Cataract Trail 0.1 mile to a junction with Simmons Trail, and continue to the left on Cataract. At a slight descent, the narrow trail skirts a grassy meadow where patches of blue and white lupine are common in spring, then begins to follow its namesake creek, here just a trickle. Huge Douglas-firs line the trail and creek, mixed through huckleberry, tan oak, California bay, and madrone. Old trail segments are occasionally visible on the opposite bank, but this trail crosses Cataract Creek only on a series of small footbridges—if you're stymied, look for a bridge; don't cross the creek without one.

Although the grade is easy, the trail is quite rocky in places, and some big boulders loom on the sides of the trail. Where Cataract Trail steps out into grassland, we saw gorgeous orange leopard lilies near the creek bed one Fourth of July weekend, and hundreds of swallowtail and California sister butterflies, dragonflies, and damselflies drifted lazily over the meadow. Back in the woods on this same hike, a powerfully sweet smell led our noses to an azalea bush in full bloom right at the trail's edge. As Cataract Trail continues downhill into a canyon, the tree cover becomes thicker and the creek swells with water feeding in from side streams. Once, on a February hike here, I saw a giant salamander eating a mouse.

At 0.8 mile, signed Ray Murphy Trail crosses the creek toward Laurel Dell Fire Road. Continue straight on Cataract Trail. This is a good stretch to look for little pink Calypso orchids in late winter. Mickey O'Brien Trail departs on the right at

1.1 mile—stick to the left on Cataract Trail as it continues to Laurel Dell. The trail passes some pit toilets and reaches a junction with Laurel Dell Fire Road at 1.2 miles. Cross the fire road and remain on Cataract Trail. Once past a few picnic tables, the trail begins to descend again along the right bank of Cascade Creek. In winter and early spring the water flows swiftly, and you'll pass the first cascade. Maples mix through the California bay and Douglas-fir in the forest, where birding is often sublime. On one winter hike I caught the orange flash of a varied thrush flitting through the woods, and watched a brown creeper earn its name—this little brown bird scrambles up tree trunks, looking for insects. At 1.4 miles, Cataract Trail meets High Marsh Trail at a signed junction. Continue on Cataract downhill a short distance to the waterfall viewpoint. After winter storms, water crashes down over huge boulders here—this is one of the most scenic waterfalls in the Bay Area. The trail (and creek) continue steeply downhill toward Alpine Lake, but for this hike, retrace your steps back uphill and turn left onto High Marsh Trail.

The trail descends through woods away from Cataract Creek, then begins to contour across steeply sloped Bare Knoll. As the name suggests, the open, sunny knob is grassy, with only a few Douglas-firs here and there. Views north are the best you'll get on High Marsh Trail, which from here on is mostly wooded and passes through no other grassland. Pass Bare Knoll Trail heading uphill to Laurel Dell Fire Road at 1.7 miles, and as High Marsh Trail prepares to head back into the woods, look on the left side of the trail for canyon live oaks. These evergreen trees are easy to pick out—their glossy oval leaves are dusted with golden powder on their undersides. Once under tree cover again, High Marsh Trail begins a campaign of rolling ups and downs, with some level interludes. From time to time the trail crests and steps out into sunny chaparral dominated by manzanita, but the majority of time you'll be hiking beneath California bay, madrone, tan oak, and Douglas-fir.

At around the 3-mile mark, unsigned Music Stand Trail heads uphill on the right—continue straight on signed High Marsh Trail. As the trail drops into a canyon surrounding Swede George Creek, look for iris in May. This part of High Marsh Trail is moist and almost completely shaded—it can be chilly here in winter, but in the summer you'll be glad for the shelter. High Marsh Trail steps across the creek (transformed into a waterfall in winter), and at 3.3 miles you'll reach a two-part junction with Swede George Trail (also known as Willow Trail). The first leg of Swede George Trail is unsigned and doubles back to the right, then climbs along the creek. To the left, Swede George and High Marsh run together briefly, then Swede George departs to the left (the High Marsh part of this junction is now signed). Continue on High Marsh. The trail begins to climb at this point, then levels out—High Marsh, on the left, is a tiny pond ringed with cattails, coyote brush, and Douglas-fir. In winter the trail becomes a bit swamped here, but by summer the trail (and sometimes the marsh) is dry. Cross Country Boys Trail departs to the right at the edge of the marsh, at 3.4 miles, but continue straight. The trail heads back into the woods. At 3.5 miles, you'll reach a junction with Kent Trail. Turn right and begin a moderate climb alternating between quiet dark woods and patches of chaparral. This narrow path is very rocky in stretches. Kent Trail meets Cross Country Trail at 4.1 miles—continue straight. We encountered a coiled and rattling rattlesnake here on a summer hike. Because it showed no interest in moving, we took a wide path around it. Kent Trail emerges from the woods and passes through a big patch of manzanita dotted with towering Douglas-fir. Here the views extend far to the north. As the trail continues uphill, bunchgrasses line the way in places.

At 4.5 miles, Kent Trail ends at the Potrero Meadows picnic area, on the right. In hot weather, the shaded tables make perfect lunch stops. Another option is Potrero Meadows proper: Turn left and, at a level grade, pass along the edge of a small, flat, grassy spot (this is the lesser of the two meadows). Once through a pocket of woods, the trail emerges to a wide, open meadow. This oasis of grassland surrounded by forest is one of Mount Tam's special places. On a winter weekday it can be surprisingly lonely, but in the thick of spring you'll likely see plenty of people in and around the meadow. (The area's name may annoy grammar sticklers—it's redundant, since *potrero* means "meadow" in Spanish.) Little carpets of flowers brighten the grass in May, when you might see buttercups, goldfields, California poppy, and Linanthus in bloom. When ready, retrace your steps back to the picnic area, then turn left onto a wide, unsigned dirt service road. Look for azaleas in bloom on the left here in early summer, as the road climbs briefly then ends at a T-junction with Laurel Dell Fire Road. Turn left and walk about 50 yards to the signed junction with Benstein Trail. Turn right.

The trail begins to climb. The initial section is very rocky and can be slippery when wet. Nestled in the woods is a little chaparral pocket of Sargent cypress and manzanita. But as Benstein Trail ascends, it becomes enveloped by a very dense forest of tan oak, chinquapin, Douglas-fir, and madrone—so thick that there is little understory vegetation. The going is steep, but the trail soon levels out a bit to the left of a manzanita thicket.

At 5.5 miles, Benstein feeds into Lagunitas–Rock Spring Fire Road. Go with the flow to the right briefly, then abandon the fire road for the path as Benstein veers off to the right. This well-cared-for segment of trail is delightful. At an easy descent, Benstein drifts downhill through madrone, Douglas-fir, and live oak. Some switchbacks drop the trail away from a fragile serpentine meadow. Milkmaids, shooting stars, and hound's tongue are common late-winter flowers along the trail. You may hear Ziesche Creek rushing in winter; you'll cross two tiny streams that head downhill to the bigger creek.

At 6 miles, a signed path heads left toward Ridgecrest Boulevard. Bear right, remaining on Benstein. The descent through madrones is still easy. Look left for a peek at a huge serpentine swale—a conspicuous greenish-blue swath of rock in a sloping grassy meadow. Benstein Trail ends at 6.3 miles. Turn left onto Simmons Trail, which sweeps across a meadow back toward Rock Spring. At 6.4 miles, turn left onto Cataract Trail and retrace your steps back to the trailhead.

MOUNT TAMALPAIS:
MATT DAVIS—STEEP RAVINE LOOP

IN BRIEF

This loop showcases the best of the Bay Area. While a number of other parks have a more pronounced wilderness vibe, Mount Tamalpais is a short drive from many parts of the North and East Bays, and San Francisco residents flock to the mountain, particularly on sunny weekends in spring.

DESCRIPTION

In the heart of summer weekends, there are so many visitors on the trails around Mount Tamalpais's Pantoll area that you might feel like a pint of blood trying to squeeze through a clogged artery. Travel is sluggish, particularly on Steep Ravine Trail, a narrow route that doesn't tolerate crowds well. Try to plan this hike for a weekday or early in the day during the off-season. The best possible time may be the thin overlap between late winter and early spring, particularly if it's been a wet winter. During that window, wildflowers bloom everywhere and the waterfalls are plump with runoff.

Steep Ravine Trail departs from a signed trailhead at the southern edge of the parking

---

Directions ———————————→

Leave San Francisco on northbound US 101 and use the Golden Gate Bridge toll plaza as your mileage starting point. Drive north on US 101 about 5.5 miles, then take Exit 445B, CA 1/Mill Valley/Stinson Beach, and drive about 1 mile on Shoreline Highway to the junction with Almonte Boulevard (look for the CA 1 sign). Turn left on CA 1 and drive about 2.5 miles to the junction with Panoramic Highway. Turn right on Panoramic and drive about 5.5 miles to the junction with Pantoll Road. Using caution, turn left into the parking lot.

GPS INFORMATION

N37° 54.195' W122° 36.250'

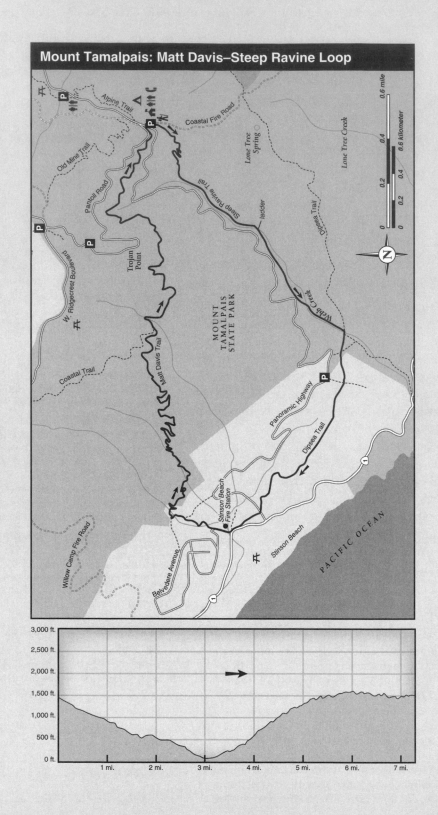

Mount Tamalpais: Matt Davis–Steep Ravine Loop

Alpine Trail

Coastal Fire Road

Old Mine Trail

Pantoll Road

Lone Tree Spring

Lone Tree Creek

Steep Ravine Trail

ladder

Dipsea Trail

W. Ridgecrest Boulevard

Trojan Point

Coastal Trail

Matt Davis Trail

MOUNT TAMALPAIS STATE PARK

Webb Creek

Panoramic Highway

Dipsea Trail

Stinson Beach Fire Station

Willow Camp Fire Road

Belvedere Avenue

Stinson Beach

PACIFIC OCEAN

0.6 mile

0.4

0.6 kilometer

0.2

0.4

0

0.2

0

3,000 ft.
2,500 ft.
2,000 ft.
1,500 ft.
1,000 ft.
500 ft.
0 ft.

1 mi.   2 mi.   3 mi.   4 mi.   5 mi.   6 mi.   7 mi.

lot. The sign warns of a 10-foot ladder, an unusual trail element, but if you're up for a 7-mile hike, descending on a little ladder shouldn't scare you.

Without any prelude, the narrow trail begins to drop into a canyon. After a few switchbacks across a steep hillside, Steep Ravine Trail hooks up with Webb Creek and follows the stream as it makes its way through a lush forest of redwood, California bay, ferns, tan oak, and Douglas-fir. Little bridges channel hikers back and forth across the creek a few times along the route. Spring wildflowers here include plants that adore moist environments, such as trillium, coast fairy bells, and stream violets.

At 0.8 mile, you'll reach the ladder. The wood can be slippery, so take it slow—I prefer to descend facing the ladder rather than facing out. Beside the ladder, a little waterfall, one of a couple along the trail, burbles soothingly. Below the ladder, trailside vegetation seems to become even more lush. Redwoods uprooted or snapped off by winter storms lie across the trail and in the streambed in places; some are notched for passage.

At 1.7 miles, the first of two junctions with Dipsea Trail departs on the left. Continue straight another 0.1 mile past an old dam on the left, then bear right, following the sign toward Stinson Beach. As Dipsea Trail begins a slight climb, a connector back to Steep Ravine veers left—keep going straight. The trail climbs through some young Douglas-fir and toyon, then reaches a junction where you'll continue straight and emerge at the edge of a meadow and another junction with a fire road. Cross the fire road, remaining on Dipsea, and watch as incredible views unfold to the north. On a clear day you'll see Stinson Beach, Bolinas Lagoon, and the forested hills of the Point Reyes peninsula.

While it's hard to top the enchantment of Steep Ravine, a spring hike through here boasts verdant grass and pockets of orange California poppy, pink checkerbloom, and blue and white lupine. Dipsea Trail descends steadily through a little coastal scrub and then a pocket of woods stretching along a creek. Gnarled moss-covered buckeyes are the star here, although California bays are more common. At 2.9 miles, Dipsea reaches Panoramic Highway. Carefully cross the road and pick up the trail on the other side.

Descending toward the town of Stinson Beach, traffic and neighborhood noise are abundant. At 3 miles, where Dipsea Trail meets CA 1, you can add an optional out-and-back to this hike by continuing across the highway and walking on city streets to the Dipsea Trail's terminus at the beach. Otherwise, carefully turn right and walk along the side of CA 1. (The other side of the street may be a better option, but you'll have to cross the road twice—if you're looking for lunch or a place to buy water, walk past the firehouse to Stinson's commercial district.) After less than 0.1 mile, turn right at the firehouse onto Belvedere Avenue. Walk up this street and, just past the WRONG WAY sign, turn right onto signed Matt Davis Trail.

Back in the woods, this narrow trail winds uphill. When you reach an unsigned T-junction, turn left, then cross a creek and, at a second junction, bear

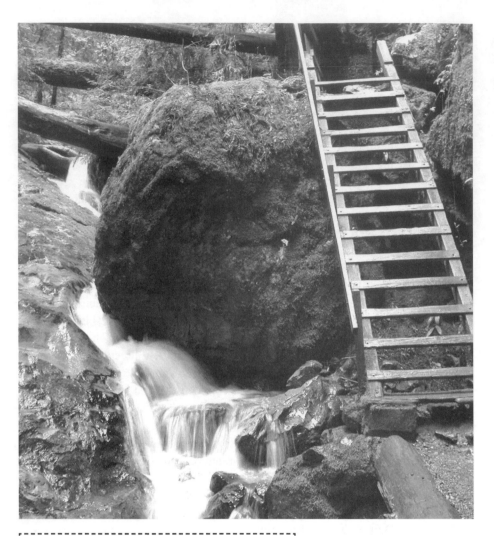

Steep Ravine's famous ladder isn't as intimidating as it looks.

right. This is the last junction for the next 2.3 miles. The sounds of town life quickly fade away and are replaced by the sounds of murmuring creek and crashing surf as the trail rises through a forest of buckeye and California bay. A bridge crosses a descending stream with less gush than Webb Creek, but the setting is incredibly pretty year-round.

After a set of steps and a switchback, Matt Davis Trail bisects a patch of chaparral. Glance over purple-flowered lupine bushes and already you have views to the ocean. The sunny interlude is short, and soon you'll ascend through a shaded woodland. The trail climbs relentlessly, but at a moderate pace. Just past another bridge a long series of steps may be the toughest stretch of the trail, especially if you have short legs.

With Table Rock Creek tumbling downhill on the left, the trail skirts a huge boulder. California bays mix through a forest of massive Douglas-firs, and ferns are a perennial star of the understory, with trilliums, iris, forget-me-nots, and milkmaids making appearances in spring. Still ascending, negotiate a few broad switchbacks and then step out of the woods into grassland. The transition is startling, particularly in late winter, when the grass is so green it practically throbs with life.

Matt Davis Trail ascends gently downslope from the ridgeline, through grassland and little pockets of trees that linger in hillside creases. Framed by tall Douglas-firs, views west take in the ocean. In late winter and spring, peruse the sides of the trail for blue-eyed grass, California buttercups, California poppies, and blue-dicks. At 5.7 miles, Coastal Trail swings sharply left from a signed junction—bear right to remain on Matt Davis Trail.

With the worst of the climbing behind you, this next segment is a pleasurable stroll at a gentle incline across the sloping grassy hillside. Bypass two quick junctions, the first with an ascending trail and the second with a descending trail; then continue straight, following the symbols for the Bay Area Ridge Trail. Prepare for more sweeping views, this time south, extending past the Headlands to San Francisco and the San Mateo County coast. You may be able to spot Northern harriers hunting from overhead.

Follow Matt Davis Trail, leaving the grassland for woods once more. Dense stands of California bay, redwood, Douglas-fir, and live oak filter the sun, creating shade that sustains a little flower favored by native-plant enthusiasts: the Calypso orchid. I saw dozens of the delicate purple flowers along the trail on one late-March hike, along with red larkspur, hound's tongue, and milkmaids.

The trail's elevation remains nearly level through here, and although trees block any views, they fail to screen the sound of traffic on Pantoll Road, just uphill to the left. You probably will cross paths with a steady flow of hikers on this part of the trail, a signal that the trailhead is growing closer with each step. Pass through an open, rocky area marked with soaring Douglas-firs, where ceanothus and chamise line the trail. Matt Davis Trail breaks off to the left, continuing toward Mountain Home Inn. Here, bear right, descend a few steps, and carefully cross the street to the Pantoll parking lot.

9 MOUNT TAMALPAIS:
MOUNTAIN HOME–MUIR WOODS LOOP

KEY AT-A-GLANCE INFORMATION

LENGTH: 4.7 miles

CONFIGURATION: Loop

DIFFICULTY: Moderate

SCENERY: Redwoods, forested canyon, and creeks

EXPOSURE: Mostly shaded

TRAFFIC: Moderate around trailhead, very heavy in the heart of Muir Woods

TRAIL SURFACE: Two short paved sections, dirt trails, and lots of steps on Lost Trail

HIKING TIME: 3 hours

SEASON: Daily, 7 a.m.–sunset. Anytime is good but summer is busiest; fall is gorgeous.

ACCESS: No fee at this trailhead; entrance to the main Muir Woods trailhead requires an $8 use fee.

MAPS: Download at tinyurl.com /mttamparkmap (no maps at the trailhead). The best map for the area is Tom Harrison Maps' *Mount Tam* topo ($9.95; tomharrisonmaps.com).

FACILITIES: Vault toilets and drinking water at trailhead

SPECIAL COMMENTS: No dogs allowed. Arrive very early for parking in summer.

CONTACTS: 415-388-2070, tinyurl .com/mttamsp

DRIVING DISTANCE: 11.7 miles from the Golden Gate Bridge toll plaza

GPS INFORMATION

N37° 54.612' W122° 34.633'

IN BRIEF

This hike starts across from Mountain Home Inn, descends on a paved service road, then winds through woods on a narrow footpath. At Van Wyck Meadow, you'll begin a steep descent following creeks into Redwood Canyon and Muir Woods, where you'll mingle with the crowds on the park's main trail. After only 0.3 mile, the hike veers off into Fern Canyon and relative solitude. A long set of steps ascends through woods into grassland, and a nearly level path makes for a quick return to the trailhead.

DESCRIPTION

Steep-sloped Redwood Canyon escaped the flying axes of the Bay Area's Gold Rush and today preserves some of the oldest and most majestic redwoods in the Bay Area. To prevent logging, William Kent began buying canyon property in 1905, then donated the land to the federal government for protection. The woods became a national monument in 1908, named in honor of conservationist John Muir. Although Muir Woods proper is quite small, the land is surrounded by Mount Tamalpais

- -

Directions ⟶

Leave San Francisco on northbound US 101 and use the Golden Gate Bridge toll plaza as your mileage starting point. Drive north on US 101 about 5.5 miles, then take Exit 445B, CA 1/ Mill Valley/Stinson Beach, and drive about 1 mile on Shoreline Highway to the junction with Almonte Boulevard (look for the CA 1 sign). Turn left and drive about 2.5 miles on CA 1 to the junction with Panoramic Highway. Turn right on Panoramic Highway and drive about 2.5 miles to a parking lot on the left side of the road, across from the Mountain Home Inn.

Mount Tamalpais: Mountain Home–Muir Woods Loop

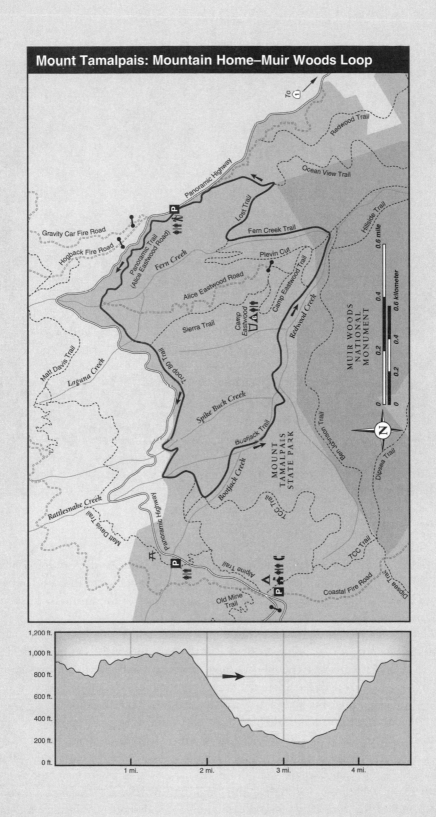

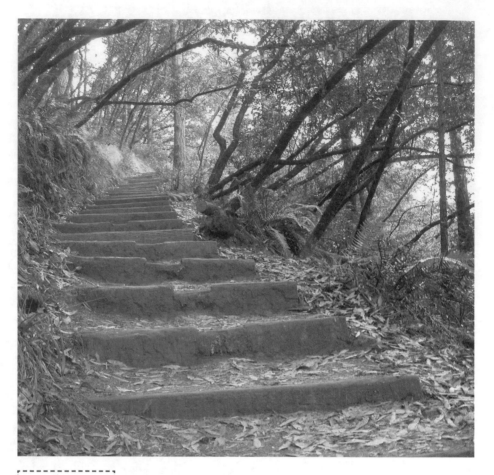

Steps on Lost Trail

State Park and Golden Gate National Recreation Area property, forming a huge greenbelt of protected redwood canyons, creeks, coastal grassland, and mixed woodland that stretches from the Golden Gate Bridge to the northern flanks of Mount Tam.

Whether you're a Bay Area visitor or a permanent resident, a trip to Muir Woods is mandatory—everyone should visit this awesome redwood monument at least once. With so many people pouring into one small canyon, Muir Woods always seems crowded, but there are ways to tour the park and still have a few quiet moments; this hike makes the most of an alternate trailhead.

Begin at the north end of the parking lot on Trestle Trail, entering Mount Tamalpais State Park. This little path drops down a flight of steps, then ends at Camp Eastwood Road. Turn right. Descending easily, the paved road, which accesses a group camp, winds through sun-drenched slopes where bush poppy and chaparral pea bloom in spring. Broom, chamise, toyon, and manzanita are common, but as the trail drops into a cool canyon, redwood, California bay, and

Douglas-fir take over. At 0.4 mile, where the road crosses Fern Creek and swings left, turn right onto Troop 80 Trail.

The narrow trail, built by Boy Scouts in 1931, ascends along Fern Creek, then veers left and climbs at an easy pace. Redwoods, Douglas-fir, and tan oak completely shade the trail, and one pocket of young redwoods is so densely packed that there is virtually no understory. At 0.8 mile Sierra Trail heads downhill on the left. Continue straight on Troop 80 Trail. Running downslope from Panoramic Highway, the forest screens views of the road, but traffic noise is steady, especially on summer weekends. Troop 80 Trail crosses creeks and damp seeps on a series of pretty bridges, winding through huckleberry patches, woods, and occasional sunny stretches of chaparral, where you might see pitcher sage and chaparral pea in bloom in spring, accompanying manzanita, coffeeberry, and chinquapin. Occasional views south encompass forested hillsides rising from Redwood Canyon.

The trail forks at 1.7 miles, with the path on the right heading to the Bootjack trailhead. Continue straight/left another 0.1 mile, through a display of false lupine (in spring) to Van Wyck Meadow. *Meadow* is a big word for this little grassy spot, but everyone seems to get a kick out of the misspelled sign that reads VAN WYCK MEADOW POP. 3 STELLAR JAYS. The meadow is a good place for a short rest before continuing into the canyon. When you're ready, head downhill to the left, on Bootjack Trail.

Stone steps begin the descent, dropping the narrow trail to the side of Bootjack Creek. Redwoods tower overhead, mixed through a lush forest of Douglas-fir and tan oak, with ferns in the understory. Look for trilliums and starflower blooming in spring. Some sections are nearly level, but the overall trend is quite steep and somewhat rocky in areas. Deer are common in this quiet part of the park, and you might see them clinging to the steeply sloped canyon walls like mountain goats, calmly munching vegetation. Bootjack Creek joins Rattlesnake Creek, plumping the stream with added water, which cascades merrily downhill.

As Bootjack Trail progresses down into the canyon, you may notice big-leaf maple, elk clover, and thimbleberry along the creek bed. The trail sweeps left and crosses a confluence of streams on a curving bridge, supported in the middle by a large boulder. Still following the creek, the grade slackens to a slight descent. At 3 miles, a path breaks off on the left, on the way to Camp Eastwood. Continue straight, following the sign toward Muir Woods. Trail traffic picks up and increases to a fever pitch as Bootjack Trail leaves the state park and ends at 3.1 miles at the main Muir Woods trail. Stay to the left, on the wide paved path, as it meanders beneath huge redwoods on the canyon floor. A trail to Camp Eastwood bends left at 3.2 miles, but continue a bit farther, to the signed junction with Fern Creek Trail. Turn left.

With a course along the banks of Fern Creek, the trail gets quieter with every step, weaving slightly uphill through redwoods and ferns, with redwood sorrel a common understory plant. At 3.6 miles, you'll reach a junction with a trail to the left leading to Camp Eastwood—turn right onto Lost Trail.

The trail starts out on an easy grade, ascending out of the canyon, but the climb soon stiffens. On a long sequence of steps, you might come to the conclusion that Lost Breath Trail would be a more appropriate name for this route. Redwoods give way to live oak, Douglas-fir, and California bay; then Lost Trail ends at 4.1 miles. Turn left onto the Ocean View Trail.

Now keeping to an easy uphill grade, the Ocean View Trail departs the wooded canyon and emerges in grassland just below Panoramic Highway. There are views north to Tam's peaks and west toward the Pacific, though the only sea I've ever seen here is a sea of trees. Stay to the left, near a boulder, and when Ocean View Trail ends at 4.4 miles, turn left onto Panoramic Trail.

The nearly level trail winds through grassland dotted with broom and acacia, two nonnative plants, and coyote brush, one of the most common native shrubs in the Bay Area. Western fence lizards scamper along the path in summer. At 4.6 miles, Panoramic Trail ends at the top of Camp Eastwood Road. You can return to the parking lot by heading down Camp Eastwood Road to Trestle Trail, or by simply walking the less than 0.1 mile along the side of Panoramic Highway to the left.

NEARBY ACTIVITIES

Instead of visiting the redwood canyons of Muir Woods, you can hike to the top of Mount Tam from this trailhead, via easily graded fire roads that follow the route of an old railroad. Gravity Car Grade begins across the street from the parking lot, and Old Railroad Grade makes the final push to the top, although you can take alternate routes on several minor footpaths.

MOUNT TAMALPAIS: PHOENIX LAKE

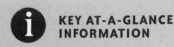

IN BRIEF

How do I love thee? Let me count the trails.

Mount Tamalpais has many trailheads and a lifetime's worth of paths. The options for hikes from here are staggering, and you can't really take a wrong step, but this gorgeous route through woods and grassland, with great views to Tam's summit, thrills me each time.

DESCRIPTION

This northern flank of Mount Tam is Marin Municipal Water District land, preserved for the primary purpose of providing water to Marin County residents. The hiker's benefit is a network of many trails and fire roads that connect to Mount Tamalpais State Park and a few small Marin County Open Space District preserves. I've loved this hike from my first visit, and it's a particularly good choice for late winter and spring, when wildflowers bloom everywhere.

From the parking lot, begin walking uphill on a broad fire road. This trail provides access to many destinations farther up the mountain and is heavily used by cyclists and runners. At an easy grade, the trail ascends

Directions

Leave San Francisco via the Golden Gate Bridge on northbound US 101, and use the Golden Gate Bridge toll plaza as your mileage starting point. Drive north on US 101 about 11 miles, then take Exit 450B, Sir Francis Drake/San Anselmo. Stay to the left, toward San Anselmo, and drive west on Sir Francis Drake Boulevard about 3.5 miles to the intersection with Lagunitas Road (at the Marin Art and Garden Center). Turn left onto Lagunitas and drive about 1 mile to the parking lot at the end of the road.

KEY AT-A-GLANCE INFORMATION

LENGTH: 4.9 miles

CONFIGURATION: Balloon

DIFFICULTY: Easy

SCENERY: Grassland, woods, lake

EXPOSURE: Nearly equal parts shade and sun

TRAFFIC: Moderate weekdays, busy weekends

TRAIL SURFACE: Dirt fire roads and trails

HIKING TIME: 2.5 hours

SEASON: Good anytime, although trails are muddy in winter.

ACCESS: Free

MAPS: Tom Harrison Maps' *Mount Tamalpais* topo ($9.95; tomharrisonmaps.com); download at tinyurl.com/mttamparkmap (no maps at the trailhead).

FACILITIES: Pit toilets at trailhead and Phoenix Lake

SPECIAL COMMENTS: Dogs welcome

CONTACTS: 415-945-1181, marinwater.org

DRIVING DISTANCE: 14.2 miles from the Golden Gate Bridge toll plaza

GPS INFORMATION

N37° 57.469' W122° 34.333'

Mount Tamalpais: Phoenix Lake

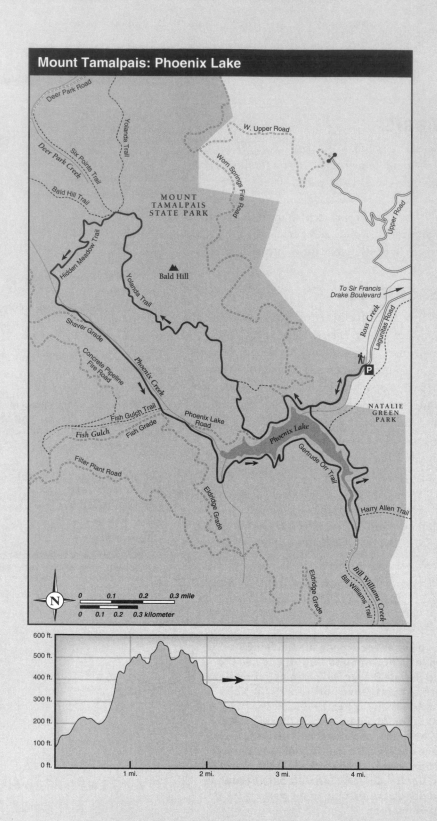

through a mixed woodland of madrone, coast live oak, buckeye, California bay, and one unpopular invasive nonnative plant called broom. Early spring flowers include California buttercups, milkmaids, and Welsh onion (another nonnative). In winter months, the water rushing downhill from Phoenix Lake is a melodious accompaniment.

The fire road passes the spillway and crests at 0.3 mile. Another fire road, the return route for this hike, heads off to the left—continue straight. After one last little hill, the fire road levels out. On the left, Phoenix Lake stretches its arms into the creases of a wooded canyon. Mature buckeye, black oak, coast live oak, and California bay provide partial shade but still permit views to the lake. Worn Springs Fire Road departs from a small cluster of redwoods on the right at 0.4 mile, offering a steep route to Bald Hill. Continue on the tour around Phoenix Lake to the next junction, at 0.6 mile, then turn right onto Yolanda Trail. This diminutive trail begins to climb at a moderate grade along a creek bed, through madrone, black oak, coast live oak, and California bay. Wildflowers emerge in these woods as early as January, when you might see hound's tongue, milkmaids, and shooting stars. In early spring, blue-dicks, buttercups, and iris are common. Yolanda crosses the creek and winds uphill into a more grassy area, somewhat overgrown with a young forest of broom. On one morning hike here, I got a little wake-up jolt when a jackrabbit came barreling down the trail toward me.

At 0.7 mile, after you pass a spur path on the right signed only with a NO HORSES symbol, the trail levels out for a few feet in a saddle between two hills, then skirts a knoll and begins a slight ascent across the flanks of Bald Hill to the right. Little pockets of shaded California bay, coast live oak, buckeye, and madrone are interspersed with long sunny stretches through grassy chaparral, with chamise, sticky monkeyflower, sagebrush, toyon, and coyote brush enjoying the western exposure.

After rainstorms in winter, mini-waterfalls gush down the slopes of Bald Hill at nearly every little fold in the hillside. A March or April hike on this stretch of Yolanda Trail is usually a very good choice for wildflower-viewing. In early spring I've seen larkspur, blue-dick, shooting star, paintbrush, popcorn flower, California poppy, blue and white lupine, and blue-eyed grass. During those soft days of late spring, grassy knolls, which extend off the trail on the left, invite a sunny snooze.

As the trail travels northwest, there are unobstructed views of Tam's summit ridgeline. Yolanda Trail then descends a bit through cool woods where a pint-sized waterfall flows well into spring. It's such a spectacular journey that I always feel a little sad to reach Six Points Junction at 1.9 miles. Yolanda Trail continues to the right; then, moving counterclockwise, there's Six Points Trail, Bald Hill Trail, and Hidden Meadow Trail. Take Hidden Meadow Trail, to the left. As it starts to descend through oaks and then grassland, the panorama revealed on the left side of the trail is one of my favorite Tam vistas. From Bald Hill to East Peak and everything in between, it's all beautiful. After a foray through grassland, the trail descends into a mixed woodland, where broom is the dominant understory plant

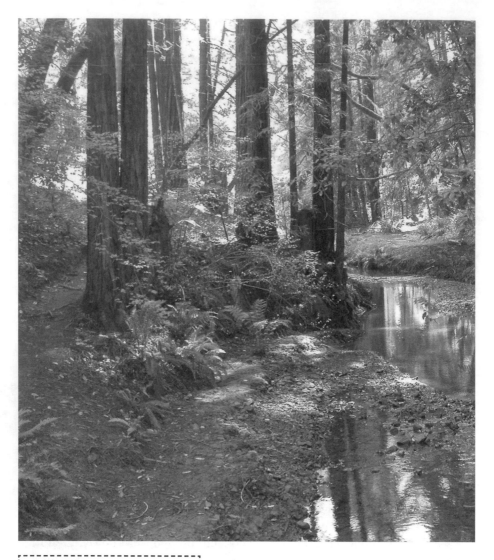

Redwoods at the edge of Phoenix Lake

(a bunch of it has been manually uprooted, but there's still plenty). A few short, tight switchbacks descend to cross a creek as it enters Hidden Meadow, a small, level, grassy shelf running between a creek on the left and an ascending hillside on the right. A forest of buckeye, California bay, and oak surrounds the meadow, and the trail winds among a few large oaks and buckeyes. Great colonies of hound's tongue linger at the fringes of the meadow in late winter.

The trail crosses another creek, then turns to accompany the water flow toward Phoenix Lake. Some young redwoods are mixed through the forest. At 2.6 miles, Hidden Meadow Trail ends at a junction with Shaver Grade. Here, turn left onto the fire road, which follows Phoenix Creek at an easy downhill grade. Be alert for bicycle traffic along this well-traveled route. The surrounding forest, where I've heard turkeys yodeling back and forth, is mostly California bay, redwood, madrone, big-leaf maple, and buckeye. At 3 miles, Shaver Grade ends at a multiple junction. Fish Gulch and Fish Grade climb off to the near right, and Eldridge Grade sets off to the far right. Continue straight; then, after about 300 feet, veer off to the right onto Gertrude Orr Trail (signed with generic water-district HIKING ONLY symbols but not named at this junction). Tall hazelnut shrubs tower above the trail, welcoming visitors into a redwood forest. The trail follows Phoenix Creek for about 150 feet, then reaches a junction just before a bridge. Turn right and cross the creek.

Gertrude Orr Trail runs along Phoenix Creek, which soon empties into the lake. Redwoods are common in the fingerlike extensions of the lake, accompanying ferns, hazelnut, creambush, and trilliums and milkmaids that bloom in early spring. In slightly sunnier stretches uphill from the shoreline, you might notice madrone, California bay, coast live oak, big-leaf maple, and black oak. The trail alternates level sections with some undulating areas where steps keep the path stable. Just past an area heavily colonized by tan oak, the trail rises, drops on a graceful flight of curving stairs, and then ends at 4.1 miles.

Bill Williams Trail heads deeper into the mountain, to the right—turn left onto a fire road, ascending at a barely noticeable rate along the eastern shore of Phoenix Lake. On the right, look for a short but pretty waterfall that's active during the rainy season; redwood, big-leaf maple, madrone, and California bay line the trail. At 4.2 miles, Harry Allen Trail sets off on the right, but continue on the fire road. Blossoms on broom and ceanothus shrubs draw hoards of bees in early spring, filling the air with a drowsy buzzing sound. Look for brilliant displays of red ribbon clarkia on the right in late spring. A bench a short distance off the trail to the left is a good spot to enjoy views that stretch across the lake to the crest of Bald Hill.

The fire road levels out above the dam, and a path leading back to Lagunitas Road departs on the right at 4.5 miles. The shallows to the left of the trail host many somewhat-tame ducks that often waddle over to quack for snacks along the shoreline. At 4.6 miles, you'll return to a familiar junction, above the spillway. Turn right and walk back downhill on the fire road.

11 POINT REYES NATIONAL SEASHORE:
BEAR VALLEY TO ARCH ROCK

KEY AT-A-GLANCE INFORMATION

LENGTH: 8.8 miles

CONFIGURATION: Out-and-back

DIFFICULTY: Moderate due to length

SCENERY: Douglas-fir forest, coastal bluff, and ocean views

EXPOSURE: Mostly shaded

TRAFFIC: Heavy

TRAIL SURFACE: Dirt fire roads and trails

HIKING TIME: 4 hours

SEASON: Good all year—beat the crowds with a winter visit.

ACCESS: Free

MAPS: Available online at nps.gov/pore/planyourvisit/maps.htm and at the Bear Valley Visitor Center, where you can also buy Tom Harrison Maps' *Point Reyes National Seashore* topo (order it online at tomharrisonmaps .com; $9.95).

FACILITIES: Restrooms and drinking water at the visitor center

SPECIAL COMMENTS: No dogs allowed. Three short interpretive trails begin at the Bear Valley trailhead, exploring the region's history, vegetation, and the effects of the 1906 earthquake.

CONTACTS: 415-464-5100, ext. 2; nps.gov/pore

DRIVING DISTANCE: 32 miles from the Golden Gate Bridge toll plaza

GPS INFORMATION

N38° 2.381' W122° 47.988'

IN BRIEF

Departing from the Bear Valley Visitor Center, a nearly level fire road ushers you through woods, a meadow, and coastal grassland. A bluff called Arch Rock, the turnaround point, rewards you with beautiful views of the ocean and shoreline. The hike returns on the same route, although more-ambitious hikers can opt for a loop to the top of Mount Wittenberg.

DESCRIPTION

Muir Woods, Big Basin Redwoods State Park, Mount Tam's Pantoll area—some Bay Area trailheads bustle with visitors from sunup to sundown. Point Reyes's Bear Valley is no exception: Every day of the year, it's inundated with nature-lovers, many of whom come just for this trail. But you can beat the crowds by arriving very early or choosing a weekday, particularly in winter, the park's quietest season.

Although a few trails begin near the visitor center, it's not hard to find Bear Valley Trail, which starts at the south edge of the parking lot—look for the steady stream of

----

Directions ⟶

Leave San Francisco on northbound US 101 and use the Golden Gate Bridge toll plaza as your mileage starting point. Drive 11 miles north on US 101, then take Exit 450B, at San Anselmo/Sir Francis Drake. Stay to the left toward San Anselmo and drive west on Sir Francis Drake Boulevard about 20 miles to the junction with CA 1. Turn right on CA 1 and drive 0.1 mile, then turn left onto Bear Valley Road. Drive about 0.4 mile, then turn left at the SEASHORE INFORMATION sign just past the red barn. Drive about 0.2 mile to the parking lots at the end of the road.

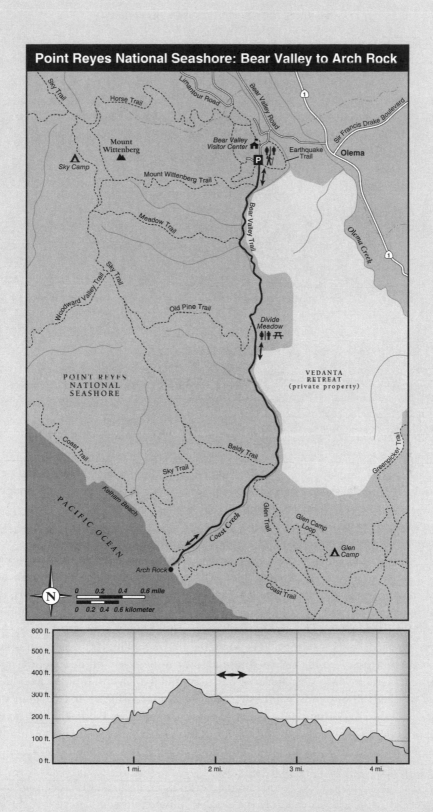

Point Reyes National Seashore: Bear Valley to Arch Rock

Sky Trail

Horse Trail

Limantour Road

Bear Valley Road

1

Sir Francis Drake Boulevard

Mount Wittenberg

Sky Camp

Bear Valley Visitor Center

Earthquake Trail

Olema

P

Mount Wittenberg Trail

Meadow Trail

Bear Valley Trail

Olema Creek

Sky Trail

Woodward Valley Trail

Old Pine Trail

Divide Meadow

VEDANTA RETREAT
(private property)

1

POINT REYES NATIONAL SEASHORE

Baldy Trail

Greenpicker Trail

Coast Trail

Sky Trail

Kelham Beach

PACIFIC OCEAN

Coast Creek

Glen Trail

Glen Camp Loop

Glen Camp

Arch Rock

Coast Trail

N

| 0 | 0.2 | 0.4 | 0.6 mile |

| 0 | 0.2 | 0.4 | 0.6 kilometer |

600 ft.
500 ft.
400 ft.
300 ft.
200 ft.
100 ft.
0 ft.

1 mi.   2 mi.   3 mi.   4 mi.

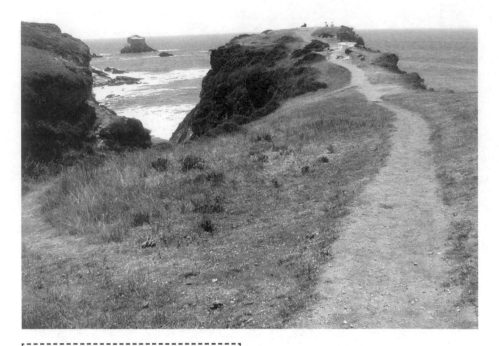

Arch Rock, a gorgeous Point Reyes destination

people. The initial section of trail runs along the edge of a meadow, but it quickly veers right and into shade. Bear Valley Trail is level, with very few blips in elevation along its length. The moist environment shelters Douglas-fir, California bay, tan oak, elk clover, creambush, red elderberry, and hazelnut.

After 0.2 mile, Mount Wittenberg Trail departs on the right, on the way to Point Reyes's tallest spot, at 1,407 feet. Stick to Bear Valley Trail at this junction and the next, with Meadow Trail at 0.8 mile. After a tour through the woods, the trail emerges at the edge of Divide Meadow at 1.6 miles. The sunny, sloping meadow, rimmed with Douglas-fir, is the turnaround point for many visitors, but more scenic delights wait for hikers down the trail. Old Pine Trail veers off uphill near the restrooms on the right—continue toward the ocean on Bear Valley Trail.

The next 1.5-mile stretch has no junctions and is a quiet part of the park. The trail descends briefly into a little shaded canyon tucked between ascending forested hillsides. At 3.1 miles, you'll reach a multiple junction. Baldy Trail begins on the right, and Glen Trail starts on the left. Here, Bear Valley Trail, in the middle, shrinks from a fire road to a trail. Cyclists who want to continue on Bear Valley Trail must leave their bikes at a rack.

Past this junction, the woods become even more lush. Coast Creek murmurs on the left and ferns cascade off the sloping hillsides. In summer you might see foxglove blooming here. Moisture-loving buckeyes sprinkled through dense stands of Douglas-fir completely shade the trail, and when you step out of the woods on a sunny day you'll be blinking like a newborn kitten. Along the trail, young Douglas-firs tower above coyote brush, sticky monkeyflower, sagebrush, and bush lupine.

Bear Valley Trail ends at a junction at 4 miles. Coast Trail picks up the baton for the final stretch to the ocean, now partially visible straight ahead. Stay to the left, following the sign for Arch Rock. At 4.2 miles, Coast Trail slips off to the left, almost unnoticed when the grasses are high in summer. The path to Arch Rock continues straight, ascending gently through a pretty mix of coastal plants, including paintbrush and lizard's-tail. Views open up to the ocean. At 4.4 miles, you'll reach Arch Rock and the end of the trail. This little bluff, jutting out over the ocean, has unfenced drop-offs, so use caution.

On a sunny day, is there a better spot for lunch anywhere in the Bay Area? If you love ocean breezes, the sound of crashing waves, the calls of sea birds, and sweeping seashore views, I think you'll be pleased. This bluff is also an excellent location for seal-watching. I lingered here on one hike, transfixed by a harbor seal bobbing up and down in the water, seeming to look right at me.

When you're ready, return to the Bear Valley trailhead. Hankering for a more strenuous hike? As you return up Bear Valley Trail, turn left on either Old Pine or Meadow Trail, then ascend on Sky Trail to Mount Wittenberg Trail, which returns to Bear Valley Trail 0.2 mile from the parking lot. The views from Mount Wittenberg are mostly obscured by a young forest of Douglas-fir, but the trails are pretty and you may see the remnants of an exotic white-deer herd.

12 POINT REYES NATIONAL SEASHORE:
ESTERO TO DRAKES BAY

KEY AT-A-GLANCE INFORMATION

LENGTH: 8 miles (8.4 miles if you continue to the "beach")

CONFIGURATION: Out-and-back

DIFFICULTY: Moderate

SCENERY: Coastal

EXPOSURE: Almost entirely unshaded

TRAFFIC: Light

TRAIL SURFACE: Dirt trails

HIKING TIME: 4 hours

SEASON: Good all year but muddy in winter.

ACCESS: Free

MAPS: Available online at nps.gov /pore/planyourvisit/maps.htm and at the Bear Valley Visitor Center, where you can also buy Tom Harrison Maps' *Point Reyes National Seashore* topo (order it online at tomharrisonmaps .com; $9.95).

FACILITIES: Pit toilets at trailhead

SPECIAL COMMENTS: No dogs allowed. Chimney Rock, at the far southwestern tip of Point Reyes, is a sublime spot for spring wildflowers.

CONTACTS: 415-464-5100, ext. 2; nps.gov/pore

DRIVING DISTANCE: 42 miles from the Golden Gate Bridge toll plaza

GPS INFORMATION

N38° 4.883' W122° 54.846'

IN BRIEF

Point Reyes has creeks; ocean and bay coastline; a lagoon; waterfalls; ponds and lakes; and an estuary, Drakes Estero, which lends its name to this trailhead. You'll descend through coastal scrub and a pocket of pines to a little bridge, then climb to a bluff where you can see the other three bays that also feed into Drakes Estero. After a bit of roller-coastering, the trail drops to ocean level, and although the official end of the trail is near the mouth of Drakes Estero, if the tide is low you can continue another quarter-mile over mudflats to glimpse Drakes Bay.

DESCRIPTION

The solitary Estero Trail departs from the parking lot through grassy coastal scrub, with coyote brush and blackberry brambles punctuating the landscape. Iris flower along the trail in spring, along with some blue-eyed grass and California buttercup. Off to the east, a steady slope rises to crest at Mount Vision. Estero

----

Directions ➞

Leave San Francisco on northbound US 101 and use the Golden Gate Bridge toll plaza as your mileage starting point. Drive 11 miles north on US 101, then take Exit 450B, San Anselmo/Sir Francis Drake. Stay to the left toward San Anselmo and drive west about 20 miles on Sir Francis Drake Boulevard to the junction with CA 1. Turn right and drive 0.1 mile, then turn left onto Bear Valley Road. After about 2 miles, Bear Valley Road ends at Sir Francis Drake; turn left. Continue on Sir Francis Drake about 7.5 more miles, and turn left at the ESTERO TRAIL sign. Drive slowly (there may be cows) for another mile to the trailhead, on the right side of the road.

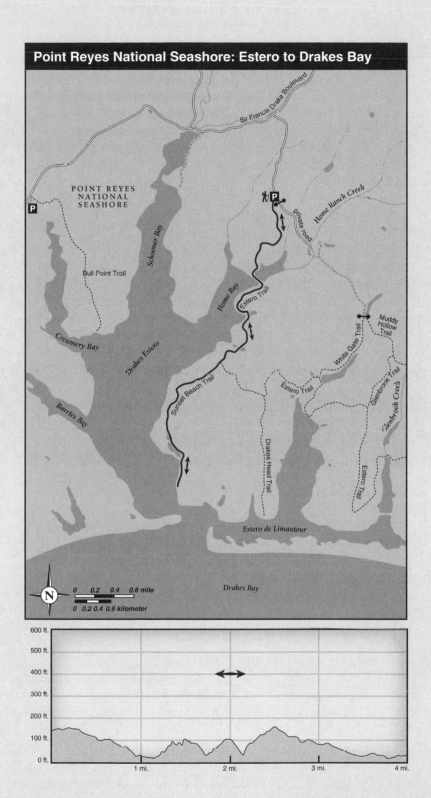

Point Reyes National Seashore: Estero to Drakes Bay

POINT REYES
NATIONAL
SEASHORE

Schooner Bay

Bull Point Trail

Home Bay

Estero Trail

Sir Francis Drake Boulevard

private road

Home Ranch Creek

Muddy
Hollow
Trail

White Gate Trail

Creamery Bay

Drakes Estero

Sunset Beach Trail

Estero Trail

Glenbrook Trail

Glenbrook Creek

Barries Bay

Drakes Head Trail

Estero Trail

Estero de Limantour

Drakes Bay

0   0.2   0.4   0.6 mile

0   0.2 0.4 0.6 kilometer

N

600 ft.

500 ft.

400 ft.

300 ft.

200 ft.

100 ft.

0 ft.

1 mi.   2 mi.   3 mi.   4 mi.

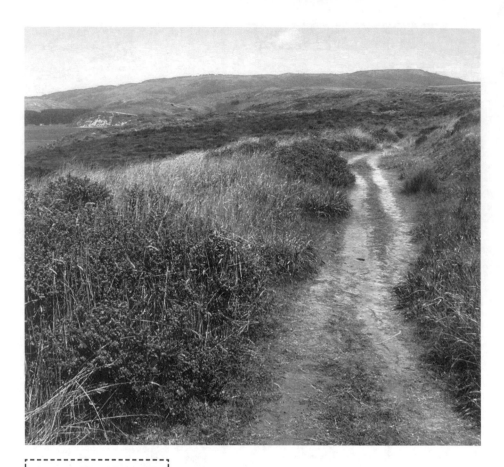

A view east from Estero Trail

Trail skirts a rounded hill, then leans right, descends, and cuts through the corner of a pine forest, where you'll hear, if not see, many birds.

This pocket of woods has an unnatural feeling to it, probably because it was planted as a grove many years ago. As the trail leaves the pines, it adopts a gentle downhill course, through more pines, coyote brush, blackberry, wild rose, and a few twinberry bushes. Estero Trail bends left and crosses the confluence of a fresh-water pond and Home Bay on a pretty little bridge.

Because Drakes Estero empties into the ocean and the entire estuary is affected by tides, the amount of water in the bay varies from slim forked threads to deep pools. On some occasions I'm happy to hike no farther than the benches at the middle of the bridge. On one of my visits here, a pair of egrets perched like sentinels on opposite sides of the viewing platform in the middle of the bridge.

At the other end of the bridge, the trail turns right and begins to climb. Quail and rabbits are commonly spotted, rushing from one cluster of vegetation to another—the sides of the trail are tangled with a variety of plants, including coyote brush, toyon, huckleberry, bush lupine, ceanothus, blackberry, sticky mon-keyflower, and sagebrush. The first crest yields impressive views of Drakes Estero, but the trail doesn't linger. Instead it drops to the shores of a tiny pond, which contributes its share of water to the estuary. A few boards cross the drainage chan-nel. This area is commonly muddy in winter, and trail conditions can be terrible if the cattle that range here have clomped through recently.

The trail climbs again through coyote brush and reaches a fence stretched across the trail (it may be open, depending on the season). Squeeze through the V-shaped stile and ascend to a hill topped with a eucalyptus tree, where daffodils bloom in late winter. Estero Trail descends again to another small pond. It's not much of a surprise at this point to begin climbing once more, but after another fence and stile the trail levels out and reaches a junction at 2.5 miles. Here, where Estero Trail bends left, continue straight onto Sunset Beach Trail.

As the trail sweeps south, short clumps of coyote brush allow views back toward the trailhead and across the Estero to feeder bays to the west. In late sum-mer, bright-yellow goldenrod seems especially showy among the drab tan-and-green brush. There's a descent, but this time it's easy. After you pass through one last cattle fence and stile, the trail reaches the edge of a small pond. According to the park maps, this is the official end of Sunset Beach Trail, at about 4 miles. From here you can see Drakes Estero emptying into Drakes Bay, but you'll get better views (and a little beach) if you continue south.

A slight path veers left, squeezes through coyote brush, poison oak, bush lupine, and sagebrush, then sets off across mudflats. If it's not too muddy, you can continue another quarter-mile to a narrow beach at a sandy point across from Limantour Spit. You may be able to see Chimney Rock, across the bay to the southwest, from here. This is one of the quietest and loneliest places in the Bay Area, where little waves lap against the shoreline and sand sings as it blows across the beach.

When you're ready, retrace your steps back to the trailhead.

13 POINT REYES NATIONAL SEASHORE:
TOMALES POINT

KEY AT-A-GLANCE INFORMATION

LENGTH: 9 miles

CONFIGURATION: Out-and-back

DIFFICULTY: Moderate

SCENERY: Coastal scrub and grassland

EXPOSURE: Full sun

TRAFFIC: Steady nearly year-round

TRAIL SURFACE: Broad sandy fire road and meandering paths, with some loose sand

HIKING TIME: 4 hours

SEASON: Spring and autumn are best.

ACCESS: Free

MAPS: Pick up the free official Point Reyes trail map at the Bear Valley Visitor Center, download it at nps .gov/pore/planyourvisit/maps.htm, or buy Tom Harrison Maps' *Point Reyes National Seashore* topo (order online at tomharrisonmaps.com; $9.95).

FACILITIES: None at the trailhead; pit toilets at nearby McClures Beach

SPECIAL COMMENTS: No dogs allowed. From this trailhead (or from a second parking lot 0.1 mile to the west), it's a 1-mile round-trip hike to McClures Beach.

CONTACTS: 415-464-5100, ext. 2; nps.gov/pore

DRIVING DISTANCE: 48 miles from the Golden Gate Bridge toll plaza

GPS INFORMATION

N38° 11.348' W122° 57.248'

IN BRIEF

Animal sightings are not uncommon in the Bay Area, but at a few locations you are nearly assured of a peek at wild creatures. One of the best spots is Point Reyes's Tomales Point. This hike is a 9-mile out-and-back trek on a remote peninsula where tule elk roam through coastal scrub and birds paddle in the ocean and soar through the skies. Bring binoculars, a hat, and a windbreaker.

DESCRIPTION

At its northwestern edge, Point Reyes tapers to Tomales Point. Pierce Point Ranch occupied the area until 1973, and the farm buildings, now historically preserved, stand near the Tomales Point trailhead. A self-guided tour through the ranch is a fine way to begin (or end) a hike. In 1978, a herd of 10 tule elk were reintroduced to the point, which was then fenced off from the rest of Point Reyes. The elk have multiplied, and the population in

---

Directions ⟶

Leave San Francisco on northbound US 101 and use the Golden Bridge toll plaza as your mileage starting point. Drive north on US 101 about 11 miles, then take Exit 450B, Sir Francis Drake/San Anselmo. Stay to the left toward San Anselmo and drive west about 20 miles on Sir Francis Drake Boulevard to the junction with CA 1. Turn right and drive 0.1 mile, then turn left onto Bear Valley Road. After about 2 miles, Bear Valley Road ends at Sir Francis Drake; turn left. Continue on Sir Francis Drake about 5.5 miles, then turn right onto Pierce Point Road. Drive about 9 miles on Pierce Point Road to the signed Tomales Point trail-head, a short distance from McClures Beach at the end of the road.

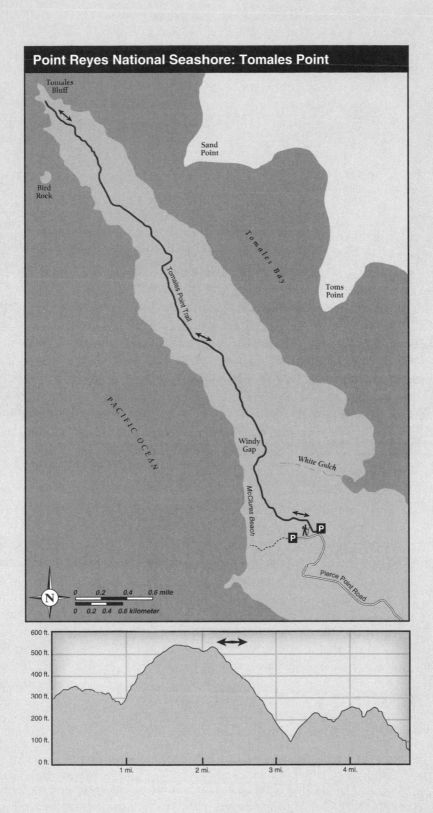

Point Reyes National Seashore: Tomales Point

Tomales Bluff

Sand Point

Bird Rock

Tomales Bay

Toms Point

Tomales Point Trail

PACIFIC OCEAN

Windy Gap

White Gulch

McClures Beach

Pierce Point Road

N

| 0 | 0.2 | 0.4 | 0.6 mile |

| 0 | 0.2 | 0.4 | 0.6 kilometer |

600 ft.

500 ft.

400 ft.

300 ft.

200 ft.

100 ft.

0 ft.

1 mi.   2 mi.   3 mi.   4 mi.

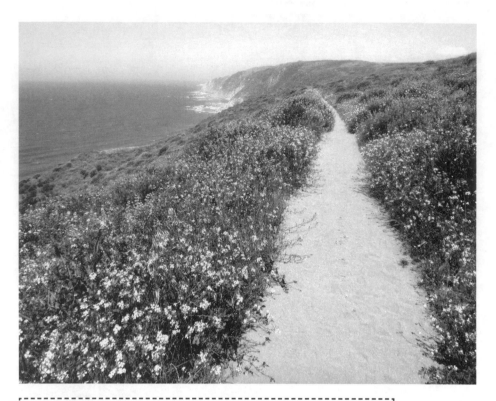

Sweet-smelling yellow bush lupines mix with fresh ocean breezes at Tomales Point.

2009 was more than 440. Other creatures you may see on the point are a variety of birds, coyotes, bobcats, and (although sightings are rare) mountain lions.

The weather plays a big part in enhancing (or ruining) hikes along the coast, and Tomales Point is no exception. Attempt a hike during one of the Bay Area's famous foggy summer days, and not only will the views be completely obscured, but the wind can chill you thoroughly. Spring and autumn are the best seasons for a visit, and note that when the elk rut (July–November), males are more aggressive and you should give them an extra-wide berth.

The trail starts at a level grade, skirting the ranch buildings before heading into a grassy coastal-scrub-plant community, dominated by coyote brush. In early spring, wild radish covers the knoll on the left, presenting a lavish display of white and lavender blossoms. Northern harriers seem to favor the point, and you might see one or two fluttering in place above the ground, looking for a meal. As the trail travels north it offers views of the coastline, which past McClures Beach gradually ascends to steep rocky bluffs. Tomales Point Trail drifts downhill to aptly named Windy Gap. If you haven't already seen elk, the sloping valley on the right is one of their favorite spots. A brief moderate ascent brings the trail up to the grassy ridgeline, dotted in some spots with wind-sculpted coyote brush. Look to the left for ocean views and right to take in the hills of Bolinas Ridge rolling up from Tomales Bay. The trail descends to Lower Pierce Point Ranch, a site now marked by a handful of cypress trees often occupied by raptors. A few salmonberry shrubs mingle through stinging nettles in a damp spot on the right.

Once again the trail begins to climb, but here vegetation begins to crowd the route. Somewhat abruptly, the path dissolves to sand at about 3.8 miles—some firmer patches of terra are ahead, but this is the trend for the rest of the trail. Navigating becomes a bit tricky, as elk paths score the area, so try to stick close to the ridgeline and keep heading northwest. Elk scat is common everywhere, and you stand a very good chance of observing *Cervus elaphus nannodes* if you keep your noise level down. On the other hand, if you're *too* quiet, you might come across a loner mostly camouflaged by the tall thick stands of lizard's-tail and yellow bush lupine. Even if you don't see them, you'll hear them—elk bellows are unlike any other animal vocalization I've ever heard. I can only describe the sound as similar to a loud, high-pitched door squeak.

The trail finally begins to descend slightly, signaling that the first leg of the hike is near its end. Be careful of unannounced sheer drop-offs on the left—the views are incredible, but the ground can be unstable near the edge. This is one of the most isolated and quiet hiking destinations on the coast, where the only sounds are the crash of the surf, the cries of the birds, and the peal of a buoy near the mouth of Tomales Bay. At about 4.5 miles, a bare spot—kind of a sandy bowl that's a bit sheltered from the wind—makes a decent rest stop, especially if you're in a group. Beyond that, a tiny path drops straight down to the tip of the point, but I don't recommend this option. After you've had your fill of this coastal gem, backtrack to the trailhead.

14 RING MOUNTAIN OPEN SPACE PRESERVE

KEY AT-A-GLANCE INFORMATION

LENGTH: 2.1 miles

CONFIGURATION: Balloon

DIFFICULTY: Easy

SCENERY: Rock-strewn grassland

EXPOSURE: Mostly unshaded

TRAFFIC: Moderate

TRAIL SURFACE: Dirt fire roads and trails

HIKING TIME: 1 hour

SEASON: Good year-round; Tiburon mariposa lilies usually bloom mid-May–early June. Trails are muddy in winter.

ACCESS: Free

MAPS: At an information signboard inside the preserve and online at tinyurl.com/ringmtnmap

SPECIAL COMMENTS: Because of the rare plants that thrive here, take special care to stay on the trails. Leashed dogs welcome.

CONTACTS: 415-473-2816, tinyurl.com/ringmountain

DRIVING DISTANCE: 10.7 miles from the Golden Gate Bridge toll plaza

GPS INFORMATION

N37° 55.254' W122° 29.657'

IN BRIEF

There's a dramatic backdrop to the spectacular views hikers enjoy on Ring Mountain. Although small and contained by Tiburon residential neighborhoods, the preserve hosts Native American petroglyphs and an incredibly rare flower.

DESCRIPTION

This 405-acre preserve sits on ultraprime real estate. A short drive from US 101, Ring Mountain offers views of San Pablo Bay, Mount Tamalpais, and San Francisco. The property was never developed because of a single flower: the Tiburon mariposa lily, which grows in a small section of Ring Mountain and nowhere else in the world.

There's no parking lot but plenty of street parking along Paradise Drive. Access the preserve from an open-space gate and stop at an information signboard for a map, which also contains the self-guided-tour key.

Begin on Phyllis Ellman Loop Trail, skirt a marshy area, and then climb through rocky grassland, coyote brush, and poison oak. These lower reaches of Ring Mountain are dominated

----

Directions ———————————→

Leave San Francisco on northbound US 101 and use the Golden Gate Bridge toll plaza as your mileage starting point. Drive north 9 miles on US 101, then take Exit 449 at Paradise Drive/Tamalpais Drive. Turn right onto Tamalpais, drive east a short distance, and bear right onto San Clemente Drive (before The Village shopping center). After a few blocks, San Clemente dumps into Paradise Drive. Continue on Paradise past Westward Drive to the preserve gate, on the right side of the road. It's about 1.5 miles from US 101.

Ring Mountain Open Space Preserve

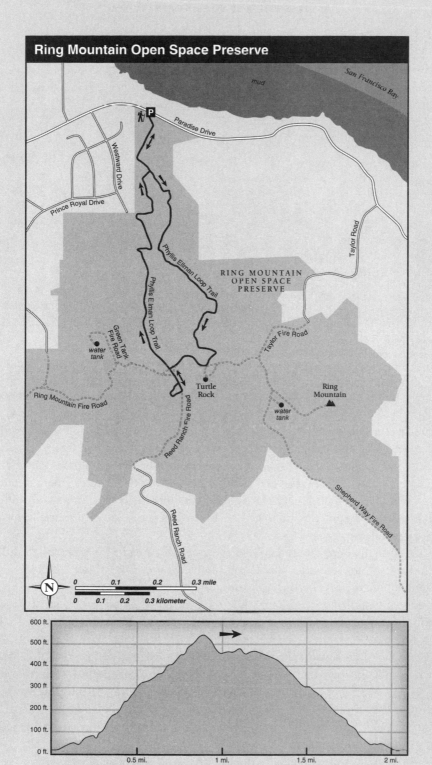

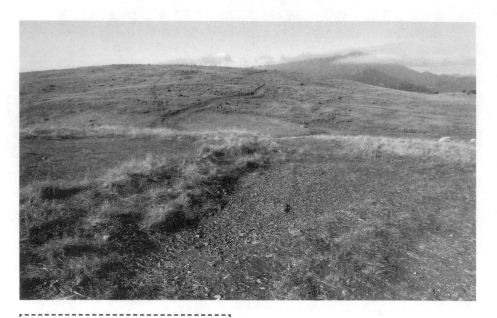

Mount Tamalpais viewed from Ring Mountain

by a damp basin, fed from little streams. In winter, near Post 1, look for osoberry, a slight deciduous shrub that produces clusters of little white nodding flowers. At 0.2 mile, the trail splits; you can hike the loop in either direction, but to follow the self-guided tour and these directions, turn left. Keeping to an easy grade, the trail travels laterally across the hillside. Toyon, coyote brush, young California bays, and some poison oak dot the grassland. Wildflowers are sprinkled across these sloping, grassy hillsides from February through late summer. The first arrivals are often milkmaids and buttercups, followed by blue-eyed grass, lupine, Ithuriel's spear, and, later still, tarweeds.

In spring, where the trail crosses the creek, look right for ninebark, a shrub with leaves that resemble blackberry and currant. Like those edible berry-producing plants, ninebark is a member of the rose family and prefers a moist yet exposed environment. Ninebark's bracts of red flowers set it apart from its kindred berry plants.

Just past Post 7, stay right, avoiding a well-trampled path that heads left and steeply uphill toward the ridge. At the next unsigned split, at 0.7 mile, stay left or you'll shortcut the loop—you should be continuing uphill. The trees get bigger and more impressive on this part of the mountain, despite the exposed location. Post 8 points out a massive coast live oak and, near Post 9, the trail winds through an incredible multitrunked California bay—one of the magical spots on the mountain.

As the trail presses on uphill, Mount Tamalpais's east peak pops up to the west. Past the creek's headwaters, the trees fade away and grassland returns, although you'll wind through one last cluster of bays and oaks near the crest. Where the first

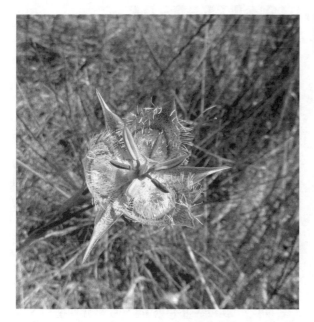

leg of Phyllis Ellman Loop Trail ends at a junction with a fire road at 0.9 mile, you'll surely want to pause and savor the views south, which extend past Richardson Bay to San Francisco. The big hunk of a rock just off the trail on the left is Turtle Rock. Turn right onto Ring Mountain Fire Road.

As the fire road follows the bare ridgeline, there are dead-on views to Mount Tam. After a brief downhill stretch, and when you reach a saddle where trails stretch out in each direction at 1 mile, turn left. A few steps down Reed Ranch Fire Road, a little unsigned path veers right. Follow this trail a short distance to Petroglyph Rock. An interpretive sign explains that the carvings still plainly visible on the boulder were made by Miwok Indians centuries ago. Where the path ends after skirting around the rock, turn left and walk back uphill on the fire road to the previous junction; then continue straight, back on Phyllis Ellman Loop Trail. Returning downhill, the long views north may distract you from the trailside display of flowers. The rocky soil along the trail sustains native wildflowers, including the Tiburon mariposa lily.

As you continue downhill, San Quentin State Prison is visible, perched on the edge of its namesake point. A gracefully canopied buckeye tree sits alone in the grassland on the right. A trail heads right and bisects the loop at 1.5 miles. Continue downhill to the left, following the route highlighted by a couple of arrow signs. In winter, before rains transform the hillsides into a verdant canvas, toyon shrubs loaded with cheerful red berries are a favorite of small birds. Where the loop closes at about 1.9 miles, stay to the left and retrace your steps back to the trailhead.

15 ROBERT LOUIS STEVENSON STATE PARK

KEY AT-A-GLANCE INFORMATION

LENGTH: 11.2 miles

CONFIGURATION: Out-and-back

DIFFICULTY: Strenuous

SCENERY: Mixed woods, chaparral, views; the highest accessible-by-trail summit in the Bay Area

EXPOSURE: First half-mile is shaded; the rest is exposed.

TRAFFIC: Moderate

TRAIL SURFACE: Dirt trail and dirt fire road

HIKING TIME: 5 hours

SEASON: Good anytime unless it's hot.

ACCESS: Free

MAPS: None at the trailhead. The Robert Louis Stevenson map (printed along with the Bothe–Napa Valley map) is available at Bothe–Napa Valley State Park, 3.5 miles south of Calistoga on the west side of CA 29, and online at tinyurl.com/rlstevensontrailmap.

FACILITIES: None

SPECIAL COMMENTS: No dogs allowed

CONTACTS: 707-942-4575, tinyurl .com/rlstevensonsp

DRIVING DISTANCE: 74.3 miles from the Bay Bridge toll plaza

GPS INFORMATION

N38° 39.162' W122° 36.002'

IN BRIEF

Mount St. Helena is the Bay Area's highest publicly accessible (by trail) peak, topping out at 4,304 feet. This trek begins uphill on a short, eroded trail, then continues to the summit on a long, sinuous, well-graded fire road. You'll find very little navigation challenge here—just a steady climb to the top, where views unfold spanning the distance from the San Francisco skyline to Mount Lassen (on a clear day).

DESCRIPTION

This long hike begins on the west side of CA 29 at the Stevenson Memorial trailhead. A few steps bring the trail up into a small, grassy meadow dotted with a few picnic tables, and then the climb begins through a mixed woodland of California bay, Douglas-fir, tan oak, madrone, and live oak. You might see red larkspur and columbine blooming in late spring, preceding pink flowers on wild-rose shrubs. Visitors have worn ugly shortcuts into the hillsides between the switchbacks here—for anyone considering following their lead, consider the erosion you will cause, not to mention the copious amounts of poison oak along the trail.

- -

Directions ⟶

Leave San Francisco via the Bay Bridge and use the toll plaza as your mileage starting point. Drive north on I-80 26 miles, then take Exit 33 onto CA 37. Drive west 2.5 miles on CA 37 to the junction with CA 29. Turn right and drive north 38 miles on CA 29 to Calistoga and the junction with CA 128/Lincoln Street. Turn right and continue another 9 miles east on CA 29 into Robert Louis Stevenson State Park, where there's roadside parking on the left side of the road (there's a larger dirt lot on the right).

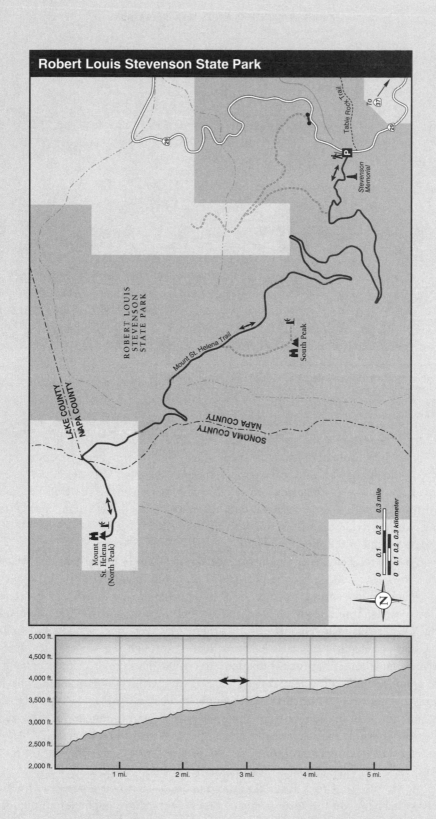

Robert Louis Stevenson State Park

To 37

Table Rock Trail

29

29

P

Stevenson Memorial

Mount St. Helena Trail

South Peak

ROBERT LOUIS STEVENSON STATE PARK

LAKE COUNTY
NAPA COUNTY

SONOMA COUNTY
NAPA COUNTY

Mount St. Helena (North Peak)

0   0.1   0.2   0.3 mile
0   0.1 0.2 0.3 kilometer

N

5,000 ft.
4,500 ft.
4,000 ft.
3,500 ft.
3,000 ft.
2,500 ft.
2,000 ft.

1 mi.   2 mi.   3 mi.   4 mi.   5 mi.

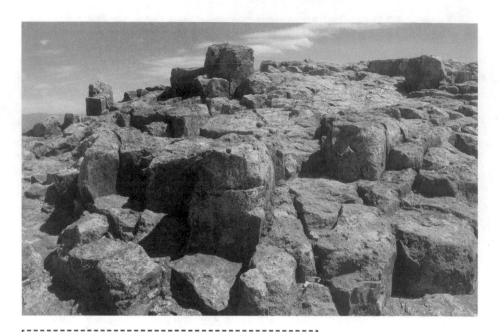

Curious rock formations cluster at the summit of Mount St. Helena.

After ascending through woods and a few pockets of manzanita, chamise, and pine, the trail reaches the Stevenson Memorial spot at 0.7 mile. Author Robert Louis Stevenson and his wife spent their honeymoon here, sleeping in a decrepit old mining building. Stevenson's slim memoir, *The Silverado Squatters*, is a vivid description of their adventures. Just past the memorial the trail becomes badly eroded, with several steep sections over exposed rock. Manzanita and knobcone pine line the last steep stretch, then the trail ends at a T-junction with Mount St. Helena Trail at 0.8 mile. Turn left.

The fire road climbs at a modest grade through sun-drenched hillsides packed with canyon live oak, knobcone pine, yerba santa, and manzanita. Bush poppy is conspicuous in late spring, when its straggly branches are crammed with gorgeous yellow flowers. Traffic from CA 29 is audible, but the noise fades as the trail bends right. Even at this relatively low elevation there are sweeping views down to Calistoga, and you might see hot-air balloons floating through the Napa Valley in the early-morning hours. Big rock formations are visible, jutting out of the mountainside uphill, and piles of little rocks line the trail with virtually no topsoil in sight. In spring, deer brush (a white-flowered ceanothus), sticky monkeyflower, paintbrush, iris, and purple bush lupine bloom along the trail. In early summer, look for red-flowered California fuchsia, a native annual flower found in rocky areas. When in *The Silverado Squatters* Stevenson writes about chaparral "thick with pea-like blossoms," he's describing chaparral pea, a shrub with vibrant magenta flowers.

At the base of a rock formation the trail bends sharply right, in the first of three switchbacks on the eastern side of the mountain. You might see chipmunks and lizards scampering across the trail and birds of prey flying overhead—be on the lookout for peregrine falcons, which nest in the park. Mount St. Helena Trail curves left on the second switchback as it gradually gains elevation. To the east are nice views of the Palisades area of the park, distinguished by dramatic, dark-red volcanic-rock formations. After the third switchback, the fire road heads north. When I hiked here on an unfortunately hot May day, I appreciated every tiny patch of shade from the occasional knobcone pine, Douglas-fir, and cluster of canyon live oak; most of the trailside vegetation is composed of chaparral shrubs.

At the 4-mile mark, the trail reaches a saddle and an unmarked junction. Look off to the right here for a peek at Lake Berryessa. The fire road doubling back to the left leads to South Peak. Continue straight on this fairly level stretch with good views toward North Peak. The trail descends gently, passing through knobcone pine, chinquapin, manzanita, toyon, and California coffeeberry. Some of the manzanita shrubs were still in bloom a few days after Memorial Day. Mount St. Helena Trail jogs left—ignore the steep path worn by shortcuts, heading straight—and begins to ascend again. Although this is a quiet part of the park, far from civilization and paved roads, keep an eye out for trucks that travel the fire roads to service the communications equipment on top of the North and South Peaks. The fire road crests at 5.1 miles, and a rough, unsigned fire road breaks off to the left—continue to the right. This spot may be the only Bay Area parkland where you can stand at the junction of three counties: Napa to the southeast, Lake to the northeast, and Sonoma to the west.

Descending slightly downslope of the hillside on the left, North Peak finally comes into view. The last push to the summit is the steepest part of the hike but offers the best views from the mountain south to the prominent Bay Area peaks, Mounts Diablo and Tamalpais. Even though it was a bit hazy on my hike, I could make out downtown San Francisco skyscrapers. The steep climb is over quickly, and at 5.6 miles you'll reach the top. With communications structures sprawling over the mountaintop, there is surprisingly little room to explore—an exposed rocky area is probably the best perch from which to gaze north, where I was stunned to see all the way to snow-topped Mount Lassen. When you're ready, retrace your steps back to the parking lot.

NEARBY ACTIVITIES

Old Faithful Geyser is a good detour on the way back to Napa Valley. Return toward Calistoga on CA 29, turn right onto Tubbs Lane, and drive about 0.5 mile to the entrance on the right. Read more about the geyser at **oldfaithfulgeyser.com,** or call 707-942-6463.

I highly recommend combining a Mount St. Helena hike with an overnight stay in one of **Calistoga**'s mineral-springs resorts. Lodging choices range from basic motels to luxurious inns—just be sure to pick a place with a heated mineral pool to soak your tired legs in after climbing the mountain.

16 SAMUEL P. TAYLOR STATE PARK

KEY AT-A-GLANCE INFORMATION

LENGTH: 6.5 miles

CONFIGURATION: Loop

DIFFICULTY: Moderate

SCENERY: Douglas-fir, California bay, big-leaf maple, and coast-live-oak woods; creek, waterfall, grassland views

EXPOSURE: The start and finish are shaded; the middle section is under full sun.

TRAFFIC: Light autumn–spring, moderate during summer camping season

TRAIL SURFACE: Dirt fire roads and trails

HIKING TIME: 3.5 hours

SEASON: Daily, 8 a.m.–sunset. Best in winter for the waterfall and in spring for the flowers. Muddy after rains.

ACCESS: Free at this trailhead

MAPS: Pick up the park map at the ranger station (when staffed), 1 mile back down Sir Francis Drake Boulevard, or download at tinyurl.com/taylorspmap.

FACILITIES: None at the trailhead; pit toilets at Devil's Gulch Horse Camp

SPECIAL COMMENTS: No dogs allowed. From the park-headquarters trailhead, you can make a 3-mile loop through redwoods on the Pioneer Tree Trail.

CONTACTS: 415-488-9897, tinyurl.com/samtaylorsp

DRIVING DISTANCE: 27 miles from the Golden Gate Bridge toll plaza

GPS INFORMATION

N38° 1.783' W122° 44.207'

IN BRIEF

From an ease-of-hiking standpoint, this 6.5-mile Barnabe Peak loop is close to perfect—like taking the escalator up and the elevator down. An easily graded path starts along a creek where salmon spawn some winters, makes a short detour to a waterfall, then ascends through wooded canyons to the high, grassy slopes of Barnabe Peak. From a viewpoint with sweeping vistas of Point Reyes, Mount Tamalpais, and Bolinas Ridge, you'll return downhill on a moderately steep fire road through grassland and back into woods.

DESCRIPTION

Samuel P. Taylor State Park's Barnabe Peak hides in plain sight. Although the 1,466-foot mountain is bare at the summit, the lower reaches of this mountain are heavily forested, obscuring views from the bottom to the top. The park's campground, picnic sites, and ranger station sit in a canyon alongside Lagunitas Creek, where hillsides covered with redwood and Douglas-fir forest ascend to Bolinas Ridge (out of the park, but part of the Golden Gate National Recreation Area). Across Sir Francis Drake Boulevard on the low slopes of Barnabe

----

Directions

Leave San Francisco via the Golden Gate Bridge on northbound US 101 and use the Golden Bridge toll plaza as your mileage starting point. Drive north on US 101 about 11 miles, then take Exit 450B, Sir Francis Drake/San Anselmo. Stay to the left toward San Anselmo and drive west on Sir Francis Drake Boulevard 15 miles, then continue past the main park entrance 1 more mile to a big dirt pullout on the left side of the road, just past the DEVIL'S GULCH sign on the right.

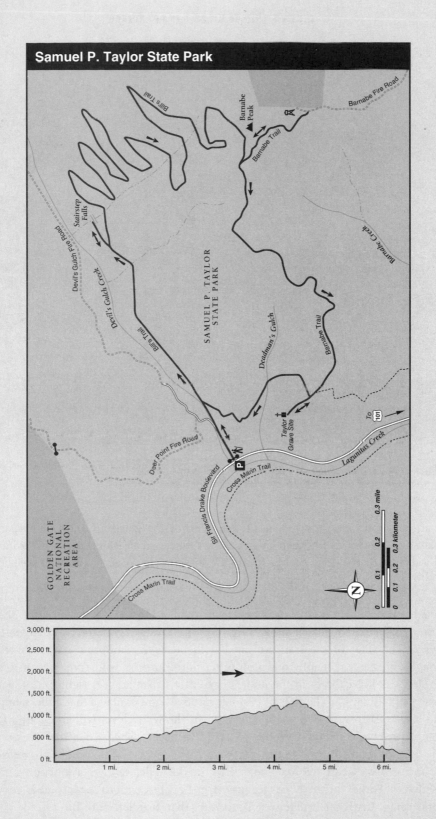

Samuel P. Taylor State Park

Bill's Trail

Barnabe Peak

Barnabe Trail

Barnabe Fire Road

Barnabe Creek

Devil's Gulch Fire Road

Stairstep Falls

Devil's Gulch Creek

Bill's Trail

SAMUEL P. TAYLOR STATE PARK

Deadman's Gulch

Barnabe Trail

Taylor Grave Site

To 101

Lagunitas Creek

Deer Point Fire Road

Sir Francis Drake Boulevard

Cross Marin Trail

GOLDEN GATE NATIONAL RECREATION AREA

Cross Marin Trail

0.3 mile
0.2
0.1
0.3 kilometer
0.2
0.1
0.1
0
0

N

3,000 ft.
2,500 ft.
2,000 ft.
1,500 ft.
1,000 ft.
500 ft.
0 ft.

1 mi.   2 mi.   3 mi.   4 mi.   5 mi.   6 mi.

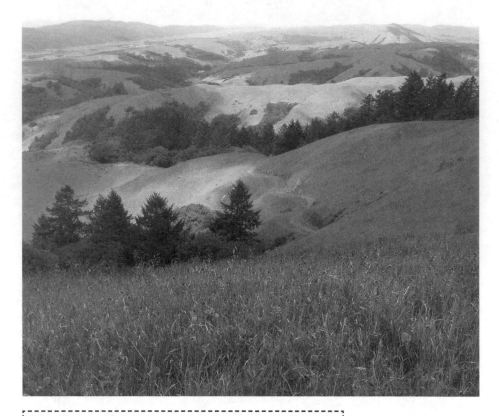

Views of West Marin's rolling hills unfold from the top of Barnabe Peak.

Peak, redwood groves thrive near the creek, while Douglas-fir, California bay, and coast-live-oak woods fill steep-sided canyons where small waterfalls run in winter and spring. At the top, near a Marin County fire lookout, wildflower displays brighten the grassland in spring.

From the pullout, carefully cross Sir Francis Drake and begin walking down a paved, gated service road signed for Devil's Gulch Horse Camp. This level road runs along one of the feeder streams for the largest waterway in the park, Lagunitas Creek. The sides of the trail are lined with buckeye, California bay, redwood, Douglas-fir, big-leaf maple, and California nutmeg, with wild rose, poison oak, hazelnut, and blackberry in the understory. After 0.1 mile, veer right onto a path signed simply TRAIL. The first of two interpretive signs explains that coho salmon and steelhead trout arrive in this creek when the water level is high enough for them to spawn, generally October–March. I've never visited when the creek was full, but in spring I always scan the water, just in case. The little path weaves around massive coast live oaks and then, at 0.2 mile, reaches a junction I call "Redwood Fork," for the huge tree just off the trail. A path to the left leads to the horse camp. Cross the bridge to a T-junction, then turn left onto Bill's Trail.

Now on the opposite bank of the creek, the trail starts a slight climb. In spring, look for columbine, woodland star, fringe cup, iris, starflower, and bleeding heart peeking out from a lush landscape of ferns, hazelnut, Douglas-fir, and California bay. This sheltered canyon is home to some very large, old trees, including some graceful mature big-leaf maples and a little cluster of eucalyptus. At 0.9 mile, the trail forks. Veer left to visit Stairstep Falls.

The path descends gradually at first, just barely clinging to the hillside. In the wettest months you'll hear the gush of water long before the path curves right and ends at the falls at about the 1-mile mark. Stairstep, as the name suggests, is a tiered waterfall with three drops totaling about 35 feet. When ready, return to Bill's Trail and turn left.

A long series of drawn-out switchbacks begins, keeping the grade incredibly easy. The first time I hiked this loop, it was so windy that tree branches crashed to the ground continuously, and I felt lucky to escape without a beaning. Usually, these woods are almost totally quiet, except for the sound of the wind through the trees and birdsong. Wildflowers begin to bloom along the trail as early as February, when the first blossoms on pink-flowering currant and milkmaids appear. Hound's tongue and checker lily are usually the next to bloom, in March; later still, you might see varieties of iris, lots of woodland star, fringe cup, starflower, and California larkspur. Banana slugs creep across the trail, in the shade of Douglas-fir, coast live oak, big-leaf maple, and California bay. Evergreen California nutmegs are very common and easy to pick out when bearing fleshy, olive-shaped arils (eaten by birds, but not edible for humans)—much different from redwood and Douglas-fir cones. Beware of poison oak, which crowds the trail in many areas.

As the trail ascends you'll cross pretty bridges and pass through woods and a few small grassy knolls. Near the end of the trail, the grassy patches are more common and bigger. Finally at 4.1 miles, just after Bridge 7, Bill's Trail emerges from the woods and ends at a fire road. Turn left.

After miles of easy hiking, the moderately steep uphill grade of Barnabe Trail is less than ideal, but the setting makes up for the climb. To the west, rolling grassy hills, dotted in spring with California poppy, buttercup, and clarkia, drift downhill and meet on the other side of the canyon a forest of evergreens, thickly covering the ascending slope. Ahead, the fire lookout at the mountaintop is conspicuous, so with the goal in site, trudge on uphill, winding through grassland and small pockets of California bay. At 4.4 miles, you'll reach a junction at a fence line and the park boundary. Ridge Trail continues to the right, descending steeply along a grassy ridge to a redwood forest.

The fire lookout sits on private property, so mind the NO TRESPASSING signs while enjoying outstanding views, particularly to the northwest, of Tomales Bay, the entire Point Reyes Peninsula, and Bolinas Ridge. Gaze south here for a rare glimpse of Kent Lake's spillway, most evident when the runoff is heavy.

When I hiked here one May, I found a sheltered spot on the slope of the peak and lunched alongside a nonplussed western fence lizard while bees browsed

Creamcups, one of the spring
flowers you might see on the
grassy hills at Samuel P. Taylor

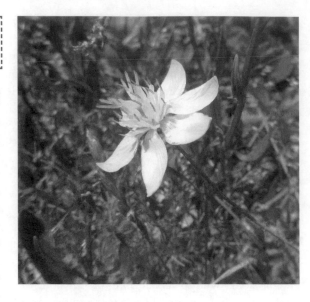

Creamcups, one of the spring flowers you might see on the grassy hills at Samuel P. Taylor

huckleberry blossoms. If you're here in spring, you may want to look through the grass downhill near the junction for such wildflowers as creamcups, California poppies, clovers, fiddlenecks, clarkia, and checkerbloom, with the best displays occurring in early May. When you're ready, retrace your steps back downhill past the junction with Bill's Trail, continuing on the fire road.

Barnabe Trail drops moderately steeply with the upper reaches of a forested canyon on the right and grassland on the left, then swings left away from the canyon into grassland and coyote brush. In spring look for paintbrush, sticky monkeyflower, blue-eyed grass, and buttercup. Other than one short uphill stretch, this is a quad-working downhill segment. At 5.9 miles, Riding and Hiking Trail departs on the left—continue straight. A white-picket-fenced plot is visible ahead—this is the grave site of the park's namesake, and the path leading to it breaks off to the left at 6 miles, a 0.1-mile out-and-back spur. Samuel P. Taylor, a Gold Rush entrepreneur, bought the area now preserved as this park and built a paper mill along the creek. It's widely reported that he named the tallest peak on his property after his mule Barnabe. (Bet his wife loved that!)

Past the grave site path, the fire road returns to woods in Deadman's Gulch, an area that's often very muddy after rains. The trail bends left and sweeps around the base of a hill. On a May hike, butterflies fluttered everywhere, landing on buttercups and blue-eyed grass flowers strewn through the grass. The path veers left back onto the fire road, which commences its moderately steep descent through the woods. At 6.3 miles, you'll reach the first bridge and junction with Bill's Trail again. Turn left and retrace your steps back to the trailhead.

SKYLINE WILDERNESS PARK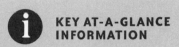

IN BRIEF

This hike starts near Skyline Wilderness's RV park, but you'll quickly leave the trappings of civilization behind on a fire road ascending through grassland and oaks to shaded woods near Lake Marie. From here a narrow path skirts sunny slopes above the lake; then you'll follow a series of paths wandering up and down grassland dotted with oaks and buckeyes.

DESCRIPTION

When Napa State Hospital decided to unload some surplus property in 1979, this land on the outskirts of Napa could easily have been developed. Local residents lobbied to preserve the property and proposed a unique plan: a volunteer-run park. Volunteers, always a huge asset to perennially budget strapped parks and preserves, manage Skyline Wilderness Park with the assistance of a few paid part-time employees. The result is a one-of-a-kind destination with miles of trails, an archery range, a disc-golf course, and a small RV park.

Begin on a trail starting at the edge of the parking lot, beneath a big coast live oak. The park is off to the left, but the Martha Walker

KEY AT-A-GLANCE INFORMATION

LENGTH: 5.8 miles

CONFIGURATION: Balloon

DIFFICULTY: Easy

SCENERY: Grassland, chaparral, lake, oaks

EXPOSURE: Some pockets of shade, but largely exposed

TRAFFIC: Light

TRAIL SURFACE: Dirt fire road and rocky trails

HIKING TIME: 3 hours

SEASON: Opens daily at 8 a.m.; closing hours vary (see Contacts, below). Good anytime but very hot in summer.

ACCESS: Cars, $5/4 people; walk-ins, $2/person; horse/bike riders, $3/person

MAPS: Pick up a trail map at the entrance kiosk.

FACILITIES: Restrooms and drinking water at the parking area

SPECIAL COMMENTS: No dogs allowed

CONTACTS: 707-252-0481, skylinepark.org

DRIVING DISTANCE: 39 miles from the Bay Bridge toll plaza

Directions

Leave San Francisco via the Bay Bridge and use the toll plaza as your mileage starting point. Drive north 26 miles on I-80, then take Exit 33 onto CA 37. Drive west 2.5 miles on CA 37 to the junction with CA 29. Turn right and drive north 7.5 miles on CA 29, then stay to the right at the junction with CA 221 (signed toward downtown Napa and Lake Berryessa). Drive north 3 miles on CA 221 (signed as Napa–Vallejo Highway) and then turn right onto Imola Avenue. Drive east 2.3 miles, then make a right into the park.

GPS INFORMATION

N38° 16.722' W122° 14.978'
2201 Imola Ave., Napa, CA 94559

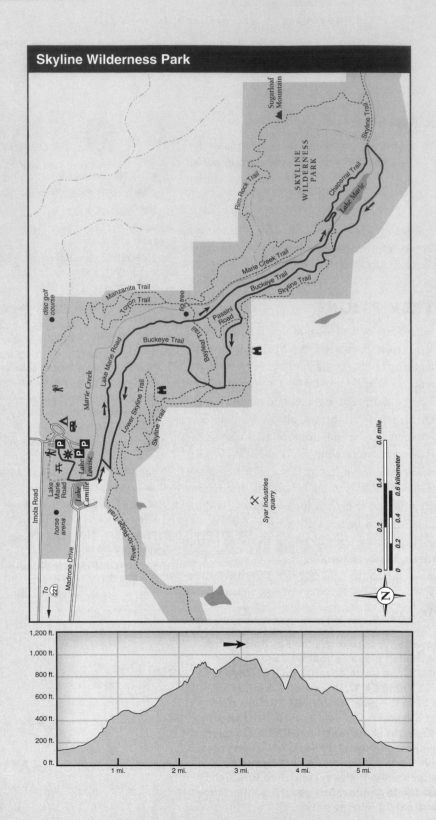

Skyline Wilderness Park

Native Habitat Garden creates a buffer between the trail and the campground. After passing some fruit and nut trees and climbing a few stairs, the trail seems to disappear in the middle of a picnic area. Stay to the right here—if you reach the Social Hall, you're headed the wrong way—passing a row of elevated concrete stands. On the far side of the picnic area, a wide trail swings in from the right, reaching a crossroads with a gravel road. Veer left onto signed Lake Marie Road.

Coast live oaks, snowberry shrubs, and blackberry vines strain against a fence that closely borders both sides of the broad dirt road. The trail sweeps left onto pavement briefly, then darts off to the right as the paved road continues straight into privately held Camp Coombs. At a level grade, Lake Marie Road skirts at a distance small lakes to the left and right, then reaches a junction at 0.3 mile. The road to the right leads to Buckeye and Skyline Trails; continue straight on Lake Marie Road.

With a grassy hillside dotted with blue oak and buckeye on the right, the fire road begins an easy climb. On a summer hike, I craned my neck to watch a hummingbird zip past overhead, then noticed a hawk soaring higher in the sky. Wild turkeys and quail also live here and are regularly spotted, even on trails and roads around the RV park. As the fire road ascends, the terrain becomes increasingly rocky, and views open up to include steep-sided Sugarloaf Mountain, the park's highest peak (not to be confused with Sugarloaf Ridge State Park, well north of Skyline Wilderness Park). Near a horse-watering trough on the left, there's a cave on the right—this is one of several mysterious old ruins throughout the park, remnants that may predate Napa State Hospital's ownership, which began in the 1870s. Easy-to-miss Lower Marie Creek Trail begins on the left, slipping down to run along the stream toward Lake Marie—continue straight on Lake Marie Road. Off in the distance to the left, look for a well-preserved stone fence dropping down the flanks of Sugarloaf Mountain, one of several stone walls in the park, constructed at an unknown date, perhaps by Chinese or Italian immigrants. Manzanita shares the hillsides with chamise and toyon as the fire road dips to a quick series of junctions at 1.2 miles.

Bayleaf Trail is the first to depart on the right. Continue straight a few more steps, where an immense fig tree on the left, heavy with fruit in late summer, is barely contained by a fence constructed to protect it. Here, an unsigned path begins on the left, leading to Lower and Upper Marie Creek Trails, Manzanita Trail, and Rim Rock Trail. Continue uphill on Lake Marie Trail, past Passini Road on the right and a path to an outhouse on the left. At a slight incline, Lake Marie Trail ducks under the shade of California bays, accompanied by varieties of fern, hazelnut, poison oak, creambush, madrone, and sticky monkeyflower. In July, you might see red-flowered Indian pink, one of the latest-blooming woodland wildflowers. On the right, the trail passes exposed rock ribs jutting out from the hillside—because no written records were kept preserving the history of the park property, it's difficult to imagine what purpose these served.

At 2 miles, just past a muddy seep beneath a wall of rock on the right, Lake Marie Road rises and an unsigned but obvious trail departs to the left. Follow this

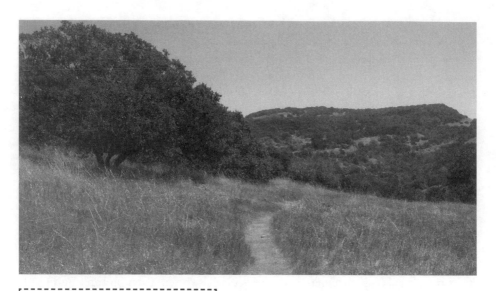

Oaks dot the grassland on Buckeye Trail.

connector trail downhill, and when it climbs to kiss Lake Marie Road goodbye one last time, stay to the left again. The trail descends through dense woods of California bay, passes a few picnic tables on the right, then climbs to Lake Marie's spillway. Here, a rustic log bench, surrounded by blooming paintbrush in spring, makes for a good lunch stop with views down to the water, where there are almost always ducks and birds to watch. This reservoir was constructed in 1908 to supply water for the hospital. Continue from the top of the dam, following the sign to Chaparral Trail, doubling back parallel to the connector from Lake Marie Road. The path runs along a thin berm, then dips to cross a creek bed and reaches a junction with Chaparral and Upper Marie Creek Trails. Turn right.

Chaparral Trail begins in the shade of coast live oak and California bay, but soon leaves these woods for sunbaked hillsides dotted with buckeye, sagebrush, sticky monkeyflower, poison oak, chamise, and coyote brush. Except for one short foray through a pocket of woods, continuous views extend downhill to the lake. Partly over exposed rock, Chaparral Trail turns right and begins a descent over a short series of switchbacks. In July, you might notice jewel-toned berries on spiny redberry shrubs, a low-growing evergreen bush often confused with ceanothus. Near the far end of the lake, the trail returns to shade beneath California bay, then reaches a T-junction with Skyline Trail at 2.7 miles. The trail to the left leads to Rim Rock Trail and the park boundary—turn right.

After crossing a feeder creek to Lake Marie, Skyline Trail begins to rise through California bay and coast live oak to a sunnier mix of buckeye, sticky monkeyflower, thimbleberry, and creambush. A connector to Lake Marie Road drops off to the right at 3.1 miles, but continue straight on Skyline, passing an old chimney and the remains of a stone house on the right. At 3.2 miles, another path heading to Lake Marie Road departs on the right, but again, stay to the left, climbing slightly to a junction with Buckeye Trail at 3.3 miles. Skyline Trail, a Bay Area Ridge Trail segment, continues uphill, keeping a course parallel to Buckeye's but at a higher elevation. Bear right.

Buckeye Trail quickly climbs into grassland before tapering off. If you visit in summer, yarrow and California poppy—the last lingering wildflowers—will be long gone, but colorful dragonflies and butterflies, including California sister and common buckeye, are abundant. To the right there are views across Marie Creek to Sugarloaf Mountain, Napa Valley, and the rugged ridges that encircle Lake Berryessa. Along the trail, a variety of trees stand in grassland, including buckeye, Oregon oak, blue oak, and coast live oak. The trail forks at 3.7 miles—stay to the right and descend through partial shade to a junction at 3.9 miles. Turn right onto Passini Road briefly, then veer left, onto the signed continuation of Buckeye Trail. Mostly keeping to exposed grassy slopes, Buckeye Trail climbs easily. The trail's namesake trees begin to shed their leaves in summer, part of an action-packed life cycle that includes bare branches and dangling poisonous chestnutlike seedpods in winter, new leaves in late winter, and sweet-smelling white blossoms in spring.

At 4.3 miles, Buckeye Trail follows a stone fence, then merges into an unsigned path from the left, connecting to Skyline Trail. Stay to the right, pass through a break in the fence into a grassy meadow, then reach a fork with a trail leading left to Skyline Trail. Veer right and descend a few yards to yet another junction, a roughly elongated X-shaped interchange with Bayleaf Trail. Turn left, then bear right, remaining on Buckeye Trail.

The trail passes through a pretty meadow, then ascends slightly to a rocky, rambling route. You may hear noise in this part of the park from a quarry operation to the west. Deciduous oaks (blue, Oregon, and black) accompany coast live oak, California bay, and buckeye as the trail sweeps across the hillsides above Lake Marie Road. At a steady descent, Buckeye Trail's final stretch runs parallel to Lake Marie Road, ending at 5.4 miles. Turn right.

The fire road descends through blue oaks, passing River to the Ridge Trail as it heads toward the Napa River on the left, before returning to the junction with Lake Marie Road at 5.5 miles. Turn left and retrace your steps back to the trailhead.

NEARBY ACTIVITIES

Skyline Wilderness Park's **Martha Walker Native Habitat Garden** is a must-stop for native-plant enthusiasts. Carefully tended by volunteers, this garden began in 1985 and is an impeccably maintained oasis, with numerous small fountains and abundant shade. There are all kinds of native plants, and benches secreted away in leafy alcoves offer perfect bird-watching spots. I saw about 20 quail and several other birds on one visit—if you're interested in providing habitat for birds and animals in your own garden, this is a great place to get some inspiration.

18 SUGARLOAF RIDGE STATE PARK

KEY AT-A-GLANCE INFORMATION

LENGTH: 6.2 miles

CONFIGURATION: Loop

DIFFICULTY: Moderate

SCENERY: Grassland, oaks, views, chaparral, creeks

EXPOSURE: Mostly full sun

TRAFFIC: Light

TRAIL SURFACE: Dirt fire roads, rocky trails, and 1 paved fire road

HIKING TIME: 3.5 hours

SEASON: Spring is best; muddy after rains and hot in summer.

ACCESS: Pay $8 fee at entrance kiosk.

MAPS: At the visitor center or entrance kiosk (when staffed), online at tinyurl .com/sugarloafparkmap

FACILITIES: Portable toilet at trailhead

SPECIAL COMMENTS: Dogs are not permitted on park trails. After rains, you'll get your feet wet crossing Sonoma Creek. Start this hike early, since there's no shade on the final push to the summit.
     Sugarloaf abuts Hood Mountain Regional Park and Open Space Preserve, a Sonoma County park with a peak 1 foot higher than Sugarloaf's Bald Mountain. More info: 707-565-2041, sonoma-county.org/parks /pk_hood.htm.

CONTACTS: 707-833-5712, tinyurl.com /sugarloafridgesp, sugarloafpark.org

DRIVING DISTANCE: 53.8 miles from the Golden Gate Bridge toll plaza

GPS INFORMATION

N38° 26.280' W122° 30.851'

IN BRIEF

Sugarloaf Ridge's Bald Mountain holds bragging rights to one of the prettiest and most serene viewpoints in the Bay Area. From a relatively diminutive height of 2,729 feet, views include every significant wine-country peak and valley. This hike starts at the edge of a sloping meadow, climbing steadily through a mixture of grassland, chaparral, and mixed woodland for 2.5 miles to the summit. The return route travels along a quiet ridge, drops steeply through gray pines and chaparral to cross Sonoma Creek, and then wanders through a meadow on the way back to the trailhead.

DESCRIPTION

At Sugarloaf Ridge, every step seems like a gift. From the get-go, the trails are quiet and the scenery is gorgeous—views from the top of Bald Mountain are icing on the cake. There's so much variety at Sugarloaf that every season has its charm. Sonoma Creek's headwaters originate here, and in winter, streams gush downhill at such a rate that you may feel transported from dry California to a more lush locale.

Directions ———————————————▶

Leave San Francisco on northbound US 101 and use the Golden Gate Bridge toll plaza as your mileage starting point. Drive about 20 miles north on US 101, then take Exit 460A onto CA 37E. Drive east on CA 37 for 7.5 miles, then turn left onto CA 121/Arnold Drive. Continue north on Arnold Drive 13 miles, then turn right onto Agua Caliente Road. After less than 1 mile, turn left onto CA 12. Continue north 8 miles, then turn right onto Adobe Canyon Road. Drive east 3 miles to the entrance kiosk, pay the fee, and then continue a short distance to the parking lot on the left.

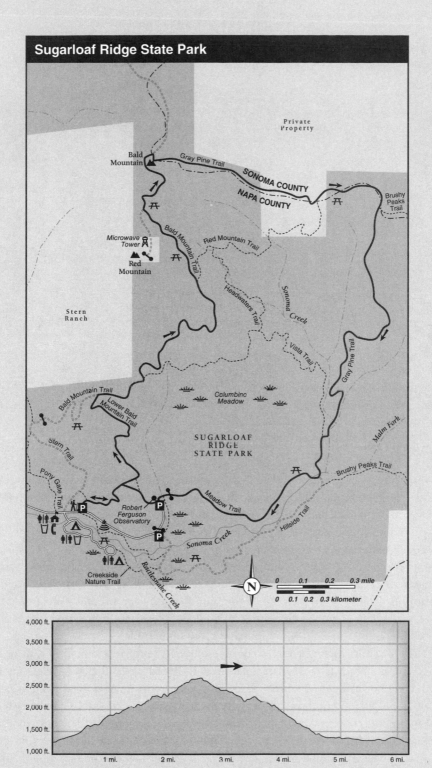

Sugarloaf Ridge State Park

Bald
Mountain

Gray Pine Trail

SONOMA COUNTY

NAPA COUNTY

Private
Property

Brushy
Peaks
Trail

*Microwave
Tower*

Bald Mountain Trail

Red Mountain Trail

Red
Mountain

Headwaters Trail

Sonoma Creek

Stern
Ranch

Vista Trail

Gray Pine Trail

Columbine
Meadow

Malm Fork

Bald Mountain Trail

Lower Bald
Mountain Trail

S U G A R L O A F
R I D G E
S T A T E   P A R K

Stern
Trail

Pony Gate Trail

Brushy Peaks Trail

Meadow Trail

P

P

Robert
Ferguson
Observatory

P

Hillside Trail

Sonoma Creek

Creekside
Nature Trail

Rattlesnake Creek

N

| 0 | 0.1 | 0.2 | 0.3 mile |
| 0 | 0.1 | 0.2 | 0.3 kilometer |

4,000 ft.					
3,500 ft.					
3,000 ft.					
2,500 ft.					
2,000 ft.					
1,500 ft.					
1,000 ft.					
	1 mi.	2 mi.	3 mi.	4 mi.	5 mi.	6 mi.

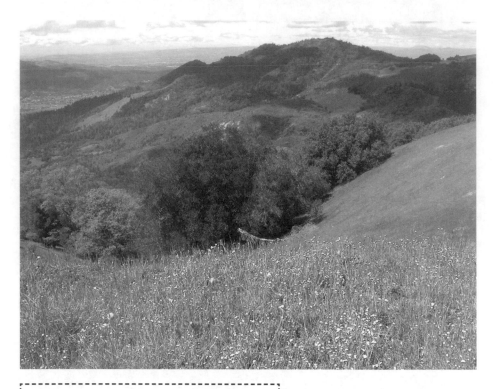

A serene wine-country vista, courtesy of Sugarloaf Ridge

Spring flowers are pretty, and the temperatures are hospitable. Summer (if you can endure the heat) brings hillsides stacked with fragrant blooming chamise. In autumn, foliage on black oaks and big-leaf maples is stunning.

Begin from the parking lot on Lower Bald Mountain Trail. At an easy grade, the rocky path begins to ascend from the valley floor, winding through grassland past a few coast live oaks, Douglas-firs, and manzanitas. Look for goldfields, buttercups, shooting stars, iris, blue-dicks, and blue-eyed grass in spring. A few small ceanothus shrubs growing close to the ground suggest the presence of serpentine soil—while it may not be obvious in this part of the park, significant serpentine swales are visible off Bald Mountain and Gray Pine Trails.

After a short foray through some trees, Lower Bald Mountain Trail returns to grassland and reaches a two-part junction with Meadow Trail at 0.2 mile. Stay to the left on Lower Bald Mountain Trail. The grade picks up as the path climbs into an open woodland composed mostly of madrone, coast live oak, California bay, and manzanita. On an April hike, I saw jackrabbits hopping up the trail. Switch-backing uphill between two creek beds, the trail gradually makes a transition to chaparral, where chamise, toyon, scrub oak, ceanothus, sticky monkeyflower, and poison oak are the most notable plants. The deep umber color of the trail surface is adobe clay. This rocky segment ends at a T-junction at 0.8 mile. Turn right onto Bald Mountain Trail.

The trail—a wide, paved road used to access communications equipment atop Red Mountain—ascends at a moderate, steady pace. Vegetation ranges from chamise, manzanita, toyon, monkeyflower, and poison oak to coast live oak and madrone. In spring, flowering purple bush lupine brightens the sides of the trail. At about the 1-mile mark, Vista Trail departs on the right, offering an early out for hikers who are discouraged by the grade. Continue uphill on Bald Mountain Trail.

In winter and early spring, the sound of running water from a creek out of sight on the right will probably accompany your hike. Bald Mountain Trail sweeps uphill through an open area where ceanothus and coyote brush are common. At one corner, water spills downhill from the left, then drops into a ravine where buckeyes nestle. California poppies, blue and white lupine, and scorpionweed bloom along the trail in May. As the trail climbs, trailside vegetation reflects the change in elevation and exposure—there's lots of chamise, ceanothus, cercocarpus, and scrub oak. At about 1.6 miles, if the day is clear, pause and look south to see Mounts Diablo and Tamalpais. Red Mountain Trail breaks off to the right at 1.7 miles, headed toward Gray Pine Trail. Continue straight on Bald Mountain Trail.

In the shadow of Red Mountain, the trail is lined with black oak, big-leaf maple, California bay, and live oak. After a swing into grassland, you'll reach a junction and saddle at 2 miles. Straight ahead, the hillside drops, then gradually rises to the flanks of Mount Hood. The pavement curves left on a dead-end spur to Red Mountain. Turn right, remaining on Bald Mountain Trail.

Now a dirt fire road, the trail adopts a moderately steep course uphill through grassland. You may notice bluish serpentine, exposed on a rock cut on the left. The grassy hillside on the right gently slips away, offering expansive views south. On an April visit, blooming popcorn flowers painted huge white swaths in spring's still-green grass. As you follow Bald Mountain Trail, sweeping around the very top of the mountain, ignore any side trails and persist to a signed junction at 2.4 miles. Here High Ridge Trail heads left on a dead-end journey. Turn right onto Gray Pine Trail. After just a few feet, Gray Pine veers left. Turn right and walk uphill a few more feet to the summit. Interpretive signs assist you in identifying the surrounding sites: In the immediate area you can see Napa Valley, Sonoma Valley, the steep hillsides of Jack London State Historic Park, and the more gently graded hillsides of Annadel State Park. On one April hike, the top of Mount St. Helena, to the north of Sugarloaf, hid in a puffy white cloud.

When visibility permits, you may also see Mount Wittenberg, the highest peak on Point Reyes (33 miles west); Snow Mountain (65 miles north and, because it's well named, easy to pick out); Mount Diablo (51 miles southeast); Mount Tamalpais (37 miles southwest); the Golden Gate Bridge (44 miles southwest); and even Pyramid Peak in the Sierra Nevada (a whopping 129 miles east). The bench at the grassy summit offers a perch for one of the most quiet and gorgeous lunch breaks in the entire Bay Area. Save for an occasional airplane, there's no outside noise. When you're ready to start moving again, return to Gray Pine Trail and begin to descend.

The first section of this trail seems poorly named, as there's nary a pine in sight. On the left, some towering black oaks make a big foliage impact in autumn, but in spring, train your gaze to the grass on the sides of the trail, where bird's-eye gilia blooms. The fire road follows just about smack on the line dividing Napa and Sonoma Counties as it descends, generally following the ridgeline. You'll see more manzanita, California bay, Douglas-fir, coyote brush, chamise, and toyon. In early April, blueblossom ceanothus flowers, followed a bit later by clematis, a trailing vine with white flowers, which drapes itself over shrubs. Although the route is downhill, there is one short uphill section. At 3.2 miles, Red Mountain Trail ventures off to the right—you could make an alternate return on Red Mountain, Headwaters, and Vista Trails. For this hike, continue straight on Gray Pine Trail.

As you descend at a slightly steep pitch, look for woodland star, buttercups, and blue-eyed grass in spring. Black oaks, chaparral, and grassland continue to line the trail, but the first of the gray pines appears as well. After one last hill climb, you'll reach the junction with Brushy Peaks Trail at 3.6 miles. Turn right, remaining on Gray Pine Trail.

By now the trailside blend of chamise, cercocarpus, ceanothus, scrub oak, manzanita, and monkeyflower should be familiar. Tall and spindly gray pine (also known as ghost pine) tower above the trail here and there—if you're hiking when it's a bit breezy, you may want to pause and enjoy the sound of the wind whispering through them. Descending off the ridge, the grade is steep and some sections are very rocky. Gray Pine Trail leaves its namesake trees behind and arcs through a grassy area, where wet-weather runoff flows down the hillsides and muddies the trail.

With your path now following a branch of Sonoma Creek, still descending but at an easy grade, madrone and coast live oak appear. After a sharp left turn, you'll cross another feeder creek. Look along the sides of the trail for golden fairy lanterns in late April and early May. Wandering along the creek through this flat creek basin during a spring hike with the sounds of rushing water everywhere, I felt like I was on an alpine vacation. Gray Pine Trail makes its first creek crossing; in the warmest months of the year you can hop over whatever water is left in the creek bed, but from winter through spring the water level is high enough that your feet (and ankles) will likely get wet. I took off my shoes and socks and waded across the cool water, and my feet felt like they'd been given a whole new lease on life. Buckeye, alder, and California bay stand near the creek, enjoying the reliable water source.

At 4.8 miles, Vista Trail feeds in from the right. Continue to the left on Gray Pine to the second creek crossing, with generally even deeper water to ford. A gorgeous mature big-leaf maple graces the stream here—if you're here in spring when the tree is clothed in fresh green leaves, you'll have to imagine it lit up with autumn foliage. Gray Pine Trail ends at 5 miles. Turn right onto Meadow Trail.

From here on out, the grade is very easy—a relaxing stroll, really. Once more you'll cross Sonoma Creek (this time on a bridge), then pass through groves of maples. A curious SATURN sign on the left is part of the Planet Walk interpretive hike that originates at Ferguson Observatory. The creek veers off to the left,

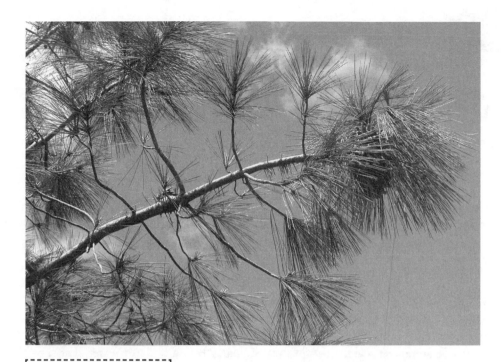

A gray pine and massive cone

continuing its journey toward Sonoma Valley, but the trail leaves the streamside to make its way through a meadow. Some chaparral thrives in a serpentine patch on the right, but grassland soon overtakes the landscape. The meadow is yet another superscenic Sugarloaf spot. This would be a good location for a bench, since both grass and trail are often damp in winter and spring.

At 5.7 miles, Hillside Trail breaks off to the left, heading back over Sonoma Creek toward the park's campground. Continue straight, through or around a gate, where you'll emerge in a parking lot. Veer right, passing Ferguson Observatory, and pick up the continuation of Meadow Trail. On a slight ascent through a rocky area, another feeder creek descends on the left. Goldfields make a big impact along the trail in spring, when they form sunny carpets in the grass. In patches of serpentine with sparse grass, you'll likely see more bird's-eye gilia. Here, on my April hike, I had another jackrabbit sighting.

At 5.8 miles, you'll reach a two-part triangle junction with Lower Bald Mountain Trail. Stay to the left and retrace your steps back to the trailhead.

19 TOMALES BAY STATE PARK

KEY AT-A-GLANCE INFORMATION

LENGTH: 2.8 miles

CONFIGURATION: Loop with a short out-and-back segment

DIFFICULTY: Easy

SCENERY: Woods, beaches

EXPOSURE: Mostly shaded

TRAFFIC: Light during off-season, moderate in summer, heavy near Heart's Desire Beach

TRAIL SURFACE: Dirt trails

HIKING TIME: 1.5 hours

SEASON: Good all year; peaceful autumn–spring

ACCESS: Pay $8 entrance fee at the ranger-station kiosk—no cash is accepted.

MAPS: At ranger station and tinyurl .com/tomalesmap

FACILITIES: Restrooms and drinking water at trailhead

SPECIAL COMMENTS: No dogs allowed. If you want to check out a nearby ocean beach, the Abbotts Lagoon trailhead is another 1.8 miles north of the Tomales Bay State Park turnoff on Pierce Point Road. From the parking lot, a nearly level path travels west along a butterfly-shaped lagoon. After 1 mile, in a gap between the two lagoon wings, the trail disintegrates in loose sand, leaving the route to the ocean up to you.

CONTACTS: 415-669-1140, tinyurl .com/tomalesbaysp

DRIVING DISTANCE: 42 miles from the Golden Gate Bridge toll plaza

GPS INFORMATION

N38° 7.874' W122° 53.462'

IN BRIEF

Most people are drawn to Tomales Bay in summer, particularly to Heart's Desire Beach, which sits just off one of the state park's parking lots. Three other beaches can be reached only by foot. Hike to one busy and one quiet beach on this 2.8-mile loop through a gorgeous woodland and along the coast.

DESCRIPTION

This little park, largely ignored by tourists who flock to the Point Reyes peninsula, is no secret with locals, who favor it for beach parties, picnics, and hikes.

Tomales Bay, a body of water that separates Point Reyes from the rest of West Marin, sits directly above the San Andreas Fault. The beaches here, more sedate than the Pacific coastline, appeal to families with kids. With beaches this pretty, it's tough to tear yourself

----

Directions →

Leave San Francisco via the Golden Gate Bridge on northbound US 101 and use the Golden Bridge toll plaza as your mileage starting point. Drive north on US 101 about 11 miles, then take Exit 450B, Sir Francis Drake/San Anselmo. Stay to the left toward San Anselmo and drive west on Sir Francis Drake Boulevard about 20 miles to the junction with CA 1; turn right and, after 0.1 mile, make the first left onto Bear Valley Road. After about 2 miles, Bear Valley Road ends at Sir Francis Drake; turn left. Continue on Sir Francis Drake about 5.5 miles, then turn right onto Pierce Point Road. Drive about 1.2 miles to the park entrance, on the right side of the road. Turn right and drive down the park road about 0.7 mile to the ranger station; stop and pay the fee, then continue about 0.9 mile to the parking lot at the end of the road (*not* the Heart's Desire lot).

Tomales Bay State Park

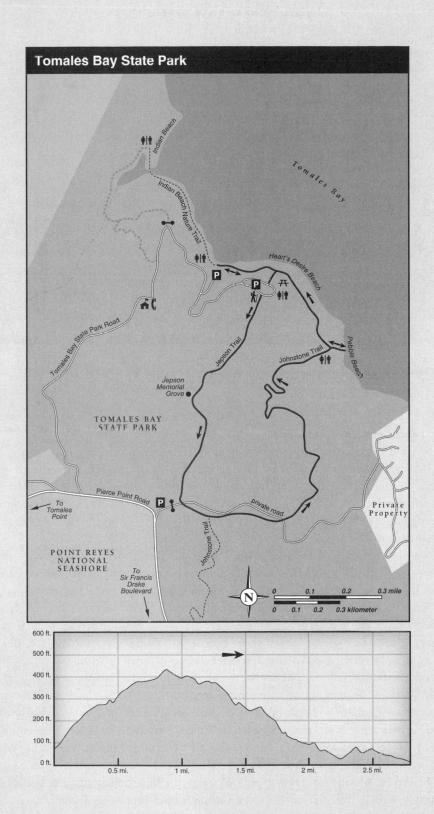

Indian Beach

Indian Beach Nature Trail

Tomales Bay

Heart's Desire Beach

P

P

Pebble Beach

Tomales Bay State Park Road

Jepson Trail

Johnstone Trail

Jepson Memorial Grove

TOMALES BAY STATE PARK

Private Property

Pierce Point Road

P

To Tomales Point

private road

POINT REYES NATIONAL SEASHORE

Johnstone Trail

To Sir Francis Drake Boulevard

N

| 0 | 0.1 | 0.2 | 0.3 mile |
| 0 | 0.1 | 0.2 | 0.3 kilometer |

600 ft.
500 ft.
400 ft.
300 ft.
200 ft.
100 ft.
0 ft.

0.5 mi.   1 mi.   1.5 mi.   2 mi.   2.5 mi.

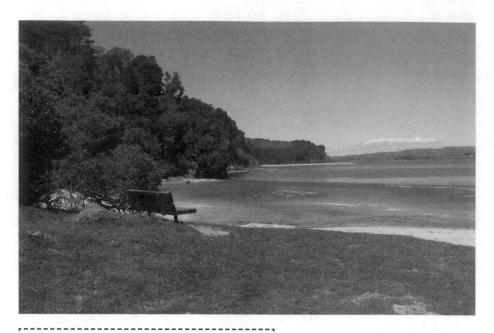

A bench invites peaceful contemplation at Tomales Bay.

off the sand. Perhaps that's why the park trails can be a quiet refuge even when the beaches are crowded.

Trails depart from the parking lots in different locations. Begin at the signed Jepson trailhead, about midway through the upper parking lot. Immediately the scenery is incredibly lush, with huge coast live oaks covered in moss while ferns, huckleberry, and California coffeeberry crowd the narrow trail. The ascent is steady but easy. You may hear deer crashing through the woods, but the foliage is so thick that it's hard to see more than a few feet into the forest.

In late spring look for tiny white flowers on yerba buena, a native herb that creeps close to the ground. Gradually Bishop pines and madrones muscle their way into the woods. In the understory, a variety of berry-producing native plants provide food for local birds and small mammals. Some of these berries, from thimbleberry, huckleberry, and currant, are palatable for humans as well. If you notice masses of a glossy-leaved shrub that seem familiar yet out of place, that's salal, a plant often used in floral arrangements; in April, you might catch it in bloom. At 0.9 mile, a path heads off to the right toward a parking area on Pierce Point Road—continue straight on Jepson Trail.

Although there's a break in the tree cover, dense stands of toyon, coyote brush, and coffeeberry still obscure any views. At 1 mile, Jepson Trail crosses a paved road that leads to a private beach. Continue straight. The same familiar vegetation lines the trail, although poison oak seems especially assertive. Honeysuckle vines dangle from shrubs, producing fragrant pink blossoms in June and pretty red berries in autumn. Jepson Trail ends at 1.1 miles. Turn left onto Johnstone Trail.

The grade remains close to level as Johnstone Trail winds through Bishop pine, coffeeberry, huckleberry, coast live oak, hazelnut, and tan oak. At 1.3 miles, the private road is crossed for the last time and the trail begins to descend easily. A bench on the left offers somewhat screened views of the bay. Madrones and manzanitas grow together in one area, inviting a comparison between these two related plants of the heath family that are common throughout the Bay Area.

Manzanitas usually grow no larger than other chaparral shrubs, while madrones can attain stately heights. Both feature reddish peeling bark; white, urn-shaped blossoms; and red, berrylike fruit. Because height comparisons can be deceiving (some manzanitas can reach 30 feet), a crucial difference is the plants' leaves. While manzanita leaves average about 1 inch in length, the madrone's are much larger, about 5 inches long.

Johnstone Trail reaches the slopes of a little canyon that drains to a creek, and you may notice moisture-loving plants along the trail, including alder, chinquapin, ferns, huckleberry, and salmonberry. Labrador tea, a shrub that looks a bit like azalea, blooms in June. A few switchbacks ease the descent, but expect some mud here in all but the driest parts of the year. Where Johnstone Trail levels and reaches a junction with a path to Pebble Beach at 2.2 miles, turn right. The path descends briefly, then ends at the beach. Not surprisingly, given the name, Pebble Beach is rocky, but it's also much quieter than sandy Heart's Desire Beach. Look across the bay for views of a series of low, rolling, grassy hills. Return to the previous junction and turn right, back onto Johnstone Trail.

Back on the main trail, California bay, coast live oak, madrone, huckleberry, ferns, and creambush line the trail. At 2.5 miles, Johnstone Trail steps out of the woods at restrooms near the trailhead. If you don't want to make the trip to Heart's Desire Beach, turn left and walk back to the parking lot; otherwise, continue straight.

After passing under some huge coast live oaks, the trail bisects a pretty group-picnic area. When the area is vacant, you can have your pick of tables, but I prefer to snack at a wooden bench overlooking the bay on the right. Keep hiking and drop down a set of steps to reach Heart's Desire Beach at about 2.7 miles. When you're ready, retrace your steps back to the junction near the restrooms, then turn right and return to the parking lot.

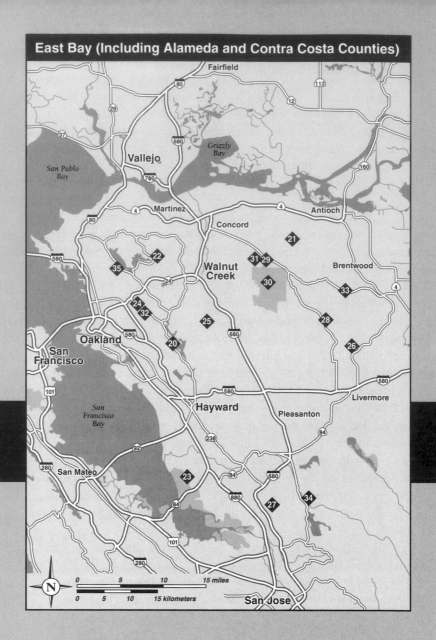

East Bay (Including Alameda and Contra Costa Counties)

Fairfield

Vallejo

San Pablo
Bay

Grizzly
Bay

Martinez

Antioch

Concord

Walnut
Creek

Brentwood

Oakland

San
Francisco

San
Francisco
Bay

Hayward

Pleasanton

Livermore

San Mateo

San Jose

0   5   10   15 miles

0   5   10   15 kilometers

N

EAST BAY
(INCLUDING ALAMEDA AND CONTRA COSTA COUNTIES)

20 ANTHONY CHABOT REGIONAL PARK

KEY AT-A-GLANCE INFORMATION

LENGTH: 5.4 miles
CONFIGURATION: Loop
DIFFICULTY: Easy
SCENERY: Grassland, woods
EXPOSURE: Mostly full sun
TRAFFIC: Moderate
TRAIL SURFACE: Dirt fire roads and trails
HIKING TIME: 3 hours
SEASON: Daily, 8 a.m.–sunset. Summer is often hot; late winter and spring are best.
ACCESS: Free
MAPS: At the trailhead's information signboard and ebparks.org/parks/maps
FACILITIES: Pit toilets at Bort Meadow; none at trailhead
SPECIAL COMMENTS: Dogs welcome ($2 fee). Trails are usually muddy through winter and early spring.
CONTACTS: 888-327-2757, ebparks.org/parks/anthony_chabot
DRIVING DISTANCE: 15.5 miles from the Bay Bridge toll plaza

GPS INFORMATION

N37° 46.653' W122° 7.501'

IN BRIEF

This loop is a circuit through the heart of Chabot, bisecting Grass Valley, climbing to a ridge, and then descending into Bort Meadow through quiet woods. I've enjoyed Chabot hikes in every season, but the park really shines in spring during wildflower season. If you're a novice flower enthusiast, this is a good, accessible place to start, with plenty of common blossoms best seen in April and early May.

DESCRIPTION

Anthony Chabot Regional Park is shaped like a foot, with long, thin toes pressing against Redwood Park and Lake Chabot settled at the heel. The East Bay Municipal Water District defines the entire eastern border of Chabot, and the western boundary is mostly residential, but a ridge blocks the bulk of the noise.

If you're unfamiliar with the area, it would be easy to consider Chabot and neighbor park Redwood as one, but it's remarkable how different two adjoining parks can be— Redwood is heavily forested, while Chabot hosts extensive grassland. The area around Lake Chabot is a warren of paths, leading to

Directions

Depart San Francisco on the Bay Bridge and use the toll plaza as your mileage starting point. About 0.5 mile past the toll plaza, bear right onto I-580 East. Drive 1.5 miles, then take Exit 19B on CA 24. Drive 3.5 miles east on CA 24, then take Exit 5 onto CA 13 south. Drive about 4 miles, then exit at Redwood Road. Turn left onto Redwood and drive uphill about 0.5 mile, to the junction with Skyline Boulevard. Continue straight on Redwood about 4.3 miles to the trailhead, on the right side of the road.

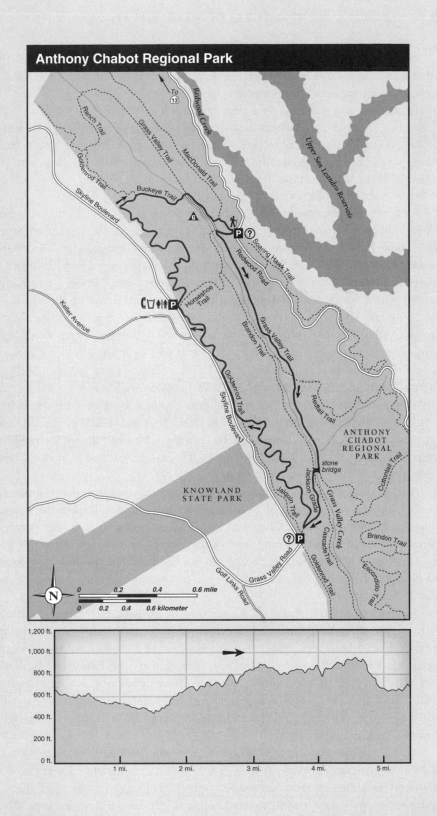

Anthony Chabot Regional Park

To 13

Redwood Creek

Upper San Leandro Reservoir

Ranch Trail

Grass Valley Trail

MacDonald Trail

Goldenrod Trail

Skyline Boulevard

Buckeye Trail

Soaring Hawk Trail

Redwood Road

Horseshoe Trail

Keller Avenue

Brandon Trail

Grass Valley Trail

Redtail Trail

ANTHONY CHABOT REGIONAL PARK

Goldenrod Trail

Skyline Boulevard

Cottontail Trail

stone bridge

Jackson Grade

Grass Valley Creek

KNOWLAND STATE PARK

Jalquin Trail

Brandon Trail

Cascade Trail

Escondido Trail

Goldenrod Trail

Golf Links Road

Grass Valley Road

N

| 0 | 0.2 | 0.4 | 0.6 mile |
| 0 | 0.2 0.4 | 0.6 kilometer |

1,200 ft.

1,000 ft.

800 ft.

600 ft.

400 ft.

200 ft.

0 ft.

1 mi. 2 mi. 3 mi. 4 mi. 5 mi.

and from a marksmanship range, golf course, picnic areas, and campsites, but the rest of the park has an undeveloped feel.

Begin from the trailhead on a paved, gated road near the information sign-board. As the service road sweeps downhill, there are views past the coyote brush and poison oak along the trail to Grass Valley on the left. At 0.1 mile, you'll reach a three-way junction. The road to the right continues to Bort Meadow, and the middle path leads to Brandon Trail, which runs parallel to Grass Valley Trail on the far side of Grass Valley Creek. Turn left onto Grass Valley Trail.

Once through a cattle gate, you'll begin a nearly level stroll along the length of Grass Valley, a narrow meadow where wildflowers are common in spring. Some oaks, coyote brush, and poison oak shrubs dot the valley, but grassland dominates the landscape, where in early April suncups, blue-eyed grass, and buttercups bloom in clusters and tiny-blossomed filaree makes a huge impact, overtaking hillsides with a purple hue. At 1 mile, Redtail Trail sets off uphill on the left. Continue on Grass Valley Trail, winding slightly downhill into a grove of eucalyptus companionably mixed through some redwoods. At 1.5 miles, Grass Valley Trail swings left toward Lake Chabot. Turn right and pass over Grass Valley Creek on Stone Bridge to a second junction, with Cascade Trail on the left and Brandon Trail on the right. Continue straight, now on Jackson Grade.

At a moderate pace, the fire road climbs through a mélange of vegetation, including eucalyptus, big-leaf maple, creambush, hazelnut, blackberry, wild rose, toyon, coast live oak, and coffeeberry. In spring you're likely to see purple bush lupine and sticky monkeyflower blooming. The ascent ends at a junction with Goldenrod Trail at 1.9 miles. Turn right.

A short distance from the park boundary, the fire road runs downslope of a hillside, within audible range of Skyline Boulevard, and you'll likely hear some vehicle and residential noise. Chaparral favors this sunny area, although eucalyptus trees have extended their range out of the canyon on the right. In spring you might see blue witch nightshade, checkerbloom, California poppy, blue-eyed grass, and blue-dick blooming beneath poison oak, toyon, broom, blue elderberry, and sticky monkeyflower.

As Goldenrod Trail veers left, a spur trail heads back to the left—continue to the right. Now, following close to Skyline Boulevard, eucalyptus trees are mostly replaced with some pines. Good views range across Grass Valley to the Upper San Leandro Reservoir watershed, managed by the East Bay Municipal Water District. At 3.6 miles, you'll approach the grounds of Chabot Equestrian Center. Follow the trail signs as a skimpy path leads left, crosses an access road, and heads back into chaparral. Horseshoe Trail sets off downhill on the right. Continue on Goldenrod Trail.

This is a good section for wildflowers, ranging from delicate, wispy woodland star to giant, sturdy cow parsnip. In May you may see owl's clover. The trail alternates between chaparral and shade, with little substantial elevation change. California poppies occupy some grassy knolls just off the trail on the right. When you reach a T-junction with a paved service road at 4.4 miles, turn right. The road skirts a water tank, then returns to dirt. Creambush, a deciduous shrub, puts forth froths of white flowers in late spring and early summer, brightening the sides of the trail. You might also notice some big-leaf maple and hazelnut. If it's a clear day, you should be able to make out Las Trampas Ridge to the east. At 4.7 miles, you'll reach a junction with Buckeye Trail. Turn right.

In a park full of fire roads, this narrow hiking-only path is a gift. Steeply sloping stairs drop the trail into a deeply shaded canyon, where coast live oak and California bay create a lush canopy. A little creek murmurs on the left, creating a moist, hospitable environment for hound's tongue and fringe cups in spring. After a bridge crosses the creek, you'll pass a shaded rest bench that is welcome on a hot day. Watch your step as the trail runs along the stream, since the ground can be unstable. Forget-me-not, one of our most charming "alien" wildflowers, covers the forest floor with a wash of light blue in late March. One last bridge transports you from woods to the edge of Bort Meadow, a wide, grassy expanse that makes a good stop for lunch or a sunny snooze. Cross the meadow to a junction on the left of the vault toilets, at about 5 miles.

The paved road (the same road on which this hike began) winds back to the parking lot, but a path to the right of a gated trail makes a nicer finish. This slight trail climbs through eucalyptus into coyote brush and poison oak. Loads of blue-eyed grass and buttercups bloom in April along the trail. There are also a few plum trees, favored by birds and the omnivorous coyote. When the trail forks at 5.3 miles, stay to the left. Coming to a crest, you'll reach a junction with Mac-Donald Trail. Turn right and walk a few feet to the parking lot.

NEARBY ACTIVITIES

The park's main trailheads surround **Lake Chabot,** around which you can hike or bike on a 12.4-mile loop; you can also spend the night at one of several campsites. Call 888-327-2757 or visit **ebparks.org/parks/lake_chabot** for more information.

21 BLACK DIAMOND MINES REGIONAL PRESERVE

KEY AT-A-GLANCE INFORMATION

LENGTH: 3.5 miles

CONFIGURATION: Loop

DIFFICULTY: Easy–moderate

SCENERY: Grassland and chaparral

EXPOSURE: Mostly full sun

TRAFFIC: Mostly moderate, but heavy near the visitor center

TRAIL SURFACE: Dirt fire road and trails; one very short trail segment is paved.

HIKING TIME: 2 hours

SEASON: Opens daily at 8 a.m.; closing hours vary (see Contacts, below). Summer is often very hot—late winter and spring are best.

ACCESS: Pay the $5 fee at the entrance kiosk.

MAPS: At the trailhead and ebparks .org/parks/maps

FACILITIES: Vault toilets and drinking water at trailhead

SPECIAL COMMENTS: Dogs welcome ($2 fee)

CONTACTS: 888-327-2757, ebparks .org/parks/black_diamond

DRIVING DISTANCE: 45 miles from the Bay Bridge toll plaza

GPS INFORMATION

N37° 57.500' W121° 51.797'

5175 Somersville Rd.
Antioch, CA 94509

IN BRIEF

Want to ramble through grassland and chaparral on one hike? This loop is a perfect tour through grassy, rolling hills as well as chamise, black sage, and manzanita-covered slopes. You'll begin in the heart of the park, climb through grassland dotted with blue oaks, follow an undulating course through chaparral, climb some more back into grassland, and then descend steadily back to the trailhead.

DESCRIPTION

Have you heard the one about the coal mine in Contra Costa County? It's no joke—from 1860 to 1906, the property we now know as Black Diamond Mines was the largest coal-mining district in California. Nearly 4 million tons of coal (black diamonds) were mined, with as many as 900 miners populating five towns in the area. When coal-mining operations ceased, underground sand mining continued until the late 1940s. The East Bay Regional Park District has preserved Black Diamond Mines as a recreational and historical park, with miles of trails laced across more than 5,700 acres of land and remnants from the mining era accessible in several locations.

Directions

Depart San Francisco on the Bay Bridge and use the toll plaza as your mileage starting point. Stay to the left, continuing northbound on I-80. Drive north on I-80 about 15 miles, then take Exit 23 onto CA 4. Drive east 25 miles on CA 4 (toward Martinez), then take Exit 26A onto Somersville Road South. Drive south 2 miles on Somersville Road into the park, continue another mile to the entrance kiosk, and then drive a little less than 1 more mile to the parking lot at the end of the road.

Black Diamond Mines Regional Preserve

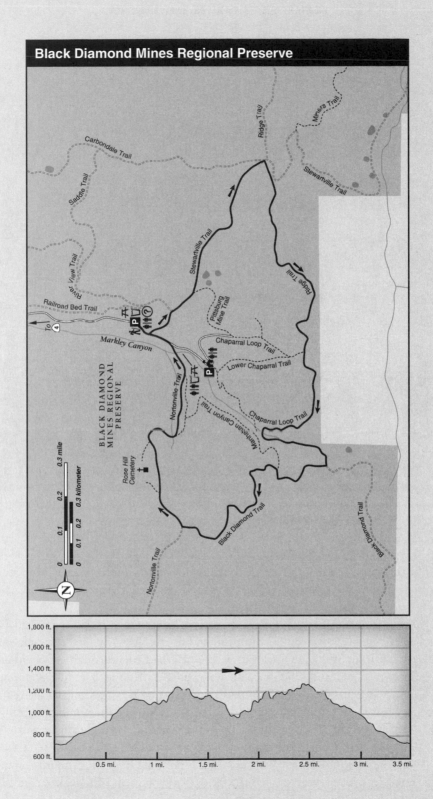

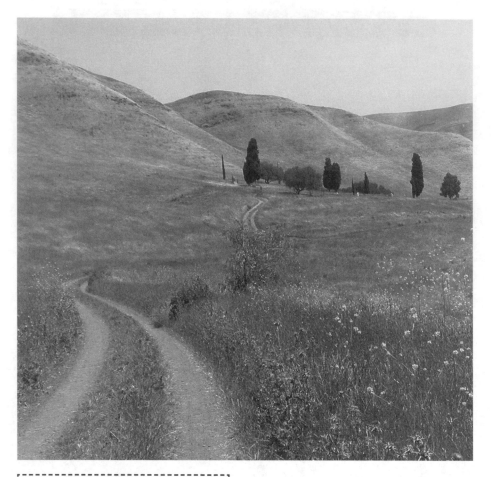

Nortonville Trail descends through grassland.

Although almost all the mine shafts, portals, and tunnels are shuttered, 200 feet of Prospect Tunnel are open for exploration, and the park's visitor center occupies the original opening to the sand mine.

Begin from the parking lot on the paved Nortonville Trail. The broad fire road ascends gently toward the visitor center, but after just 220 feet, turn left onto Stewartville Trail. Still gaining elevation, the fire road cuts through grassland and then reaches a gate and junction with Railroad Bed Trail at 0.1 mile. Continue straight on Stewartville Trail. The trees that tower above the trail here—tree of heaven, black locust, and pepper tree—were planted during the mining era. At 0.2 mile, Pittsburg Mine Trail begins on the right. Continue straight on Stewartville Trail. A long, steady climb begins, through grassland where you might see fiddle-necks and lupines in March. The trail crests at 0.6 mile, reaching a multiple junction. Look back to the west for views of the park's prominent bald peak, 1,506-foot Rose Hill. Turn right onto Ridge Trail.

Off in the distance to the southwest, you'll get a peek at the top of Mount Diablo. At a nearly level grade, the trail skirts a knoll on the left. Buckeye and blue oak sprawl through grassland along the trail—this is a good spot for wildflowers all spring long. Early in the season, smatterings of shooting stars, blue-dicks, lupines, and buttercups are common, but an even better display occurs in late April, when Ithuriel's spear, owl's clover, and big, cheerful California dandelions heavily freckle the grassland like rainbow sprinkles. Sticking downslope from the ridgeline, the trail rises a bit steeply into a dramatically different landscape of manzanita, Coulter pine, yerba santa, and sagebrush. At 1.1 miles, the trail crests at a little bare spot on the left—a wonderful place for a break, offering good views of Mount Diablo and Black Diamond's valley, downhill to the left. On a mid-May hike here, I admired a bountiful display of gorgeous mariposa lilies mixed through paintbrush. Ridge Trail begins to descend, enclosed by thick stands of chaparral. When the trail bends left, views open up to the north, encompassing rock forma-tions in the foreground and Antioch in the distance. Quite a few bush poppy shrubs are mixed through chamise and manzanita—look for bush poppy's bold yellow flowers in spring. Ridge Trail descends somewhat steeply over slippery bare sandstone, then ends at a junction at 1.4 miles. Lower Chaparral Trail sets off to the right, skirting a rock formation on the way downhill toward the visitor-center area. Continue straight on Chaparral Loop Trail.

To the west, past a low-slung sandy knoll, a prominent reeflike hill rises, with rocks jutting out at an angle. The trail rises to a power tower, then begins a descent. One long straight stretch is an aromatic alley, with sweet smells wafting from manzanita blossoms (winter), black sage and pitcher sage flowers (spring), and a froth of chamise blooms (summer). A few live oaks mingle with pine and yerba santa as Chaparral Loop Trail drops on steps and some steep grades into Manhattan Canyon. In mid-May, I've seen dozens of fairy lanterns blooming along the trail. Just after a bridge crosses the canyon at 1.7 miles, you'll reach a junction, with the trail to the right closing Chaparral Loop. Turn left, following the sign toward Manhattan Canyon Trail.

After a brief, winding climb through chamise and 6-foot-tall manzanitas, you reach a second junction. Manhattan Canyon Trail, to the right, leads downhill back toward the trailhead. The trail straight ahead is a connector to Black Dia-mond Trail. Turn left onto Manhattan Canyon Trail.

On a slope just uphill from the canyon floor, the narrow trail ascends through live oaks, pine, sticky monkeyflower, toyon, and manzanita. Somewhat abruptly, the canyon widens into a grassy bowl near the park boundary. Blue oaks dot the hill-sides as Manhattan Canyon Trail veers right and climbs steeply, ending at a junction with Black Diamond Trail at 2 miles. A bench to the right just before the junction is a good place to catch your breath. Turn right onto Black Diamond Trail.

Trailside vegetation is a mixture of grassland, pine, manzanita, and blue and live oak. Look off to the right for views back to Chaparral Loop and Ridge Trails. After a brief level interlude, the fire road begins to descend easily into chaparral, where you might see ceanothus, black sage, yerba santa, chamise, and pitcher sage. At 2.2 miles, the connector to Manhattan Canyon Trail departs on the right. Continue straight on Black Diamond Trail, ascending at a moderate grade back into grassland. On the far side of a cattle gate beneath a power tower, there are sweeping views to Stewartville Trail. By mid-May, the tips of high hills rising up to the northeast begin to fade from green to dull brown, drained of color. In early spring, shooting stars bloom in staggering numbers along the trail, in the grassy breaks between clusters of blue and live oaks. Black Diamond Trail begins to descend easily, offering views northwest to Suisun Bay on clear days. At 2.8 miles, Black Diamond Trail ends at a junction with Nortonville Trail. Turn right.

Nortonville Trail loses elevation at a moderate grade, dropping along the side of a sloping valley to the right of Rose Hill. Owl's clover is common in the short grass of early spring, but by mid-May billowing mustard plants and thistles take over. You may see and hear red-winged blackbirds in this part of the park.

At 2.9 miles, a path departs on the left, leading to Rose Hill Cemetery, the final resting place for some of the residents of the mining era. This is an optional detour—a path returns to Nortonville Trail less than 0.1 mile downhill. Nortonville Trail sweeps right and begins a return to the main park area with tree of heaven lining the route. At 3.2 and 3.4 miles, two forks of Manhattan Canyon Trail depart on the right. Continue straight on Nortonville Trail to a junction at 3.5 miles. Turn right here if you'd like to tour the visitor center (open weekends). Otherwise, turn left and follow Nortonville Trail another 0.1 mile back to the parking lot.

BRIONES REGIONAL PARK

IN BRIEF

This hike reminds me of Goldilocks and the Three Bears: It's not too long and not too hard, but just about right for most people. Briones is a happy combination of soft, rolling hills; grassy valleys dotted with oaks; seasonal lagoons; and tree-lined creeks. Visiting the heart of the park, this loop climbs along an old ranch road to a viewpoint and then descends past black oaks on the way back to the trailhead.

DESCRIPTION

How can a park with so many cows have so many flowers? The meeting of lush flora and hungry bovids seems a contradiction, but it somehow works at Briones, home to one of the best spring wildflower displays in the Bay Area. I also love the park in autumn, when the tall and tawny-colored grass is complemented by a riot of orange black-oak leaves. Is there a bad time to visit? Not really, although the trails do get muddy after a typical winter storm's deluge.

Start from the parking area on Old Briones Road, initially a paved route. Along the

Directions ──────────────▶

Depart San Francisco on the Bay Bridge and use the toll plaza as your mileage starting point. About 0.5 mile past the toll plaza, bear right onto I-580 East. Drive 1.5 miles, then take Exit 19B onto CA 24. Drive 7 miles east on CA 24, then take Exit 9 at Moraga/Orinda. Turn left and drive north on Camino Pablo Road for about 2 miles, then turn right onto Bear Creek Road. Drive on Bear Creek about 4.4 miles to the park entrance on the right side of the road. After passing the entrance kiosk, continue straight to the parking lot.

KEY AT-A-GLANCE INFORMATION

LENGTH: 4.4 miles

CONFIGURATION: Balloon

DIFFICULTY: Easy

SCENERY: Grassland

EXPOSURE: Full sun

TRAFFIC: Moderate

TRAIL SURFACE: Dirt fire roads

HIKING TIME: 2.5 hours

SEASON: Opens daily at 8 a.m.; closing hours vary (see Contacts, below). Late winter and spring are best.

ACCESS: Pay $5 fee at entrance station.

MAPS: At the trailhead's information signboard and ebparks.org/parks /maps

FACILITIES: Pit toilets at trailhead

SPECIAL COMMENTS: Dogs welcome ($2 fee)

CONTACTS: 888-327-2757, ebparks .org/parks/briones

DRIVING DISTANCE: 16.4 miles from the Bay Bridge toll plaza

GPS INFORMATION

N37° 55.627' W122° 9.350'

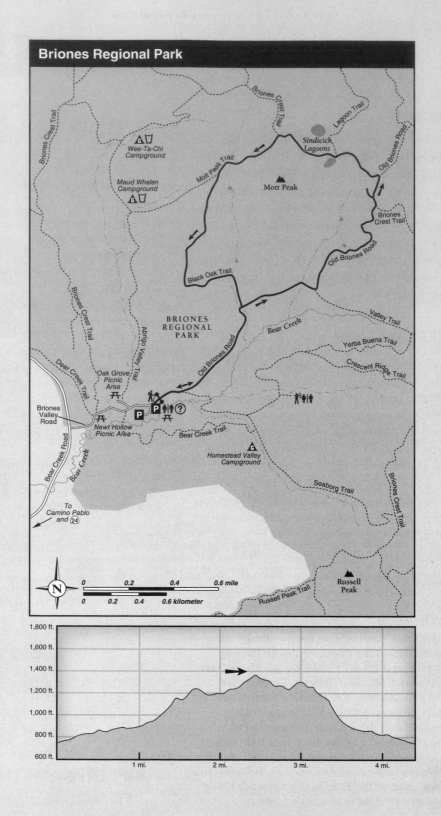

Briones Regional Park

Briones Crest Trail

Wee-Ta-Chi Campground

Maud Whalen Campground

Mott Peak Trail

Mott Peak

Sindicich Lagoons

Lagoon Trail

Old Briones Road

Briones Crest Trail

Black Oak Trail

Old Briones Road

BRIONES REGIONAL PARK

Abrigo Valley Trail

Old Briones Road

Bear Creek

Valley Trail

Yerba Buena Trail

Crescent Ridge Trail

Deer Creek Trail

Oak Grove Picnic Area

Briones Valley Road

Newt Hollow Picnic Area

Bear Creek Trail

Bear Creek Road

Bear Creek

Homestead Valley Campground

Seaborg Trail

Briones Crest Trail

To Camino Pablo and (24)

0   0.2   0.4   0.6 mile

0   0.2   0.4   0.6 kilometer

N

Russell Peak Trail

Russell Peak

1,800 ft.
1,600 ft.
1,400 ft.
1,200 ft.
1,000 ft.
800 ft.
600 ft.

1 mi.   2 mi.   3 mi.   4 mi.

flat, wide trail, the vegetation is an ordinary mix of young coast live oak, blue elderberry, and coyote brush. At 0.2 mile, Homestead Valley Trail breaks off to the right. Continue straight on Old Briones Road, now pavement-free. Once through a gate, you'll enter cattle range, skirting a hill on the left. On one hike, I noticed a little cow figurine nestled in the grass along the trail—a homage or an ironic statement? Either way, it made me laugh. The trail rises slightly, following a creek bed on the right into a little shaded woodland of California bay and coast live, valley, and black oak. Great yellow drifts of California buttercups sprawl beneath the trees in early spring.

Black Oak Trail sets off uphill on the left at 0.7 mile. This trail is your return route, much more steeply pitched than easy Old Briones Road, so continue straight. A grassy valley on the left gently rises toward Briones's highest peaks. You'll pass a corral as the trail sticks to an easy grade, but Old Briones Road begins to climb just past a junction with Valley Trail on the right, at 1.1 miles.

You might find a variety of flowers along the trail in late winter and spring, with buttercups often the first to bloom, blazing the way for fiddle-necks, lupines, California poppies, and blue-dicks. Buckeye and California bay are common, particularly in the damp creases of the hillsides. Old Briones Road climbs at an easy grade, offering pretty views down into the valley and up to grassy hills on the left. At 1.7 miles, the trail approaches a junction, fence, and crest. Just before a gate, veer left on a slight path, and walk uphill a few yards to a bench.

This bench is perhaps the perfect lunch destination if you're alone or with one other person (no one volunteers to sit on the grass in a cow-grazed park). There are 360-degree views of the park and the surrounding area, including Mount Diablo to the southeast. In late April and early May, the hillsides just downslope from the bench show off dense, colorful patches of creamcups, California poppy, and lupine. If the flowers aren't blooming, you could easily while away some time watching hawks and kestrels soaring over the valley below.

When you're ready, walk back down the path, then turn left, pass through the gate, and make another left. After a few steps the trails fork again, this time at one end of a big triangular junction. Stay to the left, on Briones Crest Trail. At a level grade, the wide fire road skirts a knoll on the left. You might notice small ponds downhill on the right—those are the Maricich Lagoons, important sources of water for the park's birds, mammals, and newts. Buttercups bloom like crazy along Briones Crest Trail in April, tinting entire hillsides lemon yellow. A cluster of coast live oaks lines the right side of the trail, interrupting the sea of grass.

Lagoon Trail begins on the right at 2.1 miles, across from one of the Sindicich Lagoons. Continue straight on Briones Crest Trail. As the trail ascends easily, good views open up downhill, to the right of another lagoon. When it's full and the sun is shining, the water makes a nice mirror, reflecting puffy white clouds drifting across the bluest skies. At 2.4 miles, Briones Crest Trail continues off to the right. Turn left onto Mott Peak Trail. After a short ascent, the fire road crests and begins to descend, skirting its namesake peak through grassland with a few

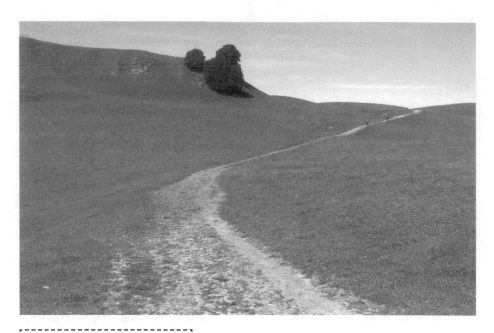

An easy ascent on Briones Crest Trail

lonely oaks sprinkled here and there. On spring hikes in this part of the park, I've seen orange patches of California poppy that were so vivid and colorful I wondered if Mother Nature played paintball. Fiddle-necks are a late-winter fixture along the trail.

Where Mott Peak Trail reaches a junction at 2.7 miles, veer left onto Black Oak Trail. Black Oak Trail roller-coasters along the ridgeline past displays of blue and white lupine. Up close in late winter's short green grass, the blooms really pop, but from a distance they make the hillsides look bruised. Black Oak bends left as the descent sharpens. In the driest months of the year, loose stones on the trail can make the descent a bit scary. I've taken the steepest section in a zigzag pattern more than once to keep from sliding. The trail runs between a beautiful oak forest on the right and a sloping, grassy hillside on the left, where a few buckeyes line a creek bed. Although they blend into the woods in spring and summer, the trail's namesake trees are easy to pick out in autumn when their leaves turn orange. Black Oak levels out on the valley floor, then ends at 3.7 miles at Old Briones Road. Turn right and retrace your steps back to the trailhead.   •

COYOTE HILLS REGIONAL PARK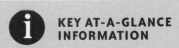

IN BRIEF

A number of parks perch on the shores of San Francisco Bay, but Coyote Hills is the whole enchilada: excellent wildlife-viewing, extensive facilities, and trails that explore not only marsh and coastline but grassland as well. You can choose a very easy hike through Coyote Hill's marsh, or stretch your legs a bit on a few short but steep paths that roller-coaster up and down grassy hills fronting the bay. This 5-mile loop does both, starting in the marsh and then traversing the hills.

DESCRIPTION

Coyote Hills is a small collection of grassy, rolling knolls rising above the bay just north of Dumbarton Bridge. The Ohlone, original inhabitants of the Bay Area who settled here more than 10,000 years ago, found this area particularly bountiful, leaving a shell mound and other historical artifacts in the marsh. The park is very popular with kids, who tour Coyote Hills on school trips guided by park staff or visit on weekends for family bird-watching. Because Coyote Hills offers many flat trails

Directions ⟶

Depart San Francisco southbound on US 101 and use the 101/I-280 split as your mileage starting point. Drive south 25 miles on US 101, then take Exit 406, CA 84 East/Dumbarton Bridge. Follow CA 84 for about 7 miles, to the eastern end of the Dumbarton Bridge, then take Exit 36 onto Paseo Padre Parkway/ Thornton Avenue (this is the first exit after the toll plaza). Turn left and drive north on Paseo Padre about 1 mile, then turn left onto Patterson Ranch Road. Drive about 1.5 miles, past the entrance kiosk and Quarry Staging Area, to the trailhead at the end of the road (near the visitor center).

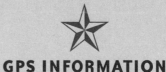

GPS INFORMATION

N37° 33.221' W122° 5.418'

8000 Patterson Ranch Rd.
Fremont, CA 94555

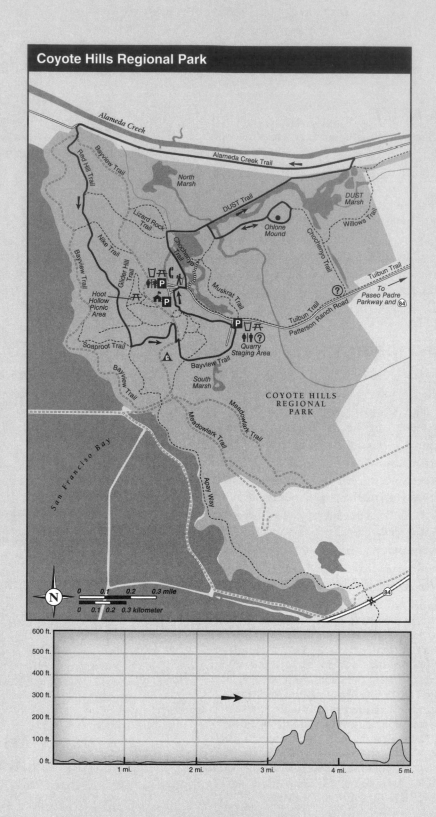

Coyote Hills Regional Park

and is a short drive from communities around Fremont, locals use the park for daily exercise. The steady foot traffic seems not to bother the park's wildlife—I've seen a fox, jackrabbits, and many birds here.

If the visitor center is open, take a quick prehike tour through exhibits highlighting Ohlone settlements and native flora and fauna. Then walk back to the parking area and cross the street to a multiple trail junction at the edge of the marsh. Bayview Trail, on the right, runs along the road back toward the park entrance. A boardwalk and Chochenyo Trail split off straight ahead into the marsh. If the marsh is relatively dry, the boardwalk can be substituted for Chochenyo's dirt path, but I've seen the boardwalk completely flooded. These two trails form a triangle, so either route is suitable to begin the hike.

Initially, the wide and flat Chochenyo Trail bisects two pools lined with cattails and reeds. After just 0.2 mile, two paths head off to the left toward Lizard Rock, and Chochenyo bends right. Continue following Chochenyo to a junction with Demonstration Urban Stormwater Treatment (DUST) Trail at 0.4 mile; then turn right for a short side trip to a shell mound, still on Chochenyo.

Dock, pickleweed, and New Zealand spinach thrive along the trail, along with thick stands of marsh plants that mostly block water views. Even if you can't see them, ducks and waterfowl may be heard splashing. Another fork comes at 0.5 mile—bear left here or you'll end up back at the trailhead. Chochenyo Trail proceeds at a level grade to a junction at 0.7 mile. At this fork, bear left.

Fences guard the shell mound on the right. This former Ohlone village site is being restored and is usually closed to the public, although naturalist-led tours can be arranged and the park often hosts shell-mound "open houses." Unless you're visiting on one of those days, you'll have to peer through the fence for a look at the historical area. Chochenyo Trail continues to the left at 0.8 mile, departing from the shell-mound area to Tuibin Trail. Because there is no direct route that connects back to DUST Trail, follow the other end of the loop to the right, back around the shell-mound site, then retrace your steps back to the junction with Chochenyo and DUST Trails at 1.3 miles. Turn right onto DUST Trail.

The marsh surrounding DUST Trail was engineered to filter polluted storm runoff before it reaches the bay. A bonus benefit is that the marsh provides wildlife habitat for ducks, geese, and more "wild" birds like herons and egrets. Plants on the side of DUST Trail range from wispy mustard, poison hemlock, and wild radish to sturdy bushes of poison oak. In summer after the plant blossoms have dried out, you might see scores of tiny birds such as bushtits and goldfinches feeding on seeds of all these plants. After a long straight stretch, DUST Trail gently curves right (a very short unnamed spur heads off to the left) as the flatlands of Fremont stretch east to a series of low, rolling hills. Where DUST Trail ends at 2 miles, turn left onto Alameda Creek Trail.

This flat, wide, paved levee trail runs along the shore of the East Bay's longest creek as it makes its way to the bay. Although the creek is really a less-than-natural managed flood channel here, Canada geese are common in and around

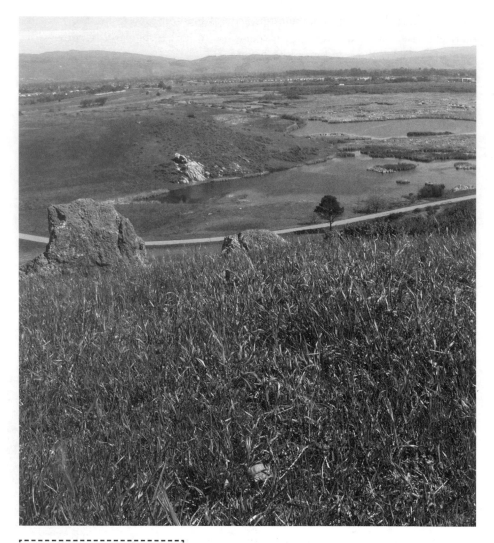

A view of the marsh from Red Hill

the creek and in the skies above the channel, and you might see birds of prey including harriers, hawks, and kestrels. A cluster of eucalyptus trees on the left punctuates the landscape and provides a little oasis of shade. Pickleweed, a ground cover often found in marshes, draws attention to itself in autumn, when it flushes a rusty red. At the hike's 3.1-mile mark, just past an Alameda Creek interpretive display, you'll reach a junction. Bear left, cross the paved Bayview Trail, and start uphill on Red Hill Trail.

Climbing moderately through grassland, the trail quickly crests. In March, orange California poppies contrast nicely with vivid green grass and blue sky—an eye-popping late-winter color palette. A steep descent commences, and at 3.6 miles Nike Trail crosses Red Hill Trail. Continue straight on Red Hill Trail.

After another sharp climb you'll reach the park's highest elevation, a mere 291 feet, where big boulders of crimson chert jut up from the grassland. Beware of poison oak nestled among the outcrops. Red Hill Trail descends slightly to a level saddle, where a barely noticeable path, Glider Hill Trail, heads downhill to the left. Proceed uphill on Red Hill Trail to yet another beautiful view, this one located on top of Glider Hill. True to its name, the hill is a good place to fly a kite or model airplane; for those without such accessories, the wind can detract from a hilltop rest break. On clear days, you can enjoy views of the Bay, Dumbarton Bridge, Mission Peak, the Santa Cruz Mountains, and Mount Diablo. As Red Hill Trail steeply descends one last time, look for jackrabbits bounding through the grass and hawks hunting overhead. At 4.1 miles, you'll reach a T-junction; turn left onto Soaproot Trail.

As the trail descends easily, look for the trail's namesake plant along the path. Soaproot has long, wavy leaves and narrow stalks that resemble asparagus (both soaproot and asparagus are members of the lily family). Ohlones dug soaproot bulbs and used them not only to make soap but to stupefy fish for easy gathering. The plant blooms May–June, but its blossoms don't open until late in the afternoon. After a sharp curve right, Soaproot Trail ends at 4.4 miles. Turn right onto Bayview Trail.

Paved Bayview Trail sweeps past Dairy Glen, a group campsite at right. Just before South Marsh, another path continues straight while Bayview Trail bends left and runs parallel to the marsh. Stay on Bayview, skirting a rocky hill on the left, then reach the fringes of Quarry Staging Area. There are a few well-worn shortcuts, but continue on Bayview almost all the way to the park road at 4.8 miles; then turn left, cross the parking lot, and head uphill on signed Muskrat Trail.

Poison oak, sagebrush, coyote brush, sticky monkeyflower, and toyon mix with grass along the narrow trail. Bush lupine is a pretty accompaniment in spring, when its sweet-smelling, purple-blue flowers emerge. Near a rock outcrop, a path (not shown on the map) doubles back to the left, but Muskrat continues straight. Veer right in front of a massive boulder, then begin a descent, with one last opportunity to gaze at the marsh as the trail drops down a set of steps. In March, you might see shooting stars in bloom on the sides of the trail. At 5 miles, the path ends within steps of the parking lot.

24 HUCKLEBERRY BOTANIC REGIONAL PRESERVE

KEY AT-A-GLANCE INFORMATION

LENGTH: 1.7 miles

CONFIGURATION: Loop

DIFFICULTY: Easy

SCENERY: Mixed woodland and chaparral

EXPOSURE: Mostly shaded

TRAFFIC: Light

TRAIL SURFACE: Narrow dirt trails

HIKING TIME: 1 hour

SEASON: Daily, 5 a.m.–sunset. Winter is best for blooming manzanitas, but any time of year is good.

ACCESS: Free

MAPS: At the trailhead's information signboard and ebparks.org/parks/maps

FACILITIES: Pit toilets at trailhead

SPECIAL COMMENTS: No dogs allowed. Learn more about Bay Area plants at the East Bay Regional Parks Botanic Garden, at Wildcat Canyon Road and South Park Drive, in Tilden Park, Berkeley. The garden is open daily except January 1, Thanksgiving, and December 25. Visit ebparks.org/parks/tilden/botanic_garden for more information.

CONTACTS: 888-327-2757, ebparks.org/parks/huckleberry

DRIVING DISTANCE: 11.5 miles from the Bay Bridge toll plaza

GPS INFORMATION

N37° 50.560' W122° 11.705'

IN BRIEF

The most visible of the East Bay's open spaces is dominated by rolling grassland, but Huckleberry Botanic Regional Preserve, in the hills above Oakland, offers a tour through a variety of vegetation, including chaparral and woods. Along this short and easy 1.7-mile loop, numbered posts and a free brochure guide hikers through a wide assortment of plants, some of which are uncommon in the area.

DESCRIPTION

This small preserve sits on an unusual deposit of shale and chert—"poor" soil that's well suited to native plants. Although surrounding neighborhoods feature grassland, forests of eucalyptus, and redwood-crammed canyons, Huckleberry is a little oasis of manzanita barrens, scads of huckleberry bushes, and a gorgeous woodland of madrone, California bay, ferns, coast live oak, hazelnut, and currant. This is an arboretum-quality collection with an ever-changing palette of colors, textures, and tastes.

Directions

Depart San Francisco on the Bay Bridge and use the toll plaza as your mileage starting point. About 0.5 mile past the toll plaza, bear right onto I-580 East. Drive 1.5 miles, then take Exit 19B onto CA 24. Drive east on CA 24 about 5 miles, and at the far side of the Caldecott Tunnel, take Exit 7A onto Fish Ranch Road, the first post-tunnel exit—stay in the right lane. Drive north on Fish Ranch Road about 1 mile, then turn left onto Grizzly Peak Boulevard. Drive 2.4 miles, then turn left onto Skyline Boulevard. Drive 0.6 mile on Skyline, then turn left into the preserve parking lot.

Huckleberry Botanic Regional Preserve

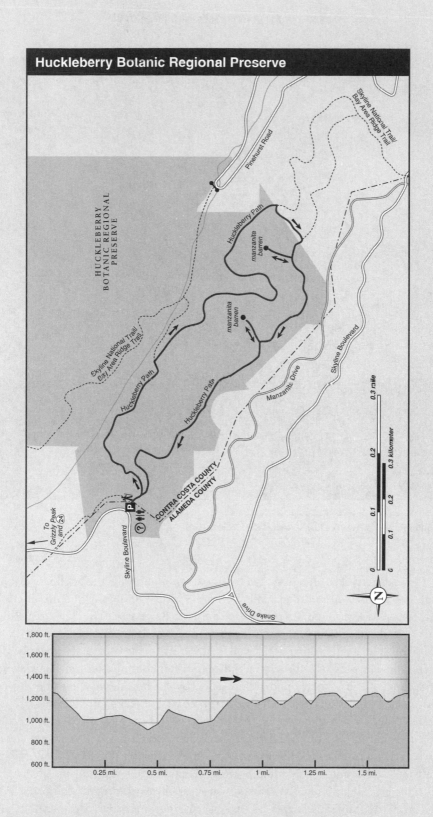

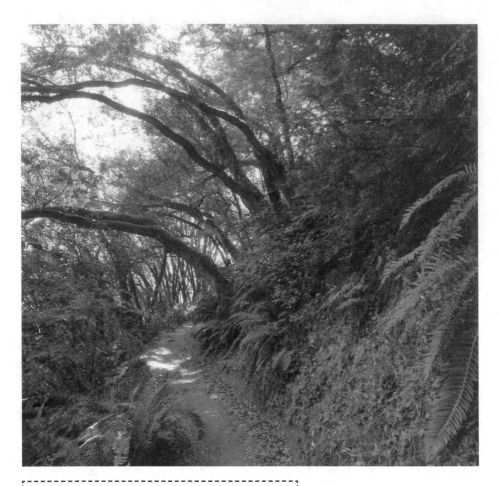

California bays arch over a lush stretch of Huckleberry Path.

Huckleberry Preserve hosts two segments of long trails: the Skyline National Trail and the Bay Area Ridge Trail. Skyline National Trail is a 31-mile multiuse path that passes through a string of six big East Bay parks. The Bay Area Ridge Trail extends more than 300 miles through nine Bay Area counties.

From the small staging area, walk a few feet to the information signboard, where you can pick up a brochure and map, then continue on the Huckleberry Path. Tangles of blackberry and creambush crowd a hillside on the right, but the trail quickly enters an area well-shaded by coast live oaks and California bays. After 200 feet, where the two legs of the loop split, bear left. A few short zigzags drop the trail into a cool, shaded canyon, where you'll make a slow and steady descent. Look for the first numbered post of the tour on the right, identifying a madrone. At 0.3 mile, the Skyline National Trail on the left heads out of the pre-serve toward Sibley Volcanic Preserve. Veer uphill to the right. California bays arch over the trail as it begins an easy ascent. The tour identifies hazelnut and sword and wood fern. A tiny-leaved, sweet-smelling plant called yerba buena hugs the ground in several places. The vegetation shifts subtly to include more coast live oak. In a few exposed areas, sticky monkeyflower and California coffeeberry bask in the sunlight.

At 0.9 mile, the Skyline Trail continues straight, while the Huckleberry Path bears right. (You can extend this hike by taking Skyline another 0.4 mile, then picking up an extension of the Huckleberry Path.) Climb to the right on Huckleberry Path. A few sets of steep stairs quickly ascend through California bay and coast-live-oak woods to a junction at 1 mile. Walk a few feet to the right, then turn right, following the sign labeled TO 6. The path ascends easily out of the woods to a sunny manzanita barren. On a clear day, views stretch to include Mount Diablo to the east. If you happen to be visiting during the manzanita bloom (generally December–February), hummingbirds and bees are common, gorging themselves on the sweet nectar from the manzanitas' small white flowers. Return to the previous junction, then turn right.

The preserve's namesake, huckleberry, dominates the trail, which winds through the towering mazelike hedges of the evergreen shrub. In August, huckleberry plants are crammed with small, dusky, blueberry-like fruit, a favorite for local birds and even coyotes, who feed from the lower branches. At 1.3 miles, bear right to another manzanita barren, where the brochure assists you in identifying canyon live oak. Retrace your steps back to the main path, then turn right. Chinquapin and silk-tassel accompany manzanita and huckleberry as the trail continues at a nearly level grade. Douglas iris blooms in clusters along the trail in spring.

At 1.7 miles, you'll return to the hike's first junction and the end of the loop. Continue straight and return to the trailhead, retracing your steps on the Huckleberry Path.

25 LAS TRAMPAS REGIONAL WILDERNESS

KEY AT-A-GLANCE INFORMATION

LENGTH: 4.6 miles

CONFIGURATION: Loop

DIFFICULTY: Moderate

SCENERY: Grassland, woods, rock formations

EXPOSURE: Nearly equal parts shaded and exposed

TRAFFIC: Light–moderate

TRAIL SURFACE: Dirt fire roads, trails, and 1 paved fire road

HIKING TIME: 2.5 hours

SEASON: Opens daily at 8 a.m.; closing hours vary (see Contacts, below). Best in spring; muddy in winter, hot in summer.

ACCESS: Free

MAPS: At the trailhead's information signboard and ebparks.org/parks/maps

FACILITIES: Pit toilets at trailhead

SPECIAL COMMENTS: Although Las Trampas is designated as a regional wilderness, the western part of the park has some decidedly domestic inhabitants: cattle, which create muddy conditions during the rainy season. If the described trails are muddy—you'll know right away— the park's eastern section (ungrazed) provides good alternative hiking.

CONTACTS: 888-327-2757, ebparks .org/parks/las_trampas

DRIVING DISTANCE: 31.8 miles from the Bay Bridge toll plaza

GPS INFORMATION

N37° 48.952' W122° 3.005'

IN BRIEF

Las Trampas (Spanish for "the traps") is like two parks in one: From the trailhead, at the bottom of a wide canyon, you can hike east to chaparral-coated Las Trampas Ridge or west to grassy Rocky Ridge. Pick this western loop in spring, after the rains have stopped, for a steady climb to Rocky Ridge, where you can enjoy sweeping views and search for wildflowers.

DESCRIPTION

Begin from the parking lot. The paved fire road is the return route—pass through a metal gate, then a cattle gate onto Elderberry Trail (which may be unsigned), to the left of the paved fire road. At a level grade, the wide trail sweeps across the grassy base of Rocky Ridge, dips to cross a seasonal creek, then runs along a corral on the left. At 0.4 mile, you'll reach a junction with a spur leading left to Bollinger Canyon Road. Turn right to remain on Elderberry Trail.

After such an easygoing intro, the subsequent climb is a bit of a shock—the trail shoots uphill, initially through a woodland of California bay, coast live oaks, and black oaks. Even when Elderberry Trail steps out into grassland, there's still no relief from the sharp

- -

Directions ———————————————→

Depart San Francisco on the Bay Bridge and use the toll plaza as your mileage starting point. About 0.5 mile past the toll plaza, bear right onto I-580 East. Drive 1.5 miles, then take Exit 19B onto CA 24. Drive east 12 miles on CA 24, then take Exit 15A south onto I-680. Drive south 10 miles and take Exit 36 onto Crow Canyon Road. Drive west (right) for about 1 mile, then turn right (north) onto Bollinger Canyon Road. Continue about 4.5 miles to the trailhead, at the end of the road.

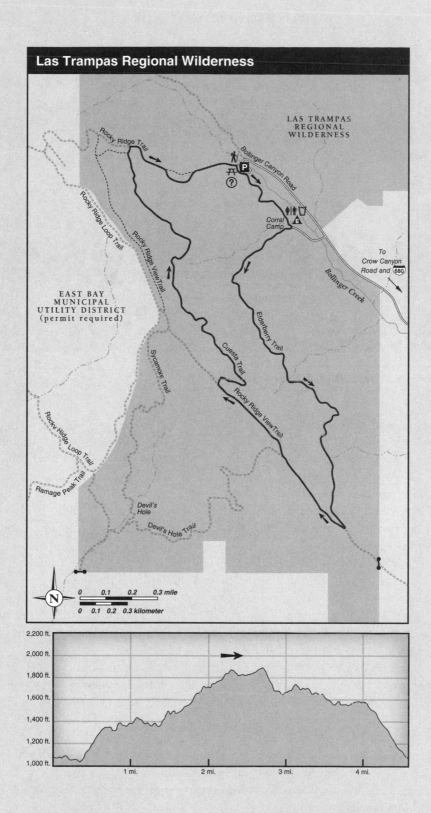

Las Trampas Regional Wilderness

LAS TRAMPAS
REGIONAL
WILDERNESS

Rocky Ridge Trail

Bollinger Canyon Road

Rocky Ridge Loop Trail

Rocky Ridge View Trail

Corral Camp

To
Crow Canyon
Road and 680

Bollinger Creek

EAST BAY
MUNICIPAL
UTILITY DISTRICT
(permit required)

Cuesta Trail

Elderberry Trail

Rocky Ridge View Trail

Sycamore Trail

Rocky Ridge Loop Trail

Ramage Peak Trail

Devil's
Hole

Devil's Hole Trail

0   0.1   0.2   0.3 mile
0   0.1 0.2 0.3 kilometer

N

2,200 ft.
2,000 ft.
1,800 ft.
1,600 ft.
1,400 ft.
1,200 ft.
1,000 ft.

1 mi.   2 mi.   3 mi.   4 mi.

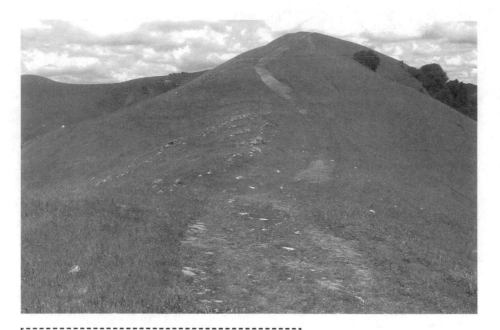

Rocky Ridge View Trail Trail climbs along its namesake ridge.

grade, which feels especially harsh in summer's heat. As you ascend, there are nice views uphill toward the ridgetop and across Bollinger Canyon to Las Trampas Ridge. The grade tapers off, and then the trail begins a campaign of brief rolling ups and downs. Paintbrush and California poppy are common in spring, blooming in sunny stretches of sagebrush and poison oak. In March, you might catch a few old fruit trees cloaked in a froth of fragrant flowers, gooseberry bushes in bloom, and buds on maple trees unfurling. Look for newts on the trail after heavy rains in winter or early spring.

Leaving the woods behind, Elderberry Trail's last stretch is a moderately steep ascent through grassland to the ridge. In mid-March the slope on the right is a kaleidoscope of flowers, including ivory-colored creamcups, purple filarees, and orange California poppies and fiddle-necks. At 1.8 miles, Elderberry Trail ends at a junction with Rocky Ridge View Trail. The segment to the left ends at the park boundary after less than 0.5 mile. Turn right.

Rocky Ridge View Trail clings to the ridgeline, ascending in fits and starts at a steep grade through grassland. Wonderful views unfold with every step uphill to Mount Diablo in the east and west all the way to the Golden Gate Bridge on clear days. Cattle seem to love this ridge, and you'll often see lots of cows hanging out up here. On a hike in March one year, I watched an unidentifiable animal running at a fast pace, back and forth on a hillside across the canyon to the left. It was too dark for a coyote, lacked the long tail of a mountain lion, but had a longer tail than a bobcat. What was this mysterious creature? I'll never know, as I forgot my binoculars that day.

Be sure to stop and examine the rock formations along the trail—the seashells are easy to pick out in these remnants of the Orinda Formation. It's hard to believe that this ridge, about 30 miles east of the Pacific, originated under the ocean. At 2.2 miles, Devil's Hole Trail departs to the left, looping through the remote part of the park where I saw that mysterious animal. Continue straight. On a breezy day the howling wind is absolutely deafening, but on a hot day you might wish for a little airflow. Rocky Ridge View Trail drops a bit off the ridgeline, then reaches a junction at 2.6 miles. Turn right onto Cuesta Trail.

This little path descends moderately through coyote brush, makes a sharp turn left, then levels out a bit, while maintaining a general downhill trend. Like Elderberry Trail, Cuesta Trail has a fair amount of elevation wobble, but it's nothing dramatic. Sheltered from the bulk of the ridge, this is an excellent wildflower trail, despite the best efforts of the park's substantial cow population. In late winter, milkmaids, shooting stars, and buttercups are common; in mid-March, mule ear sunflowers bloom along with California poppies, creamcups, and loads of purple bush lupine, all nicely accented against the green grassland. Some small pockets of California bay nestle in the crooks of the hillsides, but otherwise the descent is under full sun. Near the 4-mile mark, Cuesta Trail ends at a junction with a paved fire road, Rocky Ridge View Trail. Turn right. (A dirt path across the road is also an option—both lead back to the trailhead.)

The descent, moderately steep and steady, is a popular out-and-back route for locals walking with their dogs. Coast live oaks overtake the grassland as the trail winds downhill. After winter rains, you may hear and see small rivulets of water draining off the mountain toward Bollinger Creek, downhill to the left. At 4.6 miles, Rocky Ridge View Trail ends at a gate back at the parking lot.

NEARBY ACTIVITIES

With herds of cattle and steady equestrian traffic, most of the park feels a bit like a private ranch, but the wilderness designation rings true in the far western section of Las Trampas and the adjacent property, a massive hunk of land managed by the East Bay Municipal Utility District (EBMUD). You can add 2.5 miles to the hike described above on a loop to Devil's Hole, through a knob of East Bay Regional Park District land on the western slope of Rocky Ridge, neighboring the EBMUD watershed. In the watershed proper, trails are open to hikers by advance permit only. With a permit, a car shuttle, and plenty of water, you could hike through Las Trampas and EBMUD lands to the Chabot Staging Area, a trek of nearly 11 miles. Get more information at **ebmud.com/recreation/east-bay-trails**.

26 LOS VAQUEROS WATERSHED

KEY AT-A-GLANCE INFORMATION

LENGTH: 4.2 miles

CONFIGURATION: Balloon

DIFFICULTY: Moderate

SCENERY: Grassland

EXPOSURE: Full sun

TRAFFIC: Quiet

TRAIL SURFACE: Dirt fire roads

HIKING TIME: 2.5 hours

SEASON: Best in spring—muddy in winter, hot in summer

ACCESS: Pay the $6 fee ($5 seniors, $4 if you live in the Contra Costa Water District) at the entrance station.

MAPS: At the entrance station and tinyurl.com/losvaquerosmap

FACILITIES: Vault toilet at the trailhead

SPECIAL COMMENTS: No dogs allowed. Some trails are closed seasonally to protect nesting golden eagles.

CONTACTS: 925-688-8225, ccwater .com/losvaqueros

DRIVING DISTANCE: 43 miles from the Bay Bridge toll plaza

GPS INFORMATION

N37° 46.375' W121° 44.425'

IN BRIEF

You'll start this hike at the County Line Staging Area and walk uphill on a hiking-only loop through cattle-grazed grassland. From a ridge at the hike's high point, views extend to the reservoir, Mount Diablo, and the suburbs of the San Ramon Valley. Bring binoculars to get a better look at the golden eagles that live in the area and are commonly spotted.

DESCRIPTION

When this Contra Costa watershed first opened to recreational use in 2001, it was an incredibly peaceful place. I expected that when a marina and interpretive center opened, it would be packed with fishermen and everyone else in the area looking for a nice picnic spot, but Los Vaqueros is still a very quiet park, particularly the southern area, where trails are open only to hikers. I don't know if it's because of the watershed's steep admission fee or if hikers don't know about this recreation area, but these trails are lonely.

The northern trailhead, Walnut Staging Area, has the denser network of multiuse trails and the watershed's interpretive center. The southern trailhead, County Line Staging Area,

---

Directions ⟶

Depart San Francisco on the Bay Bridge and use the toll plaza as your mileage starting point. About 0.5 mile past the toll plaza, bear right onto I-580 East. Drive about 16 miles south and at the CA 238 split, stay to the left on I-580. Continue east about 21 miles, then take Exit 55 at Vasco Road. Turn left and drive north about 5 miles, then turn left onto Los Vaqueros Road (look for a small brown watershed sign) and continue to the County Line Staging Area, just past the entrance station.

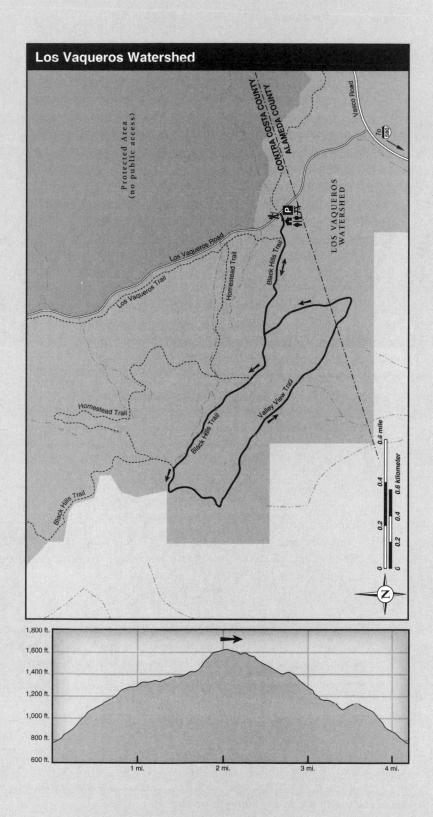

Los Vaqueros Watershed

Protected Area
(no public access)

CONTRA COSTA COUNTY
ALAMEDA COUNTY

Vasco Road

To 580

LOS VAQUEROS
WATERSHED

Los Vaqueros Road

Los Vaqueros Trail

Homestead Trail

Black Hills Trail

Homestead Trail

Black Hills Trail

Black Hills Trail

Valley View Trail

0.2 mile

0.4

0.6 kilometer

0.2   0.4

0   0

1,800 ft.
1,600 ft.
1,400 ft.
1,200 ft.
1,000 ft.
800 ft.
600 ft.

1 mi.   2 mi.   3 mi.   4 mi.

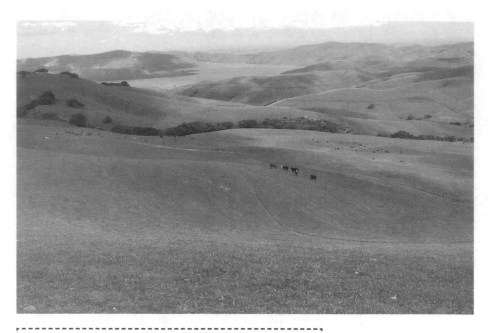

A distant glimpse of Los Vaqueros Reservoir from Valley View Trail

is off the road to the marina. There is no vehicle through-route inside the park from the north to the south.

The trails of Los Vaqueros (which translates from Spanish to "the cowboys") wander through a typical East Bay landscape of oak, grassland, and chaparral foothills. The watershed property abuts two East Bay Regional Park District preserves, Morgan Territory and Round Valley. This 4.1-mile loop barely scratches the surface of the Los Vaqueros watershed, but it is a good introduction, particularly when spring wildflowers flourish on a windy, treeless ridge.

On my first visit to the park in July 2000, I saw golden eagles before I even got out of the car. From mid-February to late June, when eagles nest in the watershed's oaks, some trails are often closed to public use (specific dates and trails change to accommodate the eagles). Spring is the most pleasant time of year at Los Vaqueros, with cool temperatures and a variety of wildflowers, but that's the season when trails are most likely to be closed. If you want a long hike, visit in summer, autumn, or winter, when the connector to Morgan Territory is open. The trails on the hike described below are not subject to closure during golden-eagle nesting.

Begin from the parking lot on Black Hills Trail. In a damp spot on the right, redwing blackbirds sit atop mustard and thistles in spring, and squirrels scamper everywhere. After you pass through a cattle gate and begin climbing on the wide fire road, look for a buckeye and some oaks in a little draw off the trail to the left—this is as close to a tree as you'll get on the entire hike.

The grade is moderately steep, and in summer there's not much to look at along the trail—just an expanse of golden grass rolling uphill to the left and downhill to the right. You may see a few blooming cardoons (thistles related to artichokes) and yellow star thistles in July. At 0.1 mile, Los Vaqueros Trail departs on the right, starting a long, rolling journey along the park road to the marina area. This trail plays a crucial role in longer loops, but unfortunately it's one of the most boring routes in the watershed. Continue uphill on Black Hills Trail.

In spring, lupine, Ithuriel's spear, filaree, and fiddle-neck bloom sparsely in the surrounding grass. As you climb you may come across some of the watershed's cattle. On one hike, I scattered the herds of cattle each time I came across them. Some stepped toward me, perhaps wondering what I was, but all of them ran (I mean *really* ran) out of sight before I got within 50 feet. For those accustomed to the bossy, elitist attitude of bovines at other East Bay parks, these shy cows are a nice contrast.

Valley View Trail, the return route for the loop, begins to the left at 0.6 mile. Continuing straight on Black Hills Trail, the grade slackens as the trail passes two small stock ponds on the right. Here are views north to chaparral-covered hillsides, with oak-dotted knolls in the foreground. At 1.5 miles, Black Hills Trail bends right, heads to a junction with Homestead Trail, then proceeds to the hills above the reservoir in the western part of the watershed, where a trail connects to Morgan Territory. When I visited one spring, Homestead Trail and Black Hills Trail from this junction to Cañada Trail were closed to protect the nesting eagles. Continue straight, now on Valley View Trail. The fire road heads toward Morgan Territory Road but then veers sharply left at 1.8 miles and begins a steep climb. When it's windy (which it seems to be all the time), you'll need to hold on to your hat. Spring brings a few flowers to the trailside grass, including blue-eyed grass, buttercups, and fiddle-necks. The trail crests, turns left, and runs along the ridgeline. Views are expansive, ranging south across the San Ramon Valley to the mountains of Sunol and the Ohlone Wilderness. Northwest, Mount Diablo is visible, and to the northeast you might see the windmills twirling near Altamont Pass.

As you make your way across the rolling ridge, the reservoir comes into view in the heart of the park. With vultures and hawks whipping overhead in the wind, you'll need a quick hand with the binoculars to identify them. Despite the steady winds and the hungry cows, wildflowers are plentiful on the north slope of the ridge in April, including loads of blue-dicks, johnny-jump-ups, California poppies, fiddle-necks, blue and white lupines, Ithuriel's spear, and filaree. Off in the distance to the west, I've seen patches of purple owl's clover bruising lush green hillsides along Morgan Territory Road.

Valley View Trail drops to a dip where a worn cow path heads off to the right. Continue straight, climbing and then descending again. The trail curves left and then leaves the ridgeline. After a steady descent, you'll reach the junction with Black Hills Trail again at 3.5 miles. Turn right and return downhill to the trailhead.

27   MISSION PEAK REGIONAL PRESERVE

KEY AT-A-GLANCE INFORMATION

LENGTH: 6.2 miles

CONFIGURATION: Out-and-back

DIFFICULTY: Strenuous

SCENERY: Grassland, views

EXPOSURE: Almost completely exposed

TRAFFIC: Moderate

TRAIL SURFACE: Dirt fire roads and trail

HIKING TIME: 3 hours

SEASON: Opens daily at 7 a.m.; closing hours vary (see Contacts, below). Spring is pleasant, winter is muddy; avoid during summer heat waves.

ACCESS: $3 parking fee

MAPS: At the trailhead's information signboard and ebparks.org/parks /maps

FACILITIES: Pit toilets at trailhead

SPECIAL COMMENTS: Dogs welcome (no fee).

Mission Peak is the western gateway to the Ohlone Regional Wilderness, a 9,156-acre area that requires an advance permit for entry ($2 if purchased in person, $4 if purchased by mail/phone/web). The Ohlone Trail makes a 28-mile journey through the wilderness, and there are backpacking campsites for hikers making the entire trip. Read more about the wilderness at ebparks.org/parks/ohlone.

CONTACTS: 888-327-2757, ebparks .org/parks/mission

DRIVING DISTANCE: 36 miles from the Bay Bridge toll plaza

GPS INFORMATION

N37° 30.262' W121° 54.500'

IN BRIEF

On this Mission Peak excursion, you'll begin at the edge of a Fremont residential neighborhood, hike up fire roads, then take a little trail straight to the summit—an ascent of more than 2,000 feet. If you've picked a clear day, the 360-degree views are inspiring, but on windy days you may want to immediately head back downhill to the parking lot.

DESCRIPTION

To get to the Mission Peak trailhead, you turn off a heavily trafficked street, drive a half-mile, then boom—you're there, at the base of a mountain. Most mountains require long drives, but heck, you can get to Mission Peak by bus!

Leaving from the parking lot, the fire road skirts a short, wide hill. Peak Meadow Trail departs to the right, but stay to the left on Hidden Valley Trail. The route ahead really stands out in late winter and early spring, when the grass is bright green. After a brief descent, the trail crosses Aqua Caliente Creek, bends left, and begins to climb. Ascending at a sharp grade through grassland, you might catch a glimpse of hang gliders drifting downhill from farther up the mountain. Hidden Valley Trail draws

---

Directions ⟶

Depart San Francisco on the Bay Bridge and use the toll plaza as your mileage starting point. Just past the toll plaza, bear right onto I-880 South. Drive about 33 miles south, then take Exit 12, Warren Avenue/Mission Boulevard. Drive northeast on Mission Boulevard, pass under I-680, and then turn right on Stanford Avenue. Drive about 0.5 mile to the trailhead at the end of the street. Park in the lot, *not* along the side of Stanford Avenue.

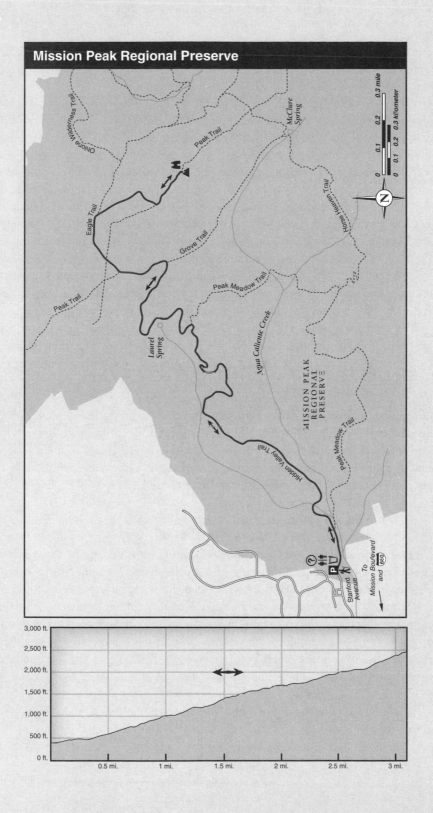

Mission Peak Regional Preserve

Ohlone Wilderness Trail

Peak Trail

McClure Spring

Eagle Trail

Grove Trail

Horse Heaven Trail

Peak Trail

Peak Meadow Trail

Laurel Spring

Agua Caliente Creek

MISSION PEAK REGIONAL PRESERVE

Hidden Valley Trail

Peak Meadow Trail

Stanford Avenue

To Mission Boulevard and 680

0.3 mile
0.1   0.2   0.3 Kilometer
0   0.1   0.2
0

3,000 ft.
2,500 ft.
2,000 ft.
1,500 ft.
1,000 ft.
500 ft.
0 ft.

0.5 mi.   1 mi.   1.5 mi.   2 mi.   2.5 mi.   3 mi.

near a wooded canyon and creek on the left, and coast live oaks along the trail offer snatches of shade. You also might notice a few islands of sagebrush, poison oak, and sticky monkeyflower floating in the sea of grassland along the trail.

City noises fade markedly as you climb, and as things quiet down, don't be surprised if you hear turkeys gobbling back and forth across the hillsides. Wild-turkey populations are on the rise in the Bay Area, and Mission Peak has its share of them. At 1.5 miles, Peak Meadow Trail departs on the right, dropping back toward the trailhead. Continue uphill on Hidden Valley Trail. Here you'll often come across some of the many cows that graze Mission Peak. Unpleasant cattle-versus-people conflicts do occur in Bay Area parks, and if you think bovines are sweet-tempered creatures, you may change your mind if a herd of them starts galloping toward you down a fire road. Sometimes the cattle seem to act completely on caprice, but there are ways to minimize conflicts: In general, give cattle plenty of room, and don't get between a mother and her calf. Be sure to close all cattle gates you encounter, and if you're hiking with a dog, either leash it or keep it close and under voice control. Cattle, like people, seem friskiest in spring.

The trail grade slackens a bit, and Mission Peak's summit gets closer with every step. You may notice rocks on the sides of the trail, and their numbers increase until, as you reach a junction at 2.2 miles, the entire steeply sloping hill-side leading to the summit is littered with rocks and boulders. At the base of the ridge, Grove Trail starts on the right. Stay to the left on Hidden Valley Trail. Mission Peak's remaining bulk rises very sharply out of a pretty little valley, but the trail ascends a gentler route. Although the slope under the summit is incredibly sharp and rocky, you may see cattle or goats grazing up there. A small herd of goats, escapees from a domesticated life, have lived elusively on the mountain for years. Still ascending at a moderate grade, the trail sweeps through grassland where fiddle-necks bloom in late winter.

At 2.3 miles, the last stretch of Hidden Valley Trail meets Peak Trail in the vertex of a big triangle-shaped junction. Stay to the right, then continue straight as a new trail heads straight uphill toward the summit (this path offers an optional ascent or descent). On the other side of a cattle gate, turn right, now on Eagle Trail. Eagle Trail ascends, sweeping right onto the northeastern side of the peak. Enjoy a nearly level stretch for the final push to the summit, which begins when you bear right onto Peak Trail at 2.6 miles. As you ascend the steep, narrow trail, look back over your shoulder from time to time to savor increasingly long views east across the Ohlone Regional Wilderness. Peak Trail jogs to the left and picks through rock outcrops as it ascends steeply. Finally, at 3.1 miles, you'll reach the top: elevation 2,517 feet.

From the summit, the entire South Bay sits at your feet. A funny little scope points out prominent natural features within visual range, including Mount Diablo to the north. Return to the parking lot the same way you came.

MORGAN TERRITORY REGIONAL PRESERVE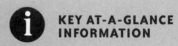

IN BRIEF

Morgan Territory's name whispers of the wilderness, evoking pioneers, wagon trains, and epic journeys. This loop rambles through a lavish landscape of grassland and oaks, drops off a ridge, then ascends on a narrow path along a creek. Morgan Territory is a good birding and wildflower-spotting preserve, so bring binoculars and field guides.

DESCRIPTION

Begin near the information signboard on Volvon Trail. After about 150 feet, Coyote Trail—the hike's return route—begins on the left. Stay to the right on Volvon. Sweeping through grassland dotted with oaks, California bay, and buckeye, Volvon is joined by Bob Walker Regional Trail, and the two paths run together. The trail meets another fire road heading to the park boundary on the right; bear left. At a slight descent, Volvon Trail meanders through a small bowl-shaped valley where johnny-tuck, California buttercups, fiddle-necks, and blue-dicks bloom in spring. Mount Diablo's twin

----

Directions ⟶

Depart San Francisco on the Bay Bridge and use the toll plaza as your mileage starting point. About 0.5 mile past the toll plaza, bear right onto I-580 East. Drive about 16 miles south, then at the CA 238 split, stay to the left on I-580. Continue east about 18 miles, then take Exit 52B onto North Livermore Avenue. Drive north on North Livermore. After about 4 miles, the road makes a sharp left and becomes Manning. Shortly after, turn right onto Morgan Territory Road. Drive about 5.5 miles on narrow, winding, one-lane Morgan Territory Road to the signed park entrance, on the right side of the road.

KEY AT-A-GLANCE INFORMATION

LENGTH: 4.7 miles

CONFIGURATION: Loop

DIFFICULTY: Moderate

SCENERY: Grassland and oaks

EXPOSURE: First leg under full sun, last leg shaded

TRAFFIC: Light

TRAIL SURFACE: Dirt fire road and trails

HIKING TIME: 2.5 hours

SEASON: Opens daily at 8 a.m.; closing hours vary (see Contacts, below). Late winter and spring are best; summer is often very hot.

ACCESS: Free

MAPS: At the trailhead's information signboard and ebparks.org/parks /maps

FACILITIES: Vault toilets and drinking water at trailhead

SPECIAL COMMENTS: Dogs welcome (no fee)

CONTACTS: 888-327-2757, ebparks .org/parks/morgan

DRIVING DISTANCE: 44.7 miles from the Bay Bridge toll plaza

GPS INFORMATION

N37° 49.118' W121° 47.741'

Morgan Territory Regional Preserve

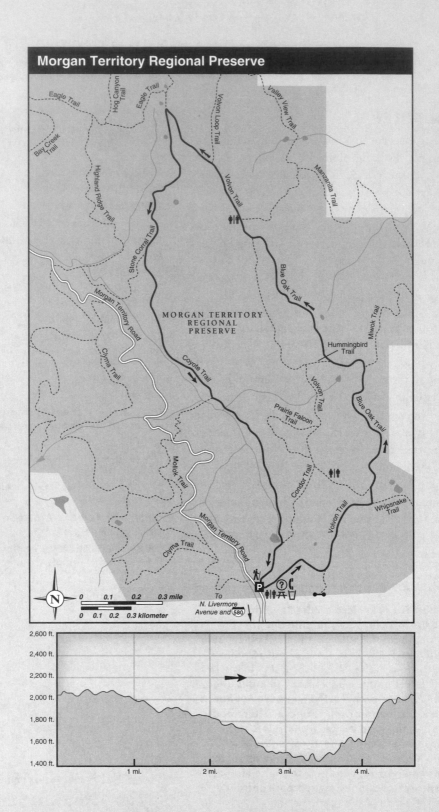

peaks loom in the distance. At 0.6 mile, a dead-end trail heads off to the right. Bear left and then, a few steps later, Volvon Trail veers left—turn right onto Blue Oak Trail.

The fire road winds gently uphill, through graceful old oaks and a few fruit and nut trees. Popcorn flower and filaree, two diminutive spring flowers, sprawl through the grass in early April. There are more sweeping views of Mount Diablo as Blue Oak Trail descends easily, but the surrounding landscape is also a visual delight—rolling, grassy hills peppered with oaks stretch in every direction.

Miwok Trail breaks off to the right at 1.2 miles, descending toward the Los Vaqueros Watershed. Continue to the left on Blue Oak Trail. In spring, carpets of goldfields appear, as blue and valley oaks begin to leaf out. Hummingbird Trail sets off to the left at 1.3 miles, connecting to Volvon Trail, but stay to the right on Blue Oak Trail. Here you can get a close look at the blue oaks lining the trail. The Volvon, a local Indian tribe, ground oak acorns into an edible mush using mortar rocks, some of which have been discovered inside this preserve. Continue straight on Blue Oak Trail, which gently rises and falls through a more wooded area domi-nated by oaks and buckeye, where blue-dicks and woodland stars bloom along the trail in spring. Other than bird cries or the soft chattering of squirrels, all is quiet. At 2 miles, Blue Oak Trail ends at a T-junction. Turn right back onto Volvon Trail.

After about 400 feet, you'll reach a cattle gate and junction with Valley View Trail. Continue straight. The trail briefly ascends to a saddle between hills. Views stretch east to the flatlands of the Central Valley. Here, 2.3 miles into the hike, you could extend your journey on a 1.2-mile loop around Bob Walker Ridge to the right. To stay on this 4.7-mile loop, continue to the left on Volvon Trail, which descends into a narrow valley. At 2.6 miles, Volvon Trail veers off to the right. Turn left onto the Stone Corral Trail.

The fire road weaves along the valley floor, where rocks are strewn through grassland. Stone Corral Trail loses some elevation and passes through a cattle gate. Ignore a well-worn path on the left and ascend a little hill to a signed junction at 3.2 miles. Turn left onto Coyote Trail.

Initially the narrow path keeps a nearly level grade as it cuts across a meadow, but at a cattle gate, Coyote Trail heads into the woods and begins to climb along a creek. The trail forks, but the two paths soon rejoin. Big-leaf maple, black oak, coast live oak, and buckeye fill the canyon, with snowberry, poison oak, cream-bush, and coffeeberry in the understory. Just past a grassy area with some manza-nita about halfway up the hill, Mollok Trail begins on the right. Continue uphill on Coyote Trail. Chinese houses, royal larkspur, and shooting stars abound in early spring. Coyote Trail crosses the creek, ascends through a boulder field, then emerges in grassland near a small pond. Bear left and skirt the pond, reaching a junction with Condor Trail at 4.6 miles. Turn right and follow Coyote Trail back the remaining 0.1 mile to Volvon Trail and the parking lot.

29 MOUNT DIABLO STATE PARK:
DONNER CANYON WATERFALL LOOP

KEY AT-A-GLANCE INFORMATION

LENGTH: 5.7 miles

CONFIGURATION: Balloon

DIFFICULTY: Moderate

SCENERY: Chaparral, grassland, oaks, waterfalls

EXPOSURE: Mostly exposed

TRAFFIC: Light

TRAIL SURFACE: Dirt fire roads and trails

HIKING TIME: 3 hours

SEASON: Best in winter and early spring

ACCESS: Free

MAPS: None at this trailhead; buy the map published by Save Mount Diablo ($12.50; savemountdiablo.org/lands _map.html) in advance, or download a free map at tinyurl.com/mtdiablo spmap.

FACILITIES: None

SPECIAL COMMENTS: No dogs allowed

CONTACTS: 925-837-2525, tinyurl .com/mtdiablosp

DRIVING DISTANCE: 27.5 miles from the Bay Bridge toll plaza

GPS INFORMATION

N37° 55.319' W121° 55.591'

IN BRIEF

This hike on Mount Diablo's northeastern slopes is the perfect antidote to winter doldrums. Spring seems to visit Donner Canyon very early, gracing the rugged hillsides with fresh grass and blooming wildflowers and shrubs, even in February. Choose a clear day after a series of storms, and you may see Donner Canyon's waterfalls.

DESCRIPTION

Rugged Mount Diablo, where temperatures soar to uncomfortable heights in summer, seems an unlikely host to waterfalls. Most of our Bay Area cascades are tucked back in forested canyons, but these falls run out in the open, dropping down rocky, steep, chaparral- and pine-covered hillsides. Although the falls aren't massive, they are pretty, and you can see them from several different perspectives along this loop. If you can arrange it, drop everything and head for this hike when snowfall accumulates on Diablo's peaks. The road to the top of the mountain is usually closed then, but since snow rarely makes a dent on the

----

Directions ──────────────────➤

Depart San Francisco on the Bay Bridge and use the toll plaza as your mileage starting point. About 0.5 mile past the toll plaza, bear right onto I-580 East. Drive 1.5 miles, then take Exit 19B onto CA 24. Drive east 12 miles on CA 24 to the I-680 split, then take Exit 15B onto Ygnacio Valley Road. Travel east on Ygnacio Valley Road about 8 miles, and turn right onto Clayton Road. Drive south on Clayton Road (which becomes Marsh Creek Road in Clayton) about 3 miles, then turn right on Regency Drive. Drive to the trailhead (with side-of-the-road parking), at the end of the road.

Mount Diablo State Park: Donner Canyon Waterfall Loop

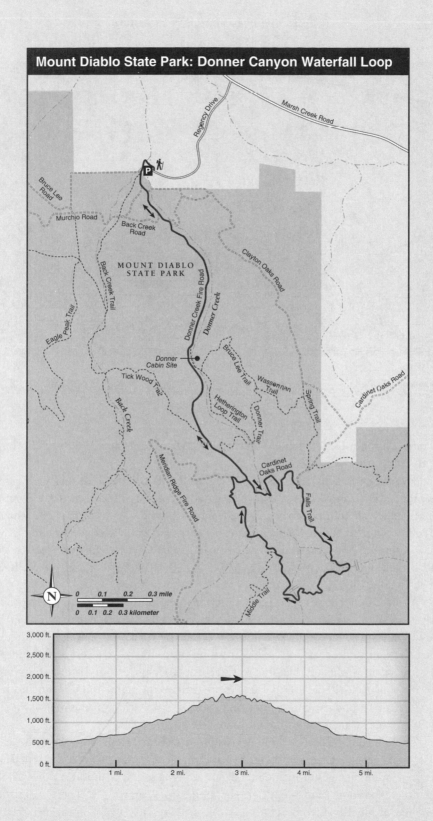

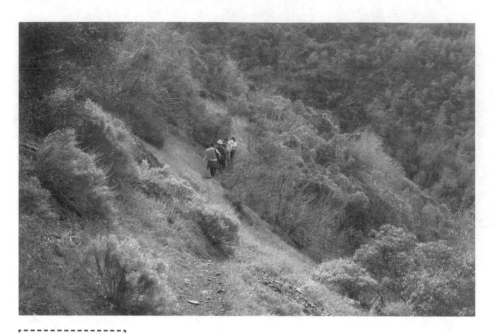

Hikers on Falls Trail

lower reaches of Mount Diablo, you can enjoy views of dusted peaks without having to trudge through snow.

The end of Regency Drive serves as a bare-bones trailhead for this hike. From the right side of the street, walk down a gated dirt fire road that ends at a T-junction. Turn left. You'll soon reach the gated park boundary and a junction. Stay to the left on Donner Canyon Road (you can choose either of two side-by-side paths, which converge down the trail). The fire road ascends just slightly, through grassland dotted with oaks and buckeye. At 0.3 mile, a trail heads right toward Back Creek Road. Continue to the left on Donner Canyon Road.

Along Donner Creek you have good views uphill to Diablo's highest peaks. Paths split off to the left (crossing the creek) and right (a path not on the map) at 0.4 and 0.5 mile—ignore these and stick to the fire road. You may see buttercups along the trail in February, as well as fresh leaves on buckeye trees. At 0.9 mile, a path breaks off to the left, heading to the Donner Cabin site, and a few steps later there's a junction with a path to Tick Wood Trail on the right. You'll reach another junction just around the corner, this one with the Hetherington Loop Trail on the left. Continue straight each time on Donner Canyon Road.

The fire road begins to climb earnestly. After heavy rains, the ascent through loose mud seems exaggerated as sticky clumps of mud cling to your boots. Trailside vegetation changes to include manzanita, yerba santa, ceanothus, poison oak, and pine. Shooting stars bloom in the understory in winter. There's another sequence of junctions from 1.1 to 1.3 miles. First Tick Wood Trail veers right, then Hetherington Loop Trail goes left. At each junction, keep going straight on Donner Canyon Road. Finally, at 1.6 miles, you'll reach an intersection that matters: Cardinet Junction. A trail to the right sets off toward Meridian Point—turn left onto Cardinet Oaks Road.

Revealing its true colors right away, the fire road descends somewhat steeply to cross Donner Creek. There's no bridge, so even though the creek is pretty small, when it's full you'll be forced to either get your shoes wet or plunge through barefoot. When I made the crossing on one February hike, the water was shockingly cold and rose up to my ankles. On the other side of the creek, Cardinet Oaks Road starts to climb at a steep grade. Switchbacks offer little relief, so if you get winded, take some time to stop and look around. There are still pines and chaparral plants along the trail, but patches of grass become more common as the trail ascends, and views back out of the canyon get better with each step. The junction with Falls Trail is quite a welcome sight at 2.1 miles. Turn right.

This is where an already scenic hike becomes spectacular. Falls Trail, just a little slip of a path, angles at a slight incline across a hillside of sagebrush, bush lupine, toyon, poison oak, pine, oaks, and grassland. The initial view of the waterfalls, even at a distance, is dramatic; water seems to appear out of thin air and gush out of creases in the hillside across the canyon. As you progress farther along the rocky trail, you'll have nice views uphill of several falls running down the side of steep Wild Oat Canyon. When Falls Trail dips to cross the creek at Wild Oat Canyon, check out the broad but short waterfall just a few feet upstream. The trail ascends sharply but then returns to a more moderate grade. Ceanothus, cercocarpus, and pines are common along the path.

Here, at the hike's highest elevation, look north for an ideal overview out of Donner Canyon and beyond. The trail descends to cross another creek, just below a small cascade (the water continues downhill to the last fall, but you have to get past it to see it). Climb uphill on the far side of the creek, then look back for my favorite view of the falls—a sheer, frothy drop that's breathtaking when the water flow is heavy. You'll cross one last creek and ascend a bit to a grassy area where hound's tongue blooms in late winter. At 3.6 miles, Falls Trail ends at a signed junction. Middle Trail heads uphill to the left, climbing steeply toward Prospector's Gap. Continue to the right on Middle Trail toward Meridian Ridge Road.

Middle Trail descends a little, through a thicket of manzanita, which fails to obscure views of the opposite side of the canyon and Mount Diablo's summit. You'll pass through an area with more dense vegetation, including toyon, chamise, and California bay, where chaparral currant blooms along the trail in February. After one last sunny stretch, Middle Trail ends at 4 miles. Turn right onto Meridian Ridge Road.

Your time on this fire road is brief—less than 0.1 mile down the trail you'll return to Cardinet Junction. Turn left and return to the trailhead on Donner Canyon Road.

30 MOUNT DIABLO STATE PARK:
MARY BOWERMAN TRAIL

KEY AT-A-GLANCE INFORMATION

LENGTH: 0.7 mile

CONFIGURATION: Loop

DIFFICULTY: Easy

SCENERY: Chaparral, grassland, views

EXPOSURE: First stretch shaded, the rest exposed

TRAFFIC: Light

TRAIL SURFACE: Initial section is paved and wheelchair-accessible; the rest is a narrow dirt path.

HIKING TIME: 0.5 hour

SEASON: Daily, 8 a.m.–sunset. Any time of year is good, but the park is hot in summer. When snow dusts the mountain, the road to the top is closed.

ACCESS: Pay $10 fee at the entrance kiosk on the way up the mountain.

MAPS: An interpretive guide is available at the trailhead; pick up the official park map at the entrance station or the Summit Museum (open daily, 10 a.m.–4 p.m.), or download at tinyurl.com/mtdiablospmap.

FACILITIES: Restrooms at the summit

CONTACTS: 925-837-2525, tinyurl .com/mtdiablosp

DRIVING DISTANCE: 35.8 miles from the Bay Bridge toll plaza

GPS INFORMATION

N37° 52.857' W121° 55.025'

IN BRIEF

Mary Bowerman Trail (formerly know as the Fire Interpretive Trail) offers perspective without perspiration. Less than a mile and gently graded, the trail makes a circuit just beneath Diablo's summit. The first section of the loop is paved and suitable for wheelchairs and strollers, but the remainder of the trail is a standard rocky mountain path.

DESCRIPTION

A drive to the top of Mount Diablo is a classic Bay Area day trip. A twisty, scenic road leads to the mountain's highest peak, which is

---

Directions

Depart San Francisco on the Bay Bridge and use the toll plaza as your mileage starting point. About 0.5 mile past the toll plaza, bear right onto I-580 East. Drive 1.5 miles, then take Exit 19B at CA 24. Drive east 12 miles on CA 24, then exit south onto I-680 (Exit 15A). Drive south 6.5 miles, then take Exit 39, Diablo Road, and turn left. Following the green PARKS signs, drive east on Diablo Road about 1 mile to the junction with El Cerro Boulevard. Turn right and continue about 3 miles on Diablo, then turn left at the stop-signed junction with Blackhawk Road onto Mount Diablo Scenic Boulevard. Drive 3.8 miles carefully uphill— as you enter the park, Mount Diablo Scenic Boulevard becomes South Gate Road—to the entrance kiosk, where you'll pay the day-use fee. (*Note:* This stretch of road is narrow; keep an eye out for bicyclists.) Continue uphill on South Gate 3.2 miles to a stop sign and junction, then turn right onto Summit Road. Keep climbing another 4 miles on Summit. Just before the road splits into two one-way segments near the summit, park in a large paved lot on the right (or continue to the summit, then drive back down to this lot).

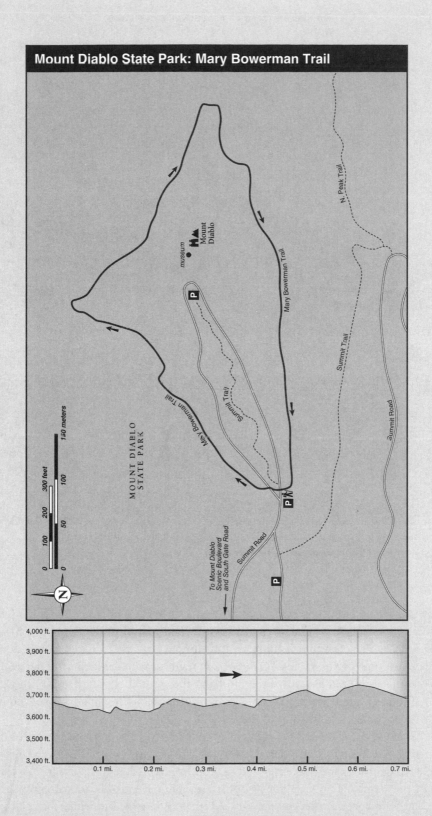

Mount Diablo State Park: Mary Bowerman Trail

N. Peak Trail

Mary Bowerman Trail

Summit Trail

Summit Road

Mount Diablo

museum

P

P

P

MOUNT DIABLO
STATE PARK

Mary Bowerman Trail

Summit Trail

Summit Road

To Mount Diablo
Scenic Boulevard
and South Gate Road

150 meters

300 feet

100

200

100

50

100

0

0

0

N

4,000 ft.

3,900 ft.

3,800 ft.

3,700 ft.

3,600 ft.

3,500 ft.

3,400 ft.

0.1 mi.   0.2 mi.   0.3 mi.   0.4 mi.   0.5 mi.   0.6 mi.   0.7 mi.

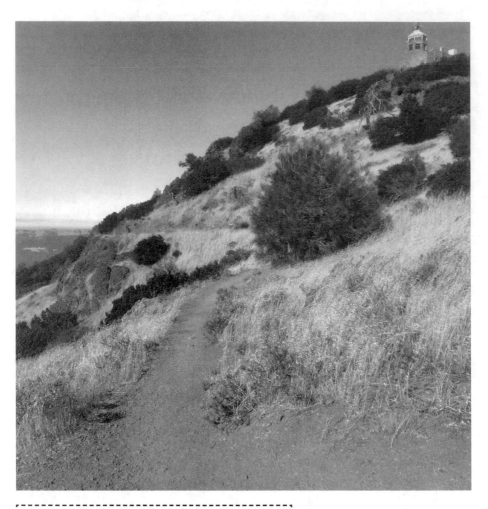

A view to Mount Diablo's summit from Mary Bowerman Trail

crowned with a stone observation tower and a little museum. On clear days, Diablo is famous for views that stretch across the San Joaquin Valley to snowcapped Sierra peaks. If you want to supplement a summit trip with a hike but you don't have much time or you're hosting out-of-town guests who are active but not really hikers, this loop trail just down the hill from the summit is perfect. Mary Bowerman Trail, a 0.7-mile circuit, features awesome views, a self-guided tour of mountain vegetation, and a fraction of the summit crowds.

Walking uphill toward the summit along the side of the park road, come to the signed trailhead on the left. Mary Bowerman Trail, marked with interpretive posts, begins under the shade of interior and canyon live oaks. Post 2 juts out from a cluster of poison oak. This deciduous plant is astoundingly variable and can grow as a vine, ground cover, or hedge. Here it's a little shrub, naked in winter but clothed again by spring with distinctive "leaves of three." Poison oak's oil, urushiol, is so strong that when any part of the plant comes into contact with clothing, the oil can survive multiple washings, reinfecting the wearer with an itchy rash.

As Mary Bowerman Trail progresses, you'll move out of the trees into a more open area, where greenstone, graywacke, and chert rocks are identified by Posts 3, 4, and 5. Look left for views north past Mitchell Canyon to northern Contra Costa County. At 0.2 mile, the pavement ends at a wooden platform. This is a great place to whip out the binoculars. Even if you can't see Mount Lassen, you'll enjoy great close-up views of Diablo's rugged North Peak.

As the trail bends right, you might notice a dramatic change in vegetation. Here chaparral plants, including ceanothus and cercocarpus, dominate with some live oaks and pines mixed through the evergreen shrubs. A fire ravaged this area in 1977, but the hillside has completely recovered and is for the most part covered with thick vegetation. I've seen mountain lion prints on the trail, but sightings of these shy creatures are not common—cougars prowl mostly at night.

The trail crosses an open, rocky hillside, then approaches Devil's Pulpit on the left. This dusky-red rock formation, composed of chert, has resisted weathering that eroded the surrounding earth. Rough paths scramble downhill to the formation and North Peak Trail, but Mary Bowerman Trail curves right as sparsely vegetated slopes roll downhill to the south. The summit buildings are visible uphill as the trail snakes through yet another plant community.

Tarantulas, which emerge from their burrows to mate in the fall, are autumn regulars on the mountain. These hairy spiders are relatively harmless, their bites being about as dangerous as wasp or bee stings. Even if you don't see them on the trails, you may spot a few crossing the park roads. Give them a wide berth and they'll ignore you—they've got more important things on their arachnid minds!

The last three posts mark juniper, yerba santa, and chamise, which crowd the trail along with some poison oak. At 0.7 mile, the trail ends across the street from the trailhead. Turn left and walk back to the parking lot.

NEARBY ACTIVITIES

The **Summit Museum–Visitor Center** is at the actual summit, a short distance from this trailhead. For more information, call 925-837-6119 or visit **mdia.org**.

31 MOUNT DIABLO STATE PARK:
MITCHELL CANYON–EAGLE PEAK LOOP

KEY AT-A-GLANCE INFORMATION

LENGTH: 7.8 miles

CONFIGURATION: Loop

DIFFICULTY: Strenuous

SCENERY: Chaparral, creek, views of the park from Eagle Peak

EXPOSURE: Almost all full sun

TRAFFIC: Moderate around the trailhead and on Mitchell Canyon Road, light farther afield

TRAIL SURFACE: Dirt fire roads and rocky trails

HIKING TIME: 4 hours

SEASON: Daily, 8 a.m.–sunset. Good anytime but summer due to the heat; exceptional wildflowers in spring.

ACCESS: Pay a $6 fee (self-register) at the entrance gate.

MAPS: Obtain the official park map at the Mitchell Canyon Interpretive Center (open weekends only) or tinyurl.com/mtdiablospmap. Better yet, order the map published by Save Mount Diablo ($12.50; savemount diablo.org/lands_map.html).

FACILITIES: Restrooms and drinking water at trailhead

SPECIAL COMMENTS: A trekking pole is handy for the Eagle Peak traverse. Check for ticks from late spring through autumn, when the grass is high. No dogs allowed.

CONTACTS: 925-837-2525, tinyurl .com/mtdiablosp

DRIVING DISTANCE: 26.7 miles from the Bay Bridge toll plaza

GPS INFORMATION

N37° 55.233' W121° 56.490'

IN BRIEF

This creek-to-peak Diablo tour begins at Mitchell Canyon and climbs on fire roads, easily then steeply, to Murchio Gap. Here the fun really begins, on a rollicking singletrack excursion over knife-edged Eagle Peak. From the exposed peak top, enjoy views of the park, then continue downhill at an often-steep grade back to the trailhead.

DESCRIPTION

Mitchell Canyon is a popular staging area for long Diablo hikes. From here you can make an all-day excursion to Diablo's summit, a 14-mile round-trip from 590 to 3,849 feet and back again—one of the Bay Area's toughest day hikes. The trek to Eagle Peak doesn't have the same cachet as the bottom-to-top hike, but I prefer the shorter loop. When the long trek to the top of Diablo nears the summit area, you'll commonly cross paths with loads of visitors around Juniper Campground and hear and see cars on a trail running parallel to Summit Road, jarring contrasts to the quiet found on most of the mountain. Peaceful and lonely,

----

Directions ——————————→

Depart San Francisco on the Bay Bridge and use the toll plaza as your mileage starting point. About 0.5 mile past the toll plaza, bear right onto I-580 East. Drive 1.5 miles, then take Exit 19B onto CA 24. Drive east about 12 miles on CA 24 to the I-680 split, then take Exit 15B onto Ygnacio Valley Road. Travel east about 8 miles on Ygnacio Valley and turn right onto Clayton Road. Drive south about 1 mile, then turn right onto Mitchell Canyon Road. Continue to the trailhead at the end of the road, about 1.5 miles.

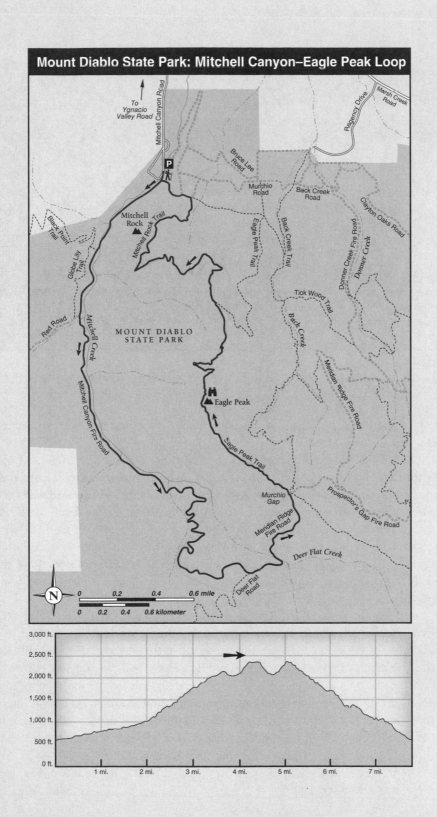

Mount Diablo State Park: Mitchell Canyon–Eagle Peak Loop

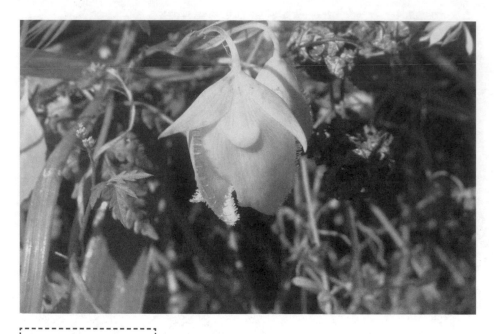

Mount Diablo fairy lantern

far from the developed parts of the park, Eagle Peak provides excellent hiking with awesome views.

Begin from the trailhead on the signed Mitchell Canyon Fire Road. As you pass through the gate, pick up the Mitchell Canyon Interpretive Guide, an excellent accompaniment to the first 2 miles of this hike. The broad fire road starts out climbing gently through grassland dotted with blue, coast live, and valley oak. At 250 feet, Mitchell Rock Trail, the return leg of this loop, begins on the left—continue straight on Mitchell Canyon Fire Road. In spring you may see sticky monkeyflower, Chinese houses, paintbrush, and Ithuriel's spear in bloom along the trail, blended through a mixture of oaks, pines, and chaparral plants, including sagebrush, California coffeeberry, poison oak, and pitcher sage.

At 0.6 mile, Black Point Trail departs on the right. Continue on Mitchell Canyon Fire Road, where the trail's namesake creek runs along to the left and pockets of riparian trees such as willow and alder are common. Swallowtail butterflies were out in abundance on a May hike, along with variable checkerspots and mylitta crescents, flitting to and fro. In spring look for Mount Diablo fairy lanterns, a yellow globe lily found only on and around Mount Diablo. On other Diablo hikes, I had seen a few of these fairy lanterns, but all along the length of the Mitchell Canyon Trail I saw dozens and dozens of them, as well as staggering amounts of wind poppy, a beautiful four-petaled orange flower.

On the right, Red Road drops down from Black Point at 0.9 mile—once again, continue on Mitchell Canyon Fire Road. As the canyon broadens slightly, views begin to unfold uphill to the left of rocky, steep-sided Eagle Peak. The fire road begins to climb with a bit more purpose, somewhat shaded by coast live oaks and a few big-leaf maples, buckeyes, and California bays. At about the 2-mile mark, the grade picks up significantly, and although there are some nearly level stretches, the climb is long and sustained. Stay alert for cyclists descending. On warm days, every bit of shade and cooling breeze is welcome.

With the creek left behind in the low reaches of the canyon, the surrounding slopes are dry and play host to many chaparral plants, with Coulter pine, sagebrush, ceanothus, goldenbush, cercocarpus, poison oak, toyon, sticky monkeyflower, and black sage prominent. There's plenty to look at along the trail, particularly in spring, when a variety of flowers bloom, including Linanthus, paintbrush, lupines, onions, mule ear sunflower, and clarkia. Views continue to open up to Eagle Peak on the left and out of the park back to the north.

The ascent, following a series of sweeping curves, seems never-ending, but abruptly the grade tapers off slightly and then the fire road sweeps right and reaches a flat on the right, at 3.4 miles. Two picnic tables provide rest spots. When you're ready, press on uphill at a moderate pace through oaks and pine to the Deer Flat junction at 3.5 miles. Deer Flat Road continues to climb toward the summit on the right, but our route, Meridian Ridge Road, swings left.

The fire road descends through oak, pine, poison oak, and California hop tree, offering a break from all that climbing. The relief is short-lived, though, for once the trail crosses Deer Flat Creek it begins to ascend steeply. Continue on Meridian Ridge Road, ascending past a grassy slope on the right, where California poppies bloom in big patches in April. The trailside vegetation shifts to chaparral, with lots of yerba santa, manzanita, pine, and chaparral pea enjoying the sunny exposure. The climb ends at Murchio Gap at 4.2 miles, where trails depart in every direction: traveling clockwise, Eagle Peak Trail begins, then Back Creek Trail, the continuation of Meridian Ridge Road, and little Bald Ridge Trail, across the road to the right. Turn left onto Eagle Peak Trail.

The slight path skirts a rock outcrop, climbing through ceanothus, chamise, yerba santa, black sage, goldenbush, and hop tree. As Eagle Peak Trail starts to descend, loose rock on the path presents a challenge—if you've brought a trekking pole, you'll definitely be glad. When you reach the saddle, you'll get a brief, level respite as the trail punches through thickets of chamise. Look to the left for a view of Mitchell Canyon Fire Road's snaking uphill route and back to the right for views of Diablo's summit area. As the trail begins to climb again, you'll enter a rocky, grassy area, where juniper and pine are common and, in early May, tons of clarkia, buckwheat, and jeweled onion brighten the grass as it begins to fade to gold. The ascent over these exposed slopes is sharp, with a couple of very rocky sections.

Finally, at 5 miles, you'll arrive at the top: 2,369 feet, unsigned but obvious. There's remarkably little real estate here, and the peak slopes drop sharply off this knife-edge ridge. You'll surely want to pause and enjoy the views, which encompass the entire northern part of the mountain, including the summit and North

Peak, as well as rolling ridges on the right and left, and hills well off into the distance. In winter, with strong binoculars, you might be able to see the waterfalls dropping out of Donner Canyon. On a May hike, I observed a horned lizard that scampered a few feet from me, almost perfectly camouflaged in the surrounding tan pebbles. Birders and butterfly enthusiasts could spend some time on this peak, watching hawks and swallowtails soaring or fluttering overhead.

The trail clings to the ridgetop, then drops off to the left, beginning a descent. There are more steep, rocky patches to traverse as Eagle Peak Trail swings through some shaded areas where you might notice currant blooming in winter. Mostly the hillsides are cloaked in an army-green coat of chamise, black sage, and toyon. Continuing down the sloping ridgeline, a second small peak is crossed, and the trail just keeps dropping. At 5.9 miles, Eagle Peak Trail swings sharply right, descending off the east side of the mountain. Here, continue straight, now on Mitchell Rock Trail.

The narrow path rises, then drops to the side of a red-rock outcrop on the right. Some pines shade the trail as you make a transition into a mixture of grassland and chaparral. Look for a good variety of flowers in spring, including California poppy, coyote mint, mariposa lily, Chinese houses, paintbrush, milkweed, owl's clover, and blue-eyed grass. Although the trend is firmly downhill, there are a few short, easy uphill stretches. The trail veers off the ridgeline into pure grassland and, other than a few forays through chaparral patches, stays that way all the way downhill. You'll pass Mitchell Rock, a pillow-basalt outcrop, on the left. By mid-May, thigh-high grass crowds the trail as it weaves downhill, reaching a junction with Coulter Pine Trail at 7.6 miles. Turn left, continuing on Mitchell Rock Trail.

After a few feet you'll reach a junction with a trail on the right leading to Bruce Lee Trail. Continue straight on Mitchell Rock Trail, and descend through blue oaks and grassland to a junction with Mitchell Canyon Fire Road at 7.8 miles. Turn right and return to the trailhead.

REDWOOD REGIONAL PARK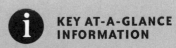

IN BRIEF

The next time you find yourself gazing east from Mount Tamalpais or the Marin Headlands, think of this: Towering above the East Bay hills in the 1800s was a row of redwoods so tall that ship captains used them to navigate through the Golden Gate into San Francisco. Although the giant trees were logged by the turn of that century, second-growth redwoods now fill canyons where rainbow trout spawn and ladybugs hibernate in the winter, wildflowers bloom in spring, and other wild creatures scamper through the woods year-round. This easy 4.1-mile loop drops into a redwood canyon and then climbs back to a nearly level trail, which returns to the trailhead.

DESCRIPTION

Redwood Regional Park is mostly just one big canyon, and although it has some neighborhood access points, most people enter from either end of the park. There are many loop options, so hikers can mix and match on

---

Directions ⟶

Depart San Francisco on the Bay Bridge and use the toll plaza as your mileage starting point. About 0.5 mile past the toll plaza, bear right onto I-580 East. Drive 1.5 miles, then take Exit 19B onto CA 24. Drive east 3.5 miles on CA 24, then take Exit 5 onto CA 13 South. After about 3 miles, take Exit 2, Lincoln Avenue/Joaquin Miller Road. At the foot of the exit ramp, make a left, take the next left, and then go straight onto Joaquin Miller. Drive uphill about 1 mile, then turn left at a light onto Skyline Boulevard (look for the brown park sign before the turn). Drive about 3 miles (you'll pass the Chabot Space Center) and turn right into the parking lot and staging area.

ⓘ KEY AT-A-GLANCE INFORMATION

LENGTH: 4.1 miles

CONFIGURATION: Loop

DIFFICULTY: Easy

SCENERY: Redwoods and a mixture of grassland and shrubs

EXPOSURE: Shaded in the canyon, partial sun on the ridges

TRAFFIC: Moderate–heavy

TRAIL SURFACE: Dirt fire roads and trails

HIKING TIME: 2 hours

SEASON: Daily, 5 a.m.–sunset. Nice year-round, although trails are muddy in winter.

ACCESS: Free from this trailhead; main park staging area requires a $5 fee.

MAPS: At the trailhead and ebparks .org/parks/maps

FACILITIES: Pit toilets at trailhead

SPECIAL COMMENTS: Dogs welcome ($2 fee)

CONTACTS: 888-327-2757, ebparks .org/parks/redwood

DRIVING DISTANCE: 13.3 miles from the Bay Bridge toll plaza

GPS INFORMATION

N37° 49.896' W122° 11.116'

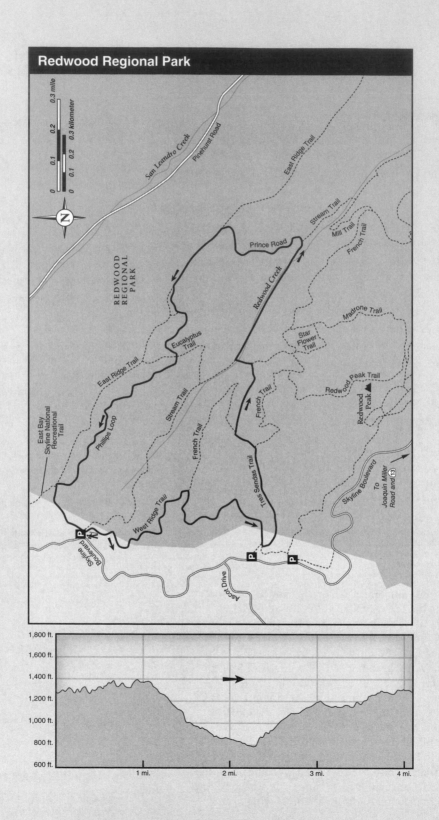

Redwood Regional Park

0.3 mile
0.2
0.1
0

0.3 kilometer
0.2
0.1
0

N

San Leandro Creek

Pinehurst Road

East Ridge Trail

REDWOOD
REGIONAL
PARK

Prince Road

Stream Trail

Mill Trail

French Trail

Redwood Creek

Eucalyptus Trail

East Ridge Trail

Madrone Trail

Star Flower Trail

Redwood Peak Trail

Redwood Peak

Stream Trail

Phillips Loop

East Bay Skyline National Recreational Trail

French Trail

French Trail

Tres Sendas Trail

West Ridge Trail

Skyline Boulevard

To Joaquin Miller Road and (13)

P

P

P

Ascot Drive

1,800 ft.
1,600 ft.
1,400 ft.
1,200 ft.
1,000 ft.
800 ft.
600 ft.

1 mi.   2 mi.   3 mi.   4 mi.

canyon and ridge trails. Hikers, equestrians, dog-walkers, runners, and cyclists frequent Redwood trails, but it's still easy to find peace and quiet, particularly on the paths closed to cyclists.

Starting from the Skyline Gate Staging Area, begin on West Ridge Trail. At a level grade, the wide fire road sweeps past some eucalyptus into a more natural setting of chaparral currant, California bay, madrone, coast live oak, toyon, hazelnut, and creambush. At 0.6 mile, French Trail sets off into the canyon on the left, but keep going on West Ridge Trail.

The sea of trees parts occasionally to reveal views southeast out of the canyon. Redwoods creep up from the canyon in places, contrasting with patches of grass and chaparral. When you reach the junction with Tres Sendas Trail at 1.1 miles, turn left and begin to descend.

The narrow trail can get quite muddy in winter when storm runoff filters downhill, plumping a little stream. It doesn't take long to make the transition from ridge to canyon at a moderate grade. In just a few minutes, you'll find yourself in the clutches of a gorge filled with redwoods, California bays, and ferns. French Trail feeds into Tres Sendas at 1.5 miles, and the two paths run together briefly, until French veers off to the left. Continue on Tres Sendas as it descends deeper into groves of redwood. Look for trilliums blooming in spring. At 1.8 miles, Star Flower Trail heads uphill on the right. Stay to the left on Tres Sendas. The trail crosses Redwood Creek and ends at 1.9 miles. Turn right onto Stream Trail.

As Stream Trail follows along Redwood Creek, fences line the trail to protect the fragile riparian environment. Here in the heart of the canyon, it's almost completely shaded all day, and the trailside vegetation is a lush tangle of ferns and blackberry vines. Moss is draped over boulders and swathed around redwood trunks. On one winter hike, I came upon thousands of ladybird beetles (also known as ladybugs) hibernating. The orange beetles looked like a pile of maple leaves from a distance, but up close I marveled at how they huddled together on branches and leaves of the understory vegetation. Observing ladybugs is a highlight of Bay Area winter hikes, and I've since seen them several other times. Stream Trail descends slightly to a junction at 2.3 miles. Turn left onto Prince Road.

As the broad trail climbs at a moderate grade out of the canyon, redwoods and California bays give way to coast live oaks and madrones; then the trees thin and coyote brush, poison oak, and blackberry dot grassland. Prince Road ends at 2.7 miles. Turn left onto East Ridge Trail.

The wide fire road follows the park boundary at a nearly level grade. Coyote brush, pine, coast live oak, and madrone seem to stand off from the trail, permitting views back across the canyon to the west ridge. Although dogs are frequent visitors to the park, there's plenty of wildlife here, and you might examine the sandy trail surface for telltale animal signs. Bobcat prints are decidedly feline, though their feet are considerably larger than those of domestic cats. Coyotes leave spadelike prints and are fond of marking their territory at junctions, leaving piles of scat as calling cards for other coyotes where deer trails and paths cross.

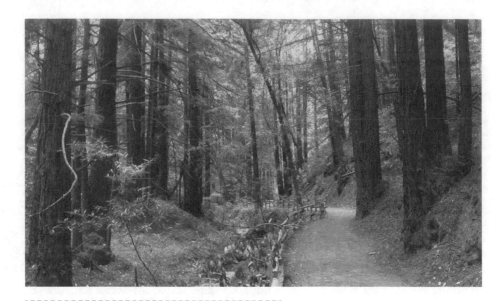

The park's namesake redwoods tower over Stream Trail.

Deer are the most common hoofed animal in the Bay Area, and their crescent-shaped prints are easy to pick out. In summer months, when the trails are dry, you might see squiggly paths left across trails by traveling snakes. At the 3-mile mark, East Ridge Trail continues to the right, while Phillips Trail swings off to the left. Either route is an option, but I prefer Phillips, so bear left.

The trail undulates a bit through coyote brush, pine, and madrone. You might hear (and see) hawks perched on tall trees nearby. Eucalyptus Trail crosses Phillips at 3.3 miles; continue straight. Eucalyptus trees, imported in the 1800s from Australia, are a common fixture in East Bay parks. Timbermen hoped the fast-growing trees would provide profitable lumber crops, but their wood turned out to be unsuitable for building purposes. Another exotic plant you might notice along the trail is cotoneaster, a landscaping shrub with glossy leaves and red berries. Unlike that of toyon, a native shrub that also bears red berries, cotoneaster's fruit is poisonous to humans, although birds eat the berries.

Phillips Trail runs downslope from the ridge on the right until the trail merges into East Ridge Trail at 3.9 miles. The trail straight across the junction leaves Redwood Park and heads north into Huckleberry Preserve on the East Bay Skyline National Recreation Trail, a 31-mile path that runs through six East Bay parks. Bear left and follow East Ridge Trail another 0.2 mile back to the trailhead.

NEARBY ACTIVITIES

Sibley Regional Volcanic Preserve (6800 Skyline Blvd., Oakland), a few miles north of Redwood Regional Park, hosts a self-guided loop through the remains of a volcano. Details: 888-327-2757, **ebparks.org/parks/sibley.**

ROUND VALLEY REGIONAL PRESERVE

IN BRIEF

Round Valley's single trailhead is on a lonely country road that winds through the eastern foothills of Mount Diablo. Hikers can take long out-and-back or shuttle hikes through this preserve and neighboring Los Vaqueros Watershed (see Hike 26), but this hike is an easy-going, three-creek, 4.1-mile tour through rolling hills of oak woods and grassland.

DESCRIPTION

Hikes at Round Valley scratch that peace-and-quiet itch. You may hear the occasional plane overhead, but traffic noise is nonexistent once you leave the trailhead, and the flanks of Mount Diablo block views of suburban sprawl to the west. This is one of those backyard get-away spots that make Bay Area life bearable for folks who love the outdoors.

Round Valley is part of a little-known mini-greenbelt. The East Bay Regional Parks District–managed Round Valley and Morgan Territory preserves abut Mount Diablo State

---

Directions ⟶

Depart San Francisco on the Bay Bridge and use the toll plaza as your mileage starting point. About 0.5 mile past the toll plaza, bear right onto I-580 East. Drive about 16 miles south and, at the CA 238 split, stay to the left on I-580. Continue east about 21 miles, then take Exit 55 onto Vasco Road in Livermore. Turn left and drive north on Vasco Road about 14 miles to the junction with Camino Diablo Road. Turn left onto Camino Diablo Road, drive about 3.5 miles, then continue left onto Marsh Creek Road. Drive west on Marsh Creek Road about 1.5 miles to the preserve entrance on the left side of the road.

KEY AT-A-GLANCE INFORMATION

LENGTH: 4.1 miles

CONFIGURATION: Loop

DIFFICULTY: Easy

SCENERY: Grassland and oaks

EXPOSURE: Mostly full sun, some partial shade

TRAFFIC: Light

TRAIL SURFACE: Dirt fire road and trails

HIKING TIME: 2 hours

SEASON: Opens daily at 8 a.m.; closing hours vary (see Contacts, below). Autumn and late winter are best—summer is often very hot.

ACCESS: Free

MAPS: At the trailhead's information signboard and ebparks.org/parks /maps

FACILITIES: Vault toilets and drinking water at trailhead

SPECIAL COMMENTS: No dogs allowed

CONTACTS: 888-327-2757, ebparks .org/parks/round_valley

DRIVING DISTANCE: 57.5 miles from the Bay Bridge toll plaza

GPS INFORMATION

N37° 52.108' W121° 45.012'

Round Valley Regional Preserve

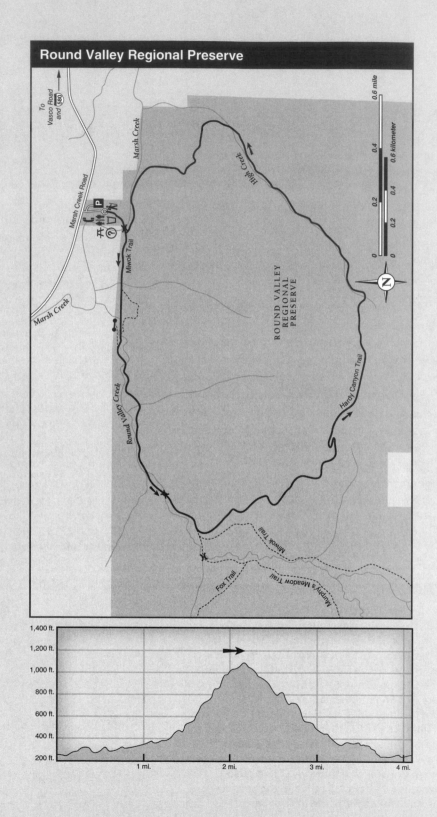

Park and Los Vaqueros Watershed (owned and run by the Contra Costa Water District), creating a huge protected block of land. The wildlife-viewing is exceptional through all these parklands; Round Valley is protected habitat for the San Joaquin kit fox, and golden-eagle sightings are frequent.

From the trailhead, follow the obvious route over a bridge to a gate and junction with Hardy Canyon Trail, the return segment of the loop. Stay to the right, on Miwok Trail. This fire road begins a moderate climb along the preserve boundary, downslope from an oak-studded hillside. After a short dip, as the trail rises again, go straight onto an unsigned but well-worn path, which shortcuts a roller-coaster stretch best suited to equestrians. The path descends and feeds back into the fire road, which meets a dead-end trail at 0.5 mile. Stay to the left on Miwok Trail.

The trail now follows along Round Valley Creek at an easy grade. Hills rise to the right and left, marked with many lovely trees, including blue and coast live oak and buckeye. There are usually quite a few squirrels scuttling about in the grassy areas off the trail, and you might see hawks sitting in trees near squirrel burrows. I've also seen golden eagles soaring above this part of the preserve in autumn. Miwok Trail ascends a bit and reaches a junction at 1.2 miles. The valley stretches south from here.

Turn left onto Hardy Canyon Trail, a narrow path that ascends through grassland and blue oak. Cattle that graze throughout the preserve seem to prefer the valley basin, but you might meet a few up in these hills as well. During the wettest months of the year, rain cascades downhill in the creases of the hillsides, where buckeyes thrive. Look for coyote and bobcat prints on the trail—as dogs are not permitted at Round Valley, all prints are most likely from wild residents of the area.

Although the grade never increases beyond moderate, you might want to stop occasionally to enjoy the northwest views, which extend beyond the boundaries of the preserve to include Mount Diablo's main and north peaks, an unusual perspective of the East Bay's tallest mountain.

Hardy Canyon Trail sticks to a course downslope from the hilltop, effectively looping around the hill. As you climb, the oaks thin a bit and grassland dominates the landscape. The trail jogs left, then right, on a little switchback around a long thin rock formation that resembles a sloping wall. After one last gentle ascent through grassland, the trail reaches a slight saddle. A rough path veers right, but the official trail almost immediately starts downhill to the left. You never reach the hilltop, but then again, with views this nice, you don't need to.

The preserve boundary is a short distance to the right, and the adjacent property is the Los Vaqueros Watershed. The two properties don't connect here, but if they did, it would create a great hiking loop opportunity (you can enter the watershed from a gate on Miwok Trail at the south end of Round Valley). As Hardy Canyon Trail descends to the east, scattered cow paths (one leading to a watering trough) make navigation a bit tricky. Aim for the crease between this hill and another to the right. Gradually you'll enter an area with a high concentration of blue and coast live oaks. After a steep little scramble down and up near a slide area, the trail

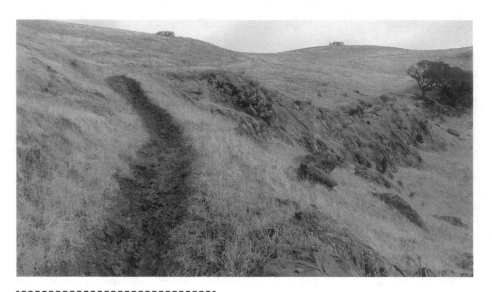

Rock formations along Hardy Canyon Trail

adopts a course along the banks of High Creek. Here, as in other parts of the park where water runs in winter and spring, buckeyes grow clustered together.

Hardy Canyon Trail climbs slightly, then descends back toward the creek. Because the creek is dry by autumn, previous ranchers maximized the flow by constructing a little dam, which still stands today, to hold back a little pool of water year-round.

At 3.3 miles, you'll reach a crucial junction, which may be unsigned. Be sure to bear left and cross the creek—the path to the right heads into private property. As you make your way gently uphill through oaks and grassland, an occasional vehicle on Marsh Creek Road may be audible. Hawks are very common in this part of the preserve, using the trees to scope out small mammals in the adjacent meadow to the right.

The trail descends into grassland, then sweeps left to reach a gate. On the other side you'll follow along yet another waterway, Marsh Creek, where cotton-wood and sycamore share their autumnal-tinted leaves in November. At 4 miles, the trail rises up to meet Miwok Trail back at the hike's first junction. Turn right and return to the parking lot.

NEARBY ACTIVITIES

In spring, the sides of **Marsh Creek Road** host a better wildflower display than the preserve, which is grazed by flower-eating cows.

SUNOL REGIONAL WILDERNESS

IN BRIEF

Sunol's jagged peaks and grassy ridges are surrounded by open space, cushioning the impact from nearby East Bay towns and highways. There's a lot of real estate here, with natural wonders that include rock formations, creeks, and even small waterfalls in winter and spring. This loop just scratches the surface of Sunol, climbing along a creek to a grassy ridge with rock formations and views galore, then descending through grassland back to the trailhead.

DESCRIPTION

Does every rose have its thorn? You may wonder at Sunol, where the bucolic splendor of rolling hills, waterfalls, and creeks is dampened by a marauding band of spunky cattle. It's easy enough to dodge their patties, and, in fact, it's best to avoid them altogether—these cows can be dangerous when they're annoyed, and they seem to get upset at the drop of a

----

Directions

Depart San Francisco on the Bay Bridge and use the toll plaza as your mileage starting point. About 0.5 mile past the toll plaza, bear right onto I-580 East. Drive 1.5 miles, then take Exit 19B onto CA 24. Drive east 12 miles on CA 24, then take Exit 15A onto I-680 south. Drive south about 25 miles, then take Exit 21A onto CA 84/Calaveras Road. Follow the brown PARKS signs: Stay in the left lane of the exit ramp, turn left, drive under the freeway, and then stay in the left lane through a stop sign to remain on Calaveras. Drive south on Calaveras about 4 miles to the junction with Geary Road, and turn left. Continue on Geary almost 2 miles to the park entrance kiosk, then continue past the visitor center to an unmarked dirt lot on the left.

KEY AT-A-GLANCE INFORMATION

LENGTH: 5 miles

CONFIGURATION: Loop

DIFFICULTY: Moderate

SCENERY: Grassland, oaks, creeks, rock formations

EXPOSURE: Mixture of shade and sun

TRAFFIC: Moderate

TRAIL SURFACE: Dirt trails and fire roads

HIKING TIME: 2.5 hours

SEASON: Opens daily at 8 a.m.; closing hours vary (see Contacts, below). Late winter and spring are best—not a good summer choice. Exceptional wildflowers in the spring.

ACCESS: Pay the $5 fee at the entrance kiosk.

MAPS: At entrance kiosk and ebparks .org/parks/maps

FACILITIES: Pit toilets at the trailhead

SPECIAL COMMENTS: Dogs welcome ($2 fee)

CONTACTS: 888-327-2757, ebparks .org/parks/sunol

DRIVING DISTANCE: 41.4 miles from the Bay Bridge toll plaza

GPS INFORMATION

N37° 30.926' W121° 49.838'

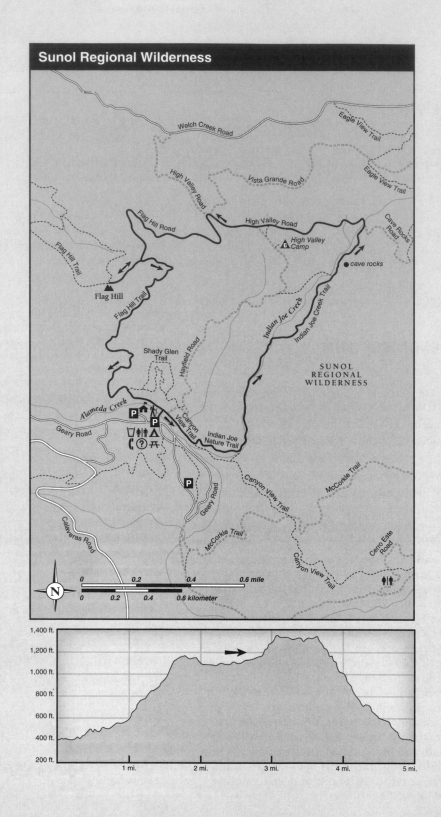

Sunol Regional Wilderness

Welch Creek Road

Eagle View Trail

Eagle View Trail

High Valley Road

Vista Grande Road

Flag Hill Road

High Valley Road

Cave Rocks Road

Flag Hill Trail

High Valley Camp

Flag Hill Trail

Flag Hill

Indian Joe Creek

cave rocks

Indian Joe Creek Trail

Shady Glen Trail

Hayfield Road

SUNOL
REGIONAL
WILDERNESS

Alameda Creek

Canyon View Trail

Geary Road

Indian Joe Nature Trail

Canyon View Trail

McCorkle Trail

Geary Road

Calaveras Road

McCorkle Trail

Cerro Este Road

Canyon View Trail

0   0.2   0.4   0.6 mile

0   0.2   0.4   0.6 kilometer

N

| | 1 mi. | 2 mi. | 3 mi. | 4 mi. | 5 mi. |

1,400 ft.
1,200 ft.
1,000 ft.
800 ft.
600 ft.
400 ft.
200 ft.

hiking boot. Some people stay away from Sunol, preferring to hike through cow-free parks, but I put up with the bovines because Sunol is that good—particularly in early spring, when flowers bloom everywhere, soft breezes ruffle fields of grass, and temperate weather encourages hikes. The optimal time to visit Sunol is from March through the end of May. Arrive earlier than that and you'll face sloppy mud. Later, the heat can be stifling—I hiked this loop once in early June, and it was so hot I had to stop and rest on a downhill stretch.

Begin by walking across Alameda Creek on a pretty footbridge. At the far side of the creek, turn right onto Canyon View Trail. This flat path follows the creek through a sparse population of buckeye, coast live oak, sycamore, and big-leaf maple. Hayfield Road sets off uphill on the left at 0.1 mile—continue on Canyon View Trail to a signed junction at 0.2 mile, then turn left onto Indian Joe Creek Trail.

The narrow path climbs slightly. Coast live oaks line the way on the left, while on the right side of the trail clusters of sagebrush frame views of oak-studded hills to the west. This little stretch features a premium blend of spring wildflowers, including wind poppy, Chinese houses, California larkspur, yellow mariposa lily, and elegant clarkia. Just before the trail bends left, at about 0.4 mile, you'll come to another connection to Canyon View Trail on the right. Stay to the left on Indian Joe Creek Trail.

Crowded by toyon, the path descends toward the banks of Indian Joe Creek. On one April hike, I saw an unlikely pair of wildflowers together—sturdy mule ear sunflowers seemingly employed as bodyguards to a huddle of delicate fairy lanterns. In autumn, thickets of snowberry dangle their ghostly white berries in the shade of coast live oaks. The trail crosses through a cattle gate and begins to climb slightly, beginning a journey out of the canyon. Sycamores appear occasionally, but coast live oaks are more common, and you might also see sagebrush, sticky monkeyflower, and California coffeeberry. As the trail cuts across a sloping, grassy hillside, there are views uphill to the park's highest ridge. Indian Joe Creek Trail crosses back and forth from one side of the creek to the other, then abruptly begins a somewhat steep ascent. Stands of coast live oak and California bay shade some of the route, while other stretches pass through little patches of grassland dotted with sagebrush. In the hottest days of summer, some of the park's cattle seek refuge from the harsh sunlight under the trees. At about the 1.8-mile mark, a trail heads left toward Hayfield Road. Continue uphill on Indian Joe Creek Trail.

Just off the left side of the trail, sycamores and buckeyes ring a basalt-rock formation known as Indian Joe Caves. The trail presses on uphill, alternating between level stretches and steep ones. Finally, at 2.2 miles, the trail ends at a junction with a fire road. Turn left onto Cave Rocks Road.

You'll cross Indian Joe Creek one last time, then begin an easy stroll through grassland on a high plain. Look for turtles in a little pond on the right. Some huge solitary valley oaks stand off to the sides of the trail, where in spring popcorn flowers and Ithuriel's spear bloom throughout the grass. Cave Rocks Road

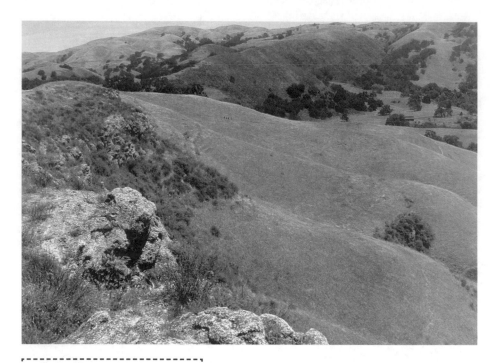

The grassy slopes of Sunol's Flag Hill

descends to a junction at 2.6 miles with Hayfield Road dropping past a barn, part of High Valley Group Camp on the left. Continue straight to the next junction at 2.8 miles, marked by a couple of valley oaks. Turn left onto Flag Hill Road.

The fire road sweeps uphill through grassland. There are competing views—look back to admire High Valley from a different perspective, and gaze off to the right for excellent views of Maguire Peaks, two rocky spires at the northern edge of the park. If you can tear yourself away from the long views, check out the sides of the trail for spring wildflowers. I've seen blue-eyed grass, fiddle-necks, lupines, and California buttercups, mostly on the downslope to the right. Flag Hill Road makes a sharp turn left and levels out considerably. If you're hiking in early June, take some time to look for mariposa lily, a stunning wildflower that looks like it was hand-painted by a watercolor master. Beetles and spiders love them, and you might see a half-dozen tiny insects crawling in the bowl of each flower. At 3.6 miles, Flag Hill Trail begins on the left. This will be the return route, but first continue straight on an unmarked but obvious path.

The trail winds along this little ridge, through rocky grassland where coyote mint, California poppy, lupines, and owl's clover bloom in spring. You'll reach the end of the path and a rock formation at about 3.7 miles. Carefully scramble onto the rocks. Once you get up there, you'll see why caution is in order: There's a steep drop-off, but the views are simply out of this world. The entire eastern section of the park seems to sit at your feet, and it's common to see vultures and hawks

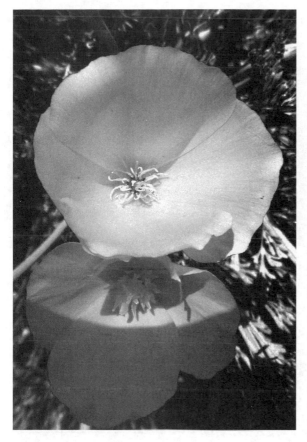

California poppies bloom at Sunol all spring long.

soaring below your perch—an unusual experience. Needless to say, this is the day's lunch-break destination.

When you're ready to move on, walk back to the previous junction, and turn right onto Flag Hill Trail. If you're suffering from a post-lunch stupor, this tiny path may be a bit of an affront. There are rocky sections, and overall the descent is quite steep. The scenery is mostly grassland with a few coast live oaks interspersed here and there. Once through a cattle gate, oaks are clustered closer together, yielding more shade. The descent is steady, and soon you'll arrive at a junction and another gate at about 4.9 miles. Shady Glen Trail goes off to the left. Bear right, remaining on the Flag Hill Trail.

After a short downhill section, the trail ends at the banks of Alameda Creek. Turn left and follow the creek back to the bridge at 5 miles. Turn right and retrace your steps back to the parking lot.

NEARBY ACTIVITIES

Del Valle Regional Park (7000 Del Valle Rd., Livermore) offers a similar, slightly tamer terrain of rolling oak savanna, plus a lake for swimming, boating, and fishing, and a campground. More info: 888-327-2757, **ebparks.org/parks/del_valle**.

35 TILDEN REGIONAL PARK

KEY AT-A-GLANCE INFORMATION

LENGTH: 3.7 miles

CONFIGURATION: Out-and-back

DIFFICULTY: Easy

SCENERY: Views of the East Bay Hills, grassland, eucalyptus forest

EXPOSURE: Mostly full sun

TRAFFIC: Heavy

TRAIL SURFACE: Paved

HIKING TIME: 1.5 hours

SEASON: Daily, 5 a.m.–sunset; good year-round

ACCESS: Free

MAPS: At the trailhead and ebparks .org/parks/maps

FACILITIES: Pit toilets at trailhead

SPECIAL COMMENTS: Dogs are permitted on this hike but prohibited on some other Tilden trails.

CONTACTS: 888-327-2757, ebparks .org/parks/tilden

DRIVING DISTANCE: 12.6 miles from the Bay Bridge toll plaza

GPS INFORMATION

N37° 54.303' W122° 14.671'

IN BRIEF

This easy hike on paved Nimitz Way hosts walkers from the very young to the very old, and every age in between. It's a favorite for anyone looking for easy yet scenic exercise, and dogs are welcome.

DESCRIPTION

Tilden Regional Park is a recreation paradise in the backyard of the East Bay communities of Berkeley and Kensington. In addition to miles of trails that connect to adjacent parks, enabling long rambles, Tilden provides exceptional opportunities for family fun, with a merry-go-round, a swimming lake, pony rides, steam trains, and picnic areas that can be reserved.

Directions ───────────────→

Depart San Francisco on the Bay Bridge and use the toll plaza as your mileage starting point. About 0.5 mile past the toll plaza, bear right onto I-580 East. Drive 1.5 miles, then take Exit 19B onto CA 24. Drive east about 5 miles on CA 24 and, at the far side of the Caldecott Tunnel, take Exit 7A onto Fish Ranch Road, the first post-tunnel exit—stay in the right lane through the tunnel. Drive north on Fish Ranch Road about 1 mile, then turn right onto Grizzly Peak Boulevard. Drive 1.4 miles, then turn right onto South Park Drive. After 1.5 miles, bear right onto Wildcat Canyon Road. Continue about 0.8 mile to the Inspiration Point trailhead, on the left side of the road.

Note: South Park Drive closes annually November–March to protect migrating newts. If it's closed on your visit, continue on Grizzly Peak to Golf Course Road, turn right, and then turn right again onto Shasta Road. Finally, bear right onto Wildcat Canyon Road and continue to Inspiration Point.

Tilden Regional Park

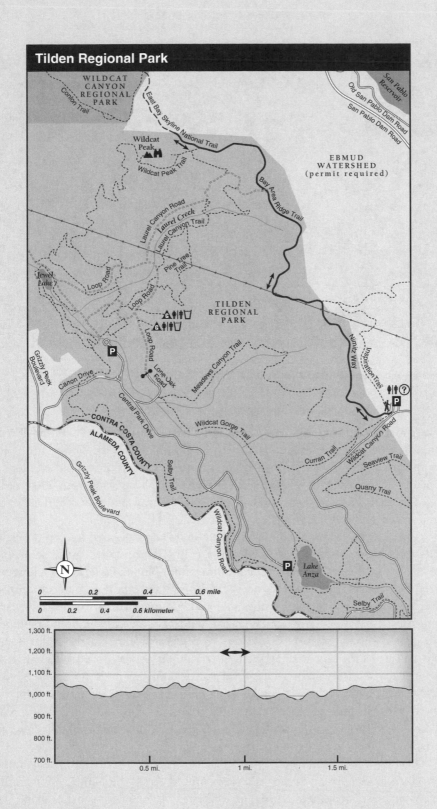

WILDCAT CANYON REGIONAL PARK

Conlon Trail

WILDCAT CANYON REGIONAL PARK

East Bay Skyline National Trail

Wildcat Peak

Wildcat Peak Trail

San Pablo Reservoir

Old San Pablo Dam Road

San Pablo Dam Road

EBMUD WATERSHED (permit required)

Bay Area Ridge Trail

Laurel Canyon Road

Laurel Creek

Laurel Canyon Trail

Pine Tree Trail

Jewel Lake

Loop Road

Loop Road

Loop Road

TILDEN REGIONAL PARK

Nimitz Way

Inspiration Trail

Grizzly Peak Boulevard

Cañon Drive

Lone Oak Road

Central Park Drive

CONTRA COSTA COUNTY

ALAMEDA COUNTY

Grizzly Peak Boulevard

Meadows Canyon Trail

Selby Trail

Wildcat Gorge Trail

Wildcat Canyon Road

Curran Trail

Wildcat Canyon Road

Seaview Trail

Quarry Trail

Lake Anza

Selby Trail

| 0 | 0.2 | 0.4 | 0.6 mile |
| 0 | 0.2 | 0.4 | 0.6 kilometer |

1,300 ft.
1,200 ft.
1,100 ft.
1,000 ft
900 ft.
800 ft.
700 ft.

0.5 mi.   1 mi.   1.5 mi.

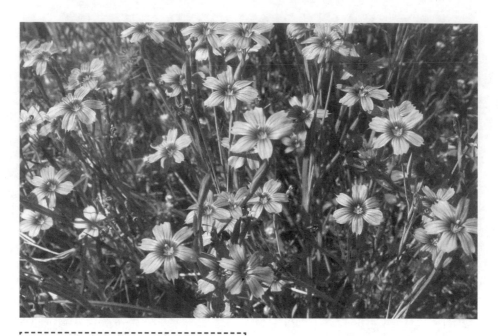

Blue-eyed grass festoons Tilden's trails in spring.

Countless future hikers have been introduced to the great outdoors at Tilden, often on an easy out-and-back excursion on Nimitz Way. With a little one strapped to a parent's chest or snuggled in a stroller, baby's first hike is one that the entire family can enjoy, with excellent facilities, a paved trail with only gentle elevation changes, plenty of rest benches along the way, and wonderful views of the East Bay and beyond.

Walk from the parking lot toward the Nimitz Gate. A gated trail on the right leads to East Bay Municipal Utility District (EBMUD) property and is accessible only by advance permit. Once through (or around) Nimitz Gate, begin hiking on paved Nimitz Way. This trail runs north for 3.5 miles to a peak in Wildcat Canyon Park, but if you're hiking with a dog and/or a child in a stroller, you'll likely want to turn back before entering cattle-grazed Wildcat Canyon. The broad multiuse trail enters weedy grassland downslope from the ridgeline to the right. Some pines tower overhead, but along the trail you might notice cardoon, a relative of the artichoke whose similarly leafy vegetation and big buds unfold to reveal pretty, thistly flowers. Expect good birding here year-round; the most commonly spotted birds include scrub jays darting from tree to tree, and vultures and red-tailed hawks perched on power lines. To get glimpses of local or migratory songbirds, you'll likely need a good pair of binoculars.

The trail undulates gently past clusters of poison oak and young coast live oak. On the left side of the trail, views unfold across the Berkeley flats to the bay, Mount Tamalpais, and San Francisco. The first of many benches along the route appears. Spring flowers include blue-eyed grass, mule ear sunflowers, check-erbloom, and yellow bush lupine, but tangles of blackberry, coyote brush, and poison oak choke out most of the grassland (and flowers) in this stretch. High-tension power lines run along the trail for a while. Around the 1-mile mark, the trail descends noticeably, then levels out again. Look for shrubby willows on the right, partly screening a seasonal boggy pond. At 1.3 miles, a trail departs on the left, heading downhill toward Tilden Nature Area, where no dogs are allowed. Continue straight on Nimitz Way.

The trail is lined with coyote brush, poison oak, diminutive coast live oak, and California bay. In summer, great clusters of sweet pea and cow parsnip draw bees and butterflies. Nimitz Way enters a eucalyptus grove where on a spring hike I saw several pipevine swallowtail butterflies fluttering through the aromatic woods. At 1.7 miles, there's a junction with a trail to Wildcat Peak on the left. This out-and-back path makes a good addition to this hike if you're hiking without a stroller. Continue a bit farther on Nimitz Way, out of the woods to a cattle guard and boundary with Wildcat Canyon Regional Park. Nimitz Way continues north, but this is the turnaround point for this hike. Enjoy views east, across the hills of Briones Regional Park, all the way to Mount Diablo, then retrace your steps back to the trailhead.

NEARBY ACTIVITIES

Tilden's northern neighbor, **Wildcat Canyon Regional Park** (5755 McBryde Ave., Richmond) provides more hiking choices on trails that climb up and down mostly grassy slopes grazed by cattle. More info: 888-327-2757, **ebparks.org/parks/wildcat.**

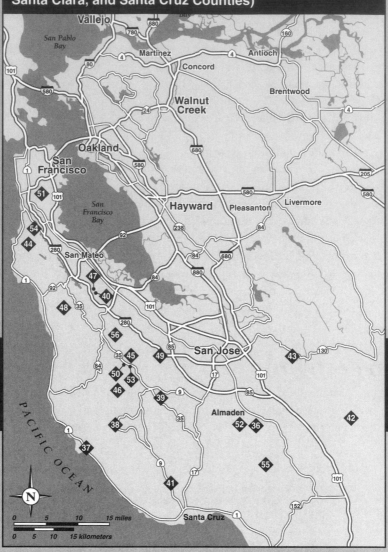

Peninsula and South Bay (Including San Mateo, Santa Clara, and Santa Cruz Counties)

PENINSULA & SOUTH BAY
(INCLUDING SAN MATEO, SANTA CLARA, AND SANTA CRUZ COUNTIES)

36 ALMADEN QUICKSILVER COUNTY PARK

KEY AT-A-GLANCE INFORMATION

LENGTH: 7.8 miles

CONFIGURATION: Balloon

DIFFICULTY: Moderate

SCENERY: Grassland, oaks, and chaparral

EXPOSURE: Mostly sunny, some shade

TRAFFIC: Quiet weekdays, steady weekends

TRAIL SURFACE: Dirt fire roads and trails

HIKING TIME: 4 hours

SEASON: Daily, 8 a.m.–sunset. Good year-round but best in spring.

ACCESS: Free

MAPS: At the trailhead's information signboard and tinyurl.com/aqparkmap

FACILITIES: Portable toilets at trailhead

SPECIAL COMMENTS: Leashed dogs welcome

CONTACTS: 408-268-3883, tinyurl.com/aqcountypark

DRIVING DISTANCE: 57 miles from the I-280/CA 1 merge at the San Francisco–Daly City border

GPS INFORMATION

N37° 10.438' W121° 49.516'

IN BRIEF

If you prefer your history laced with fresh air, Almaden Quicksilver is an ideal hiking destination. This nearly 4,000-acre park, a former mercury mine, hosts trails that wind past mining artifacts, shuttered shafts, and former settlements. In addition to the mining remnants, there are plenty of natural wonders here: scads of wildflowers, gorgeous oaks scattered in grassland, and a healthy animal population.

DESCRIPTION

On a typical day at Almaden Quicksilver, oak leaves whisper in the breeze, rattlesnakes bask in the sun, wildflowers bloom with abandon, and coyotes scamper across grassy hillsides. It's hard to believe that the park once teemed with human activity as the most productive mine in California history. For decades, the Ohlone Indians used cinnabar, a dark-reddish, cinnamon-colored mineral, for pigment, trade, and religious ceremonies. When the Ohlone showed Andrés Castillero, a Mexican mining engineer, the cinnabar deposits in 1845, he heated the mineral to release its stored mercury, and soon applied for and received mineral rights to the land, although he never set

Directions

Drive south from San Francisco on I-280 and use the CA 1/19th Avenue merge as your mileage starting point. Drive south on I-280 about 36 miles, then take Exit 12B onto CA 85 South. After about 12 miles, take Exit 6, Almaden Expressway; drive south on Almaden Expressway about 4 miles, then turn right onto Almaden Road. Drive on Almaden about 3 miles to the Hacienda trailhead, on the right side of the road.

Almaden Quicksilver County Park

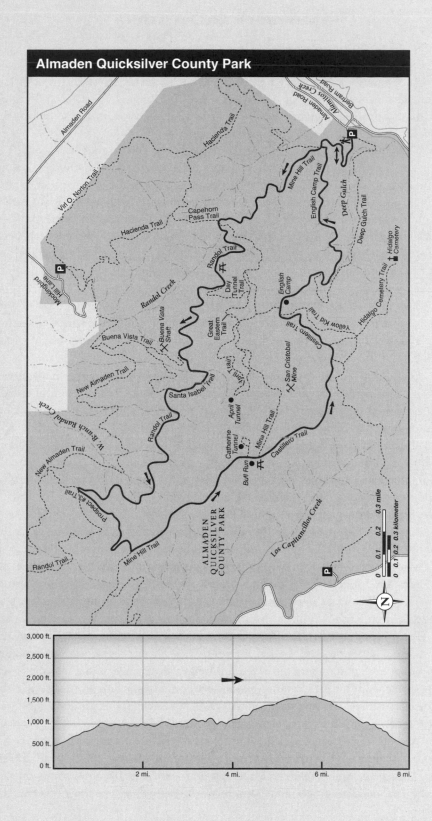

up mining operations. A private firm then retained mining rights in 1846. When full-scale operations commenced, settlements, including schools and stores, sprang up on the hillsides. Workers from all over the world mined, crushed, and heated cinnabar to produce mercury, which, although highly toxic, was essential in the processing of gold and silver, and in hat production.

Mine ownership changed throughout the years, and mining ceased in 1927 when the New Almaden Corporation went bankrupt. Piecemeal mining picked up again from 1928 to 1972, but the mines closed for good when mercury use declined and the health risks of the element became known. Santa Clara County bought the land in the early 1970s, and after a thorough cleanup, opened Almaden Quicksilver County Park in 1975. Keep in mind that although the park has been "rehabilitated," some hazards still exist: Mice in the park may harbor hantavirus, ramshackle buildings are unstable, and the land surrounding old shafts and mines can still shift. Stick to the trails to stay out of trouble here.

This hike climbs on an old mining road, passes a few mine shafts, then ascends to a grassy ridge. From there it's an easy stroll around the park's tallest hill and a steady descent through manzanita, black sage, and toyon back to the trailhead.

Begin from the trailhead on Mine Hill Trail, an old mine road that's now a dirt fire road, which ascends at a moderate clip through coast live and blue oak, California bay, and coyote brush. At 0.4 mile, the Hacienda Trail leaves on the right and English Camp Trail begins on the left—continue straight on Mine Hill Trail. In spring, you might see a variety of wildflowers along the trail, including milkmaids and blue-dicks. As the trail continues to climb, views to the surrounding mountains unfold and expand. A windy little flat called Capehorn Pass is marked by a junction and a picnic table at 1.1 miles. Turn right, pass the picnic table, and then turn left onto Randol Trail.

Angling across the hillside, Randol Trail is nearly level. If you look past the chamise and sagebrush lining the trail, you might begin to notice remnants of mining days. A gigantic pile of tailings on the right marks the spot of Day Tunnel, at 1.6 miles. Interpretive panels feature photos of the area during the mining boom. Day Tunnel Trail heads uphill on the left just past the sealed tunnel site, but stay to the right on Randol Trail.

Before long, debris piles around Buena Vista Shaft come into view on the right. At 2.2 miles, Randol Trail veers right while Santa Isabel continues straight/ left. Either trail is an option, but Randol is longer. Bear left onto Santa Isabel Trail.

Spring wildflowers, including shooting stars and baby blue-eyes, thrive in the shade of coast live oaks and California bays. Santa Isabel Trail ends at Randol Trail at 2.6 miles. Bear left to once again pick up Randol Trail.

Without major elevation fluctuations, the trail is an easy stroll. You'll pass through cool shaded canyons and more-exposed areas as Randol Trail travels west. Chaparral shrubs including black sage and manzanita occupy a sunny hillside on the left, delighting bees and hummingbirds with their blossoms. Finally, the trail reaches grassland and a junction at 3.8 miles. Turn left here onto Prospect #3 Trail.

At a fairly steep grade, the narrow path traverses a sloping meadow dotted with gorgeous mature blue and black oaks. A bountiful display of blossoms spreads through the grass in March—look for Linanthus, johnny jump-ups, and popcorn flower. Prospect #3 Trail veers into the woods, still climbing but now under the shade of black and coast live oaks. The trail emerges from the woods and ends at a junction at 4.3 miles, where you'll turn left onto Mine Hill Trail.

If you need an excuse to stop and catch your breath, a pause to admire the views is justifiable. The prominent mountain to the west is Mount Umunhum, the highest peak in the Sierra Azul range. Mine Hill Trail ascends, slightly downslope from the ridgeline, through oaks and grassland. Just past a brief shaded stretch, a trail to Catherine Tunnel branches off to the left at 5 miles. Continue straight on Mine Hill Trail, which tapers off to a level grade and reaches a junction at Bull Run. A picnic table on the right is a popular rest stop for mountain bikers. Stay to the right, now on Castillero Trail.

After a short level segment, the fire road begins a descent. On the exposed sunny hillsides along the trail you might see California coffeeberry, sagebrush, and poison oak, as well as nonnative broom and pampas grass. Keep an eye out for rattlesnakes if the weather is warm. A large complex of old mining structures is visible downhill on the right. At 5.7 miles, a trail to Hidalgo Cemetery heads off on the right. Continue straight on Castillero Trail.

Follow a steady but easy descent to the 6.1-mile mark, where you'll reach a multiple junction at the edge of English Camp. A few buildings still stand where hundreds of miners and their families lived in the late 1800s. Consult the park map and wander around if you wish—there are interpretive signs throughout the area. When you're ready, head downhill past the barns on English Camp Trail.

Winding downhill through grassland, continue straight at a junction at 6.3 miles; Deep Gulch Trail, on the right, is an alternate return route to the trailhead. As the descent sharpens a bit, the trail turns to follow a wooded canyon. Quiet hikers might surprise a bobcat loping along the trail, which is lined with toyon, black sage, manzanita, and sticky monkeyflower. Off in the distance to the right, a tall brick chimney stands at the site of a mining furnace. Other than one brief uphill section, it's all downhill from here to the accompaniment of a string of power lines. English Camp Trail ends at a junction at 7.3 miles. Turn right and descend back to the trailhead, once again on Mine Hill Trail.

NEARBY ACTIVITIES

Visit the **Almaden Quicksilver Mining Museum** (21350 Almaden Rd., New Almaden) to learn more about the history of mercury mining here. Call 408-323-1107 or visit **tinyurl.com/aqmuseum** for more information.

37 AÑO NUEVO STATE PARK

KEY AT-A-GLANCE INFORMATION

LENGTH: 4 miles

CONFIGURATION: Balloon

DIFFICULTY: Easy

SCENERY: Coastal views, seals, sea lions

EXPOSURE: Full sun

TRAFFIC: Moderate

TRAIL SURFACE: Dirt fire roads and trails; some loose sand

HIKING TIME: 2 hours

SEASON: Park is open daily, 8 a.m.–sunset. Seal-viewing area is open daily, 8:30 a.m.–midafternoon. During seal-breeding season, it can be difficult to secure reservations for the guided walks (see below); late spring and summer are great times to visit.

ACCESS: Pay the $10 parking fee at the entrance kiosk. April–November, obtain a free permit on-site to walk through the wilderness area. During seal-breeding season, mid-December–late March, the protection area is accessible only via docent-guided walks ($7), and you must preregister. For reservations, call 800-444-4445 or visit anonuevo.reserveamerica.com.

MAPS: At entrance kiosk and tinyurl.com/anonuevospmaps

FACILITIES: Restrooms and water at trailhead

SPECIAL COMMENTS: No food or dogs

CONTACTS: 650-879-2025, tinyurl.com/anonuevosp

DRIVING DISTANCE: 48.5 miles from the I-280/CA 1 merge at the San Francisco–Daly City border

GPS INFORMATION

N37° 7.184' W122° 18.441'

IN BRIEF

Although this park was created to protect elephant seals and other marine mammals, Año Nuevo is an incredibly restorative destination for humans as well. On this hike you can enjoy fresh sea air, views of the shoreline and mountains, and birdcalls. If you're lucky and the season is right, you might glimpse seals and sea lions basking on the sandy beaches.

DESCRIPTION

Año Nuevo Point was named by Spanish explorer Sebastian Viscaino to commemorate the day he first sailed past the point in 1603, on New Year's Day. At that time, a tribe of Ohlone Indians lived in the area, grizzly bears roamed along the coast and through the forested slopes of the Santa Cruz Mountains, and hundreds of thousands of elephant seals swam through the waters off the point. By the late 1800s, the grizzlies were gone and the elephant seals had been hunted nearly to extinction, primarily for their oil-rich blubber. Although their population numbered fewer than 100 when the U.S. and Mexican governments gave northern elephant seals protected status in the 1920s, they slowly began a comeback. Seals were first sighted on Año Nuevo Island in 1955, and in 1961 the first pup was

Directions

Drive south from San Francisco on I-280 and use the CA 1/19th Avenue merge as your mileage starting point. Drive 14 miles south on I-280, then take Exit 34 onto CA 92 West. Drive west 8 miles to the junction with CA 1. Turn south (left) and drive about 28 miles south to the park entrance on the right side of the road, just north of the Santa Cruz County border.

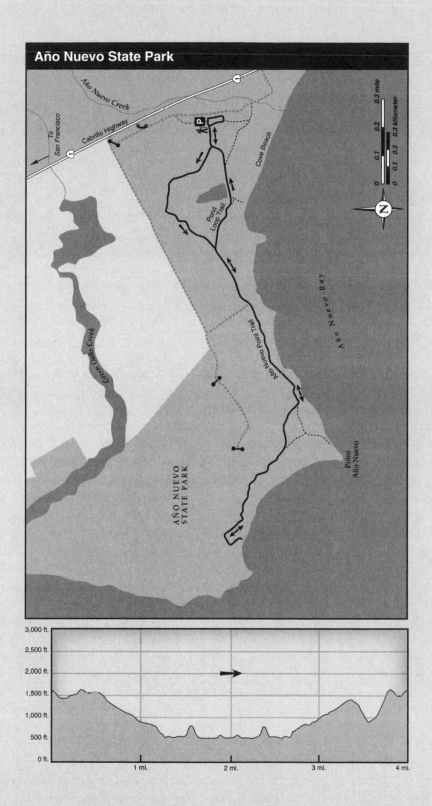

Año Nuevo State Park

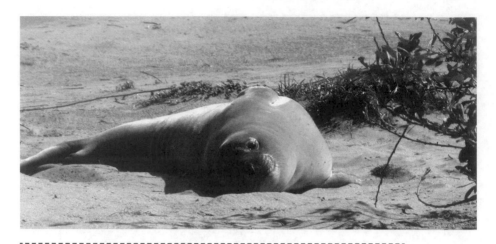

Visitors are prohibited from disturbing wildlife at Año Nuevo, but this curious seal was relaxing just a few feet off the trail. I tiptoed past.

born there. Seals moved onto the mainland to breed. In 1971, the point and island were purchased by the state of California, and a reserve was established. Since then the elephant seal population has continued to flourish, and sea lions and harbor seals have found both the mainland and island hospitable for breeding and migratory rest stops. Año Nuevo State Park now hosts the largest mainland breeding colony of northern elephant seals in the world.

Begin from the parking lot on the Año Nuevo Point Trail. After about 90 feet, you'll reach a T-junction. Turn right toward the wildlife area—if you prefer to tour the visitor center first, turn left, then return to this spot.

The first of a sporadic series of interpretive signs appears, this one telling the tale of the schooner *Point Arena,* which was bashed into bits against the rocks at Pigeon Point in 1913. A piece of the ship stands off to the side of the trail, with an old porthole nicely framing an ocean view. Pond Loop Trail sets off to the left here—this is the path for the hike's return leg, so stay to the right. Año Nuevo Point Trail keeps a nearly level grade as it travels through a plant community of coyote brush, poison oak, California coffeeberry, toyon, blackberry brambles, and grasses. A few shrubby Douglas-firs seem out of place in this coastal environment. In late summer and early autumn, yellow goldenrod is conspicuous in a sea of tawny dry grass and army-green shrubs. The ocean is audible but not visible. At 0.7 mile, Pond Loop Trail feeds in from the left. Continue straight.

The trail resembles a city boulevard, straight and wide. If you pause to look back to the east, patches of stark white soil sharply contrast to Chalk Mountain's surrounding dense forest. You'll reach the border of the wildlife-protection area at 0.9 mile. In a little exhibit building, interpretive displays describe Steller sea lions, harbor seals, California sea lions, and elephant seals. If you're visiting during the restricted season, this is the trailhead for docent-led walks; the rest of the year (with your wildlife permit in hand), proceed on Año Nuevo Point Trail.

Gorgeous ocean views unfold as the trail runs along the coast. To the west, the remains of a lighthouse constructed in 1890 are visible on abandoned Año Nuevo Island. Guide wires remind visitors to stay on the trail. As if to emphasize the point, coyote brush, bush lupine, and blackberry form protective thickets along the trail—then the shrubs thin and a boardwalk channels visitors over a damp area. Just past an exhibit about whales, the trail shifts to loose sand and dunes appear, dominating the landscape. At 1.4 miles, a path heads left toward the South Point, but stay to the right, toward the North Point seal overlook.

Past this area, the trail network is fluid and may be changed (or closed) with no advance notice to protect the seals; simply follow the guide wires and signs to stay on course. There's a tremendous amount of loose sand to climb through, so if you've ever wanted your own Lawrence of Arabia moment, you've come to the right place. From the top of the dunes the surroundings are scenic and peaceful, with the sounds of the ocean and barking seals, birds swooping overhead, and stunning mountains just to the east. You'll pass a few side paths heading off to the left—optional out-and-backs, assuming they're open. After the trail crosses a boardwalk, coastal plants including bush lupine, ragwort, coyote brush, beach primrose, sand verbena, sea rocket, and shrubby willow stabilize the dunes somewhat.

At 2 miles, the trail curves sharply left and then ends at a viewpoint above the beach. Docents can answer questions and help you identify whatever mammals are present. When I visited one year in autumn, a few elephant seals were romping in the water, building calluses on their chests for the fierce competition of mating season, which generally begins in December. When you're ready, return to the junction of Año Nuevo Point Trail and Pond Loop Trail at 3.3 miles, then turn right.

Pond Loop Trail makes its way through grasses dotted with coyote brush. The visitor center, an old barn, is visible in the distance. A few steps bring the trail down to the shores of a pond and a junction at 3.6 miles. The trail on the right descends to Cove Beach—continue straight on Pond Loop Trail, skirting the shores of the little pond, where you might see white pelicans either in the water or overhead. At 3.8 miles, a trail heads south to the reserve boundary and New Years Creek. Continue to the left, climbing slightly. The trail levels out and returns to the junction with Año Nuevo Point Trail. Bear right and, when you reach the next junction, either turn left to return to the parking lot or continue straight to the visitor center.

NEARBY ACTIVITIES

Año Nuevo's inland section hosts a trail connection to **Big Basin Redwoods State Park** (see next hike). A good guide to this area, known as Cascade Ranch, is the *Trail Map of the Santa Cruz Mountains: Map 2*, published by the Sempervirens Fund ($8; call 650-949-1453 to order).

Costanoa Lodge, a few miles north of Año Nuevo in Pescadero, has accommodations ranging from campsites to canvas-walled "tent bungalows" to hotel rooms, in a natural coastal setting. Call 650-879-1100 or visit **costanoa.com** for more information.

38 BIG BASIN REDWOODS STATE PARK:
WATERFALL LOOP

KEY AT-A-GLANCE INFORMATION

LENGTH: 11 miles

CONFIGURATION: Loop

DIFFICULTY: Strenuous

SCENERY: Redwoods, waterfalls, creeks

EXPOSURE: Mostly shaded

TRAFFIC: Very heavy around park headquarters, otherwise moderate

TRAIL SURFACE: Dirt trails, with 1 short, steep downhill scramble over rocks at Silver Falls

HIKING TIME: 6 hours

SEASON: Good all year—waterfalls are at their peak in late winter and spring.

ACCESS: Pay the $10 fee at the entrance station or park headquarters.

MAPS: At park headquarters and tinyurl.com/bigbasinmap

FACILITIES: Restrooms and drinking water at the trailhead

SPECIAL COMMENTS: Dogs are not permitted on trails.

CONTACTS: 831-338-8860, tinyurl .com/bigbasinsp

DRIVING DISTANCE: 65.7 miles from the I-280/CA 1 merge at the San Francisco–Daly City border

GPS INFORMATION

N37° 10.319' W122° 13.340'

21600 Big Basin Way
Boulder Creek, CA 95006

IN BRIEF

Redwoods, creeks, and waterfalls—that's what this loop is all about. Nestled in California's oldest state park, this popular hike begins at the Big Basin park headquarters and follows undulating Sunset Trail downhill through forested canyons to a series of three dramatic waterfalls. The return leg, a segment of Skyline to the Sea Trail, rises along murmuring creeks back to the trailhead.

DESCRIPTION

There is one main parking lot, in front of the massive REDWOOD TRAIL sign, and secondary lots across from the park store. Begin on a path to the left of the Campfire Center, following the signs to Skyline to the Sea Trail. After crossing Opal Creek on a little bridge, you will reach a T-junction with Skyline to the Sea Trail. Turn right toward Dool and Sunset Trails.

At a level grade, the broad trail runs along Opal Creek, through the outskirts of the park-headquarters area. Noise from vehicles

- -

Directions ➝

Drive south from San Francisco on I-280 and use the CA 1/19th Avenue merge as your mileage starting point. Drive south on I-280 about 36 miles, then take Exit 12, CA 85 South. After about 4.5 miles, take Exit 14 onto Saratoga Avenue. Drive west about 2 miles into Saratoga and the junction with Saratoga–Sunnyvale Road, then continue straight on CA 9/ Big Basin Way. Drive uphill on CA 9 for about 7 miles to Saratoga Gap (the junction of CA 9 and CA 35), then continue straight on CA 9. Drive downhill 6 miles on CA 9, then turn right onto CA 236. Proceed on this narrow, winding road for 8.5 miles to the park headquarters (left) and parking lots (right).

Big Basin Redwoods State Park: Waterfall Loop

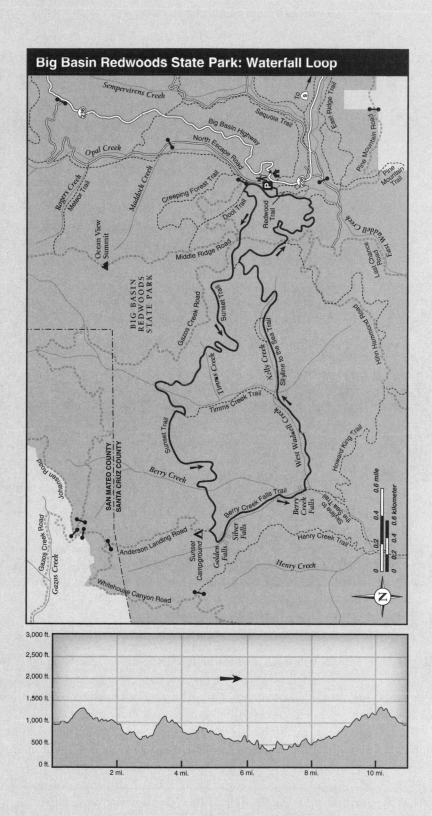

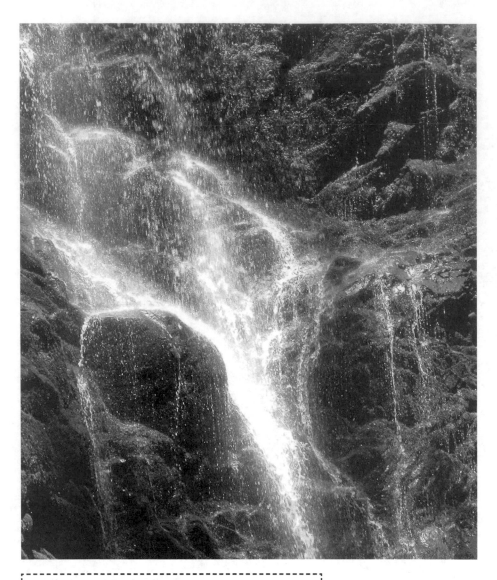

Five-finger ferns and moss thrive in the spray of Berry Creek Falls.

and park visitors fades with each step through redwood, huckleberry, and tan oak woods. After about 0.3 mile, Skyline to the Sea continues north on its way to Castle Rock, but turn left, onto Dool Trail. The trail rises easily through forest, then reaches a junction with Sunset Trail, at about 0.4 mile. Turn left.

Sunset Trail begins to climb through woods where madrone are prominent. Many of the trees along the trail have been charred by fire, and some of the huge redwoods have burned-out trunks. Early settlers confined poultry in these hollowed-out trees, which became known as "goose pens." At 0.9 mile, Sunset Trail crests at the junction with Middle Ridge Road. Continue across the fire road on

Sunset Trail, which begins an easy descent. Winding down into a redwood canyon, you might see milkwort and California harebell in summer, and in a short grassy stretch, lingering blossoms of Ithuriel's spear and vetch.

At 1.1 miles, a connector to Skyline to the Sea departs on the left, but continue straight on Sunset Trail. A few coast live oaks give way to a forest dominated by redwood and tan oak. The trail ascends gently, crosses a knoll, and drops through woods where trilliums, redwood violets, western heart's ease, and fairy lanterns bloom in spring. At West Waddell Creek, a pretty stream graced with a few big-leaf maples, the trail rises again. Timms Creek Trail begins at 3.9 miles, heading off to the left as Sunset Trail makes a sharp right turn. Timms Creek Trail, which leads to Skyline to the Sea Trail, is the bail-out route for hikers who are ready to return to the trailhead.

Continue on Sunset Trail, climbing steadily. Sunset Trail crests near a huge fallen redwood, then begins to descend through very quiet woods. After crossing Berry Creek, the path ascends again, and soon steps out of the woods to bisect a swale of chaparral. Manzanita covers the chalky white hillsides to the left and right, and these low-slung shrubs, mixed through occasional knobcone pines, permit views south to the forested canyon surrounding the waterfalls. Bush poppy's cheerful yellow flowers stand out in a sea of green in early summer, preceding the bloom of chamise and fruit on huckleberry shrubs.

As Sunset Trail leaves the chaparral, live oak, California nutmeg, and Douglas-fir bridge the transition back into redwood and tan oak. At 5.5 miles, the trail to Sunset Camp breaks off to the right; continue straight, now on Berry Creek Falls Trail. The sound of rushing water increases as the trail descends. Then, on the right, Golden Falls comes into view. A short switchback drops the trail to the side of the fall, where water slides down a sloping wall of tawny sandstone. The water rushes to a second, short drop, then pools at the top of Silver Falls. As the water shoots straight down 50 feet in a single gasp, the trail clings to the side of the cliff, descending rock stairs. The guide wire on the right is essential: Take special care when the water flow is heavy, for the steps will be slippery.

Berry Creek Falls Trail reaches the base of Silver Falls, then levels out and follows the creek. When the creek is low, you can jump across to the right and walk a few feet to get a close look at the falls. This interlude between waterfalls is my favorite spot on the hike—West Berry Creek burbles along the trail and sunlight filters through the redwoods to an understory of ferns, where starflower, trilliums, and redwood sorrel brighten the forest floor in spring and butterflies float through the air in summer. Just past the confluence of West Berry and Berry Creeks, the trail crosses the stream and rises to overlook the top of Berry Creek Falls, a 60-foot drop distinguished by gorgeous ferns and moss covering the rocks around the water flow. There are wonderful views to the falls as the trail descends to a viewing platform near the base of the falls; if it's not crowded, this is an ideal location for lunch. Past the platform, the trail descends to a junction at 6.7 miles. Turn left onto Skyline to the Sea Trail.

A bridge crosses the confluence of Berry and West Waddell Creeks, and then Skyline to the Sea Trail climbs somewhat sharply to a bench where you have one last view to Berry Creek Falls. I lunched here on one hike and enjoyed not only the waterfall view but the entertainment provided by a band of marauding Steller's jays, perched on a nearby fence hoping for bread crumbs. Past the bench, Skyline to the Sea Trail begins a rollicking course of short ups and downs along West Waddell Creek. Azaleas and big-leaf maples line the stream as the trail crosses the water for the south bank, where you may notice salal and wild rose in the understory of tan oak and redwood. Past some big boulders sitting in the creek bed at 7.9 miles, Timms Creek Trail crosses the creek on the left, at the confluence of West Waddell and Kelly Creeks.

Continue straight on Skyline to the Sea Trail, still climbing, here at a more straightforward uphill pace. The trail wanders through a beautiful redwood forest where clintonia, a lily with magenta flowers, blooms in late spring. Later, in summer, orchids unfurl, including the native reddish-striped and -spotted coralroots and purple-green helleborine, a Eurasian floral import. Skyline to the Sea Trail forks, with the left leg crossing the creek—either path is an option, as they reconnect shortly.

Past the rejoining, Skyline to the Sea Trail crosses Kelly Creek, then begins to climb out of the canyon, away from the creek. The forest remains quiet and shaded, and you might see banana slugs along the trail, particularly in cool, damp weather. At 9 miles, the connector to Sunset Trail heads uphill to the left; continue straight on Skyline to the Sea Trail. The ascent mellows as you reach the hike's highest elevation, more than 1,300 feet.

Skyline to the Sea Trail crosses Middle Ridge Fire Road at 9.5 miles, then descends through redwoods scarred by fire. At the 10.6-mile mark, bear left at a fork toward park headquarters. At 10.9 miles, you'll return to the hike's first junction. Turn right, cross Opal Creek, and return to the trailhead.

NEARBY ACTIVITIES

This is the most popular Big Basin hike (the short Redwood Trail loop is really just a walk), although you have scores of other possibilities. The website **bigbasin.org** has some brief descriptions of hiking options, along with an online trail map. One of my favorite hikes is the out-and-back trek to **Buzzard's Roost,** a sandstone outcrop with incredible views of the park.

CASTLE ROCK STATE PARK

IN BRIEF

Castle Rock is an appropriate and majestic name for a park with so much natural beauty. Starting at the crest of the Santa Cruz Mountains, this hike descends into an evergreen forest; winds through chaparral and oak; passes massive boulders and smaller sandstone formations; offers fabulous, sweeping views west; and stops at a waterfall before returning uphill toward the trailhead. On the return leg, a brief detour visits the park's namesake rock formation.

DESCRIPTION

Hikers love Castle Rock, and for good reason. It's beautiful year-round and has a few little extras that elevate it to the top tier of Bay Area parks and preserves. One bonus is a variety of vegetation, with woods, chaparral, and oak savanna. A second feature is Castle Rock Falls, less than 1 mile from the parking lot. This 70-foot waterfall nearly disappears in the driest months of the year, but winter storms send plenty of water rushing down in a single fall. The third and perhaps most unusual Castle

---

Directions ⟶

Drive south from San Francisco on I-280 and use the CA 1/19th Avenue merge as your mileage starting point. Drive south on I-280 about 36 miles, then take Exit 12 onto CA 85 South. After about 4.5 miles, take Exit 14, Saratoga Avenue. Drive west about 2 miles into Saratoga and the junction with Saratoga–Sunnyvale Road; then continue straight, now on CA 9/Big Basin Way. Drive uphill on CA 9 for about 7 miles to Saratoga Gap (the junction of CA 9 and CA 35), turn left onto CA 35, and drive south about 2.5 miles to the park entrance, on the right side of the road.

KEY AT-A-GLANCE INFORMATION

LENGTH: 5.5 miles

CONFIGURATION: Figure-eight

DIFFICULTY: Moderate

SCENERY: Chaparral, waterfall, woods, sandstone formations, oaks

EXPOSURE: Nearly equal parts shade and sun

TRAFFIC: Quiet in winter, moderate in spring, summer, and autumn

TRAIL SURFACE: Dirt trails, with quite a few short scrambles over sandstone rocks

HIKING TIME: 3 hours

SEASON: Good all year, but skip it when the Bay Area gets a cold snap— it sometimes snows in this part of the Santa Cruz Mountains.

ACCESS: Pay $8 fee at the kiosk in the parking lot (self-register if kiosk is unstaffed).

MAPS: Available for $2 when the entrance kiosk is staffed; download a free map at tinyurl.com/castlerock spmap.

FACILITIES: Pit toilets near the trailhead

SPECIAL COMMENTS: No dogs allowed

CONTACTS: 408-867-2952, tinyurl .com/castlerocksp

DRIVING DISTANCE: 54 miles from the I-280/CA 1 merge at the San Francisco– Daly City border

GPS INFORMATION

N37° 13.840' W122° 5.750'

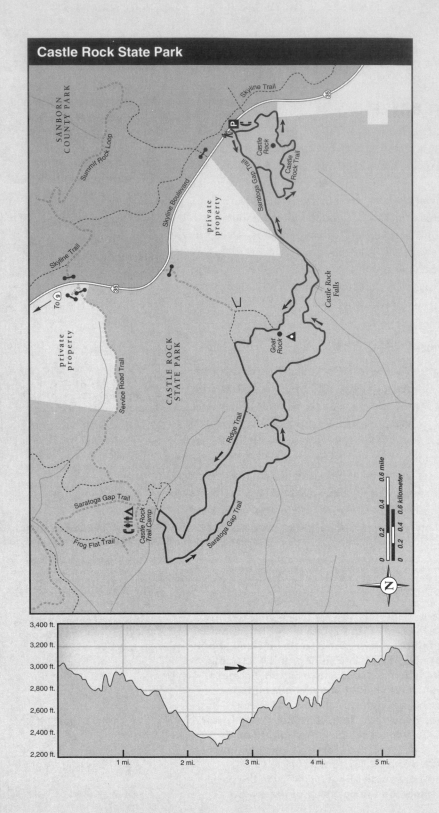

Castle Rock State Park

Rock attribute is the tafoni-sandstone formations. Although a few other locations in this part of the Bay Area have these formations, Castle Rock's are the biggest and best, with interesting clusters on the trail around the park's namesake feature, Castle Rock, and also along Saratoga Gap and Ridge Trails. The park permits low-impact climbing, so you may see climbers on the largest rock formations.

Start from the parking lot on Saratoga Gap Trail. Under deep shade, the narrow trail descends, squeezed on both sides by hillsides heavily forested with tan oak, madrone, and Douglas-fir. Look for pink-flowering currant on the right, blooming in March and April. The trail crosses a seasonal creek twice, then reaches a junction at 0.2 mile with Castle Rock Trail. Stay to the right on Saratoga Gap Trail.

The trail loses elevation steadily but moderately, following a creek bed that channels water from a confluence of smaller streams. When you arrive at the junction with Ridge Trail at 0.7 mile, you'll cross the creek on a tiny footbridge. Note the giant Douglas-fir in the crook between the two trails—easily the size of a mature redwood. Stay to the right, on Ridge Trail.

The narrow path winds a bit uphill, passing a massive white boulder. Moss-covered live oaks give way to sunny chaparral composed of ceanothus, manzanita, yerba santa, chamise, pitcher sage, toyon, and sticky monkeyflower. Deciding where to cast your gaze is tough, with sweeping views west, rocks and roots strewn about the trail, and weird rock outcrops visible uphill on the right. These odd pockmarked boulders are some of the park's most visible tafoni formations, the sandstone slowly shaped by exposure to rain and temperature change. Winter rains seep into the rocks, dissolving calcium carbonate; then summer's low humidity draws moisture containing the mineral to the rock's outer shell. Over time, the rocks develop interior weak spots and break from the inside out, creating dimples, holes, and small caves.

You'll encounter the first of the hike's two rock scrambles here, where the trail is very rocky and the route seems to disappear. At the first, the trail climbs, then drops off to the left. At the second, ascend to the right, picking your way uphill until the rocks give way to more tame terrain. The trail bends right under a buckeye at the base of Goat Rock, and a set of steps brings the trail to the upper reaches of the rock formation and a junction at 1.2 miles. The path heading right leads to an interpretive shelter. Bear left and, after a few feet, follow the trail off to the left to Goat Rock overlook. This mellow path passes through oak grassland, then ends at a viewpoint surrounded by live and black oak, manzanita, ceanothus, and chamise. Two interpretive signs help you identify landforms visible in the distance, including Monterey Bay, the Butano Range, and Big Basin's Eagle Rock. Return to the previous junction and bear left, following the sign toward Ridge Trail and the campground.

I've seen the sides of the trail, beneath madrones, California bays, and black oaks, torn up—a telltale sign that wild pigs have passed through. Feral pigs are troublesome residents of the Bay Area, and in this part of the Santa Cruz Mountains you don't have to look far to see the evidence of their bad behavior. The pigs, descended from escaped domestic swine and boars imported for hunting, dig

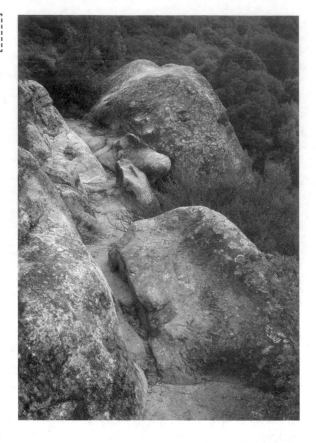

Hikers squeeze through sandstone boulders on Saratoga Gap Trail.

through topsoil searching for roots and acorns. Mountain lions and coyotes kill some piglets, but adults can tip the scales at more than 300 pounds and have no predators (except the automobile). Some parks have begun a campaign of trapping and euthanasia, but the pig problem is nonetheless spreading throughout the Bay Area. The path winds slightly uphill through grassland and trees, where baby blue-eyes blooms in April. At 1.4 miles, you'll reach a T-junction. Turn left onto Ridge Trail.

Madrones, black and live oaks, and Douglas-firs form a sparse forest along the trail as it descends easily. A little path veers off to the left, leading to a bird-observation lookout, a short out-and-back option (there are better views to come, however). At 1.7 miles, a shortcut to Saratoga Gap Trail breaks off to the left. Continue straight on Ridge Trail.

As the trail descends downslope from Varian Peak, thick stands of madrone, tan oak, and live oak close off views. Just past a spot with a rock formation and some manzanita, Ridge Trail passes beneath some towering knobcone pines. The ridgeline thins, and the trail makes a transition from a course downslope of the ridge to the top of the ridge. Woods prevail until there's a sudden break in the tree cover, and you'll step out to the edge of a cliff. Eye-popping views unfold to the west, across miles of forested ridges. The trail heads back into a forest now dominated by madrone, descending to a junction at 2.5 miles. Castle Rock Trail Camp is a short distance down the trail to the right. Turn left onto Saratoga Gap Trail.

At a mostly level grade, the trail winds through a forest where, after heavy rains, you may hear water tumbling down Craig Springs Creek on the right. Saratoga Gap Trail bends left and changes its character completely. Under the dappled shade of live oaks, the trail passes beneath a rock outcrop, then descends a short segment of very steep steps cut into a boulder. A metal guide wire bolted into the rock is helpful—there's a steep drop-off on the right. Saratoga Gap Trail ascends slightly through chaparral. As it weaves through (and sometimes over) sandstone outcrops, the views west are outstanding. Along the trail, manzanita and two varieties of ceanothus (wartleaf and buckbrush) bloom in late winter and early spring, while yellow bush lupine, paintbrush, and lizard's-tail flower later, in early summer. Other common plants include chamise, yerba santa, and toyon. A few California bays and live oaks shade the trail every once in a while. Watch out for poison oak, which is very common on the fringe of the trail. As the trail skirts Varian Peak, vegetation shifts to grassland and black oaks. The connector leading back uphill to the Ridge Trail starts at 3.5 miles. Continue straight on Saratoga Gap Trail.

Once past a little bunch of buckeyes in a gully on the right, you'll climb back into chaparral and get a good look ahead to steep, rock-studded hillsides near Goat Rock. But there's a little surprise in a damp crease along the trail: a grove of California bay and a pocket of redwood. The tour through this cool oasis is short-lived, and Saratoga Gap Trail rises back into chaparral. Keep your eyes open for tafoni with visible caves on the left side of the trail. There seems to be a "wow" with every step—hawks soaring overhead, flowers blooming at your feet, and, always, the view. The trail squeezes between two boulders, marking a transition to a woodland of California bay, tan oak, live oaks, and Douglas-fir. A pile of little boulders similar to the rock piles on the way to Goat Rock must be picked through. Waterfall-lovers may quicken their steps when they begin to hear the sound of rushing water. Hop onto an observation platform on the right for a look down to Castle Rock Falls. This 70-foot sheer drop is at its best after days of heavy rain, but it trickles even in summer. The route continues uphill, following the creek. At 4.5 miles, you'll return to the junction of Saratoga Gap and Ridge trails. Turn right, and head back uphill.

When you reach the junction with Castle Rock Trail again, turn right. The trail ascends gently through a forest of tan oak, madrone, and Douglas-fir, to Castle Rock. Unlike the largest tafoni formations toured so far on this hike, Castle Rock is not perched out in the open but nestled among the trees. Does it resemble a castle? It's surely big enough to house a family of Lilliputian elves, and it doesn't take too much imagination to see jutting pieces of rock as gargoyles, eroded into waves and cascades. The trail opens to fire-road width and passes another large rock formation on the right. Soon after, bear left, following the sign toward the parking lot. An easy descent finishes the hike, returning you to the trailhead.

NEARBY ACTIVITIES

Two other parks in the Santa Cruz Mountains feature sandstone formations. **Sanborn County Park** (16055 Sanborn Rd.; 408-867-9959, **tinyurl.com/sanborncounty park**) sits on the east side of CA 35/Skyline Boulevard, across from Castle Rock, and **El Corte de Madera Creek Open Space Preserve** (650-691-1200, **openspace.org /preserves/pr_ecdm.asp**) is on the west side of CA 35, about 18 miles north of this Castle Rock trailhead.

40 EDGEWOOD COUNTY PARK AND NATURAL PRESERVE

KEY AT-A-GLANCE INFORMATION

LENGTH: 3.1 miles

CONFIGURATION: Balloon

DIFFICULTY: Easy

SCENERY: Mixed woodland, serpentine grassland, wildflowers

EXPOSURE: Mixture of shaded woods and exposed grassland

TRAFFIC: Moderate year-round; heavy during spring peak

TRAIL SURFACE: Well-maintained dirt paths

HIKING TIME: 1.5 hours, plus more time to search for wildflowers

SEASON: Opens daily at 8 a.m.; closing hours vary (see Contacts, below). Good year-round but exceptional March–May.

ACCESS: Free

MAPS: At the trailhead's information signboard and tinyurl.com/edgewood map

FACILITIES: Restrooms, drinking water, and picnic area at trailhead

SPECIAL COMMENTS: No dogs allowed

CONTACTS: 650-368-6283, tinyurl .com/edgewoodparkandpreserve

DRIVING DISTANCE: 21.7 miles from the I-280/CA 1 merge at the San Francisco–Daly City border

GPS INFORMATION

N37° 28.387' W122° 16.690'

IN BRIEF

This hike ascends gently through coast-live-oak and California bay woodlands, then traverses grassland where hikers visiting in spring may see drifts of flowers. On the return leg of the loop, a tiny waterfall in a wooded canyon charms visitors after heavy rainstorms.

DESCRIPTION

Edgewood County Park is a little jewel of a park surrounded by a bustling highway, a busy county road, and residential neighborhoods. Thousands of commuters zip past this park every day on I-280, and between the traffic noise and the hum of suburban living, there's no confusing Edgewood with the wilderness. However, the park hosts an incredible wildflower display in spring and shelters a community of animals including hawks, coyotes, deer, and jackrabbits.

Edgewood's chaparral-coated hillsides, serpentine grassland, and oak-forested canyon were nearly lost in a series of threatened developments from the 1960s to 1993, when the parcel became a San Mateo County nature preserve and park. An Edgewood advocacy group works tirelessly to preserve habitats for endangered plants and butterflies, and docent-led hikes offered by volunteers during the

----

Directions

Drive south from San Francisco on I-280 and use the CA 1/19th Avenue merge as your mileage starting point. Drive south on I-280 about 20 miles, and take Exit 29 onto Edgewood Road. Turn left and drive east on Edgewood Road about 1 mile, and turn right into the park. There's overflow parking in a paved lot right off Edgewood Road, plus a smaller parking lot inside the park gates.

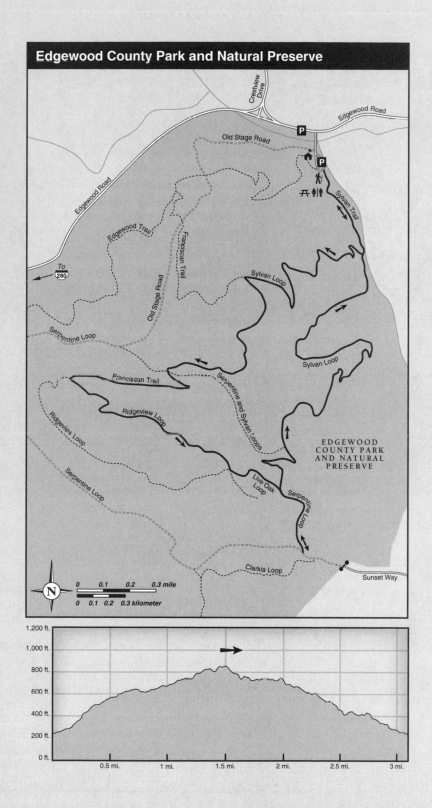

Edgewood County Park and Natural Preserve

Crestview Drive

Edgewood Road

P

Old Stage Road

P

Sylvan Trail

Edgewood Road

Edgewood Trail

Franciscan Trail

To 280

Old Stage Road

Sylvan Loop

Serpentine Loop

Sylvan Loop

Franciscan Trail

Serpentine and Sylvan Loops

Ridgeview Loop

Ridgeview Loop

EDGEWOOD
COUNTY PARK
AND NATURAL
PRESERVE

Serpentine Loop

Live Oak
Loop

Serpentine Loop

Serpentine Loop

Clarkia Loop

Sunset Way

N

| 0 | 0.1 | 0.2 | 0.3 mile |
| 0 | 0.1 | 0.2 | 0.3 kilometer |

1,200 ft.

1,000 ft.

800 ft.

600 ft.

400 ft.

200 ft.

0 ft.

0.5 mi.   1 mi.   1.5 mi.   2 mi.   2.5 mi.   3 mi.

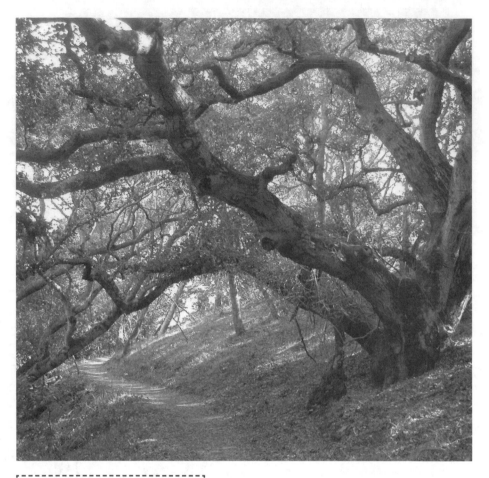

A sprawling namesake on Live Oak Trail

park's "high season" are a great way to learn about the creatures that thrive throughout the park's 467 acres. Because bicycles and dogs are not permitted in the park and horse traffic is limited to a few trails, Edgewood is very hiker-friendly and is a good destination for a family hike with small kids.

Begin at the parking lot, following the signs for Sylvan Loop Trail (not the paved service road). Along this nearly flat path, which runs parallel to the park boundary, grow a few plum trees, which flower in late winter and fruit in early summer. A few other "exotic" plants, including acacia and a palm tree, are mixed with native buckeye, California bay, and coast live oak.

After about 0.2 mile, Sylvan Loop Trail forks. Here, bear right and climb up the canyon's shoulder on a series of switchbacks, mostly shaded by mature coast live oaks and California bays. Shooting stars and hound's tongue bloom in the understory in spring, and in winter you may see birds picking berries off toyon shrubs. Poison oak is abundant, but it blends in with other benign plants from autumn to spring when it loses its leaves, so beware of bare-branched shrubs. At 0.7 mile, Sylvan Trail crests, emerges from the woods, and reaches a junction. Turn left.

Under partial cover of coast live oak and California bay, the trail skirts a hilltop on the right. From a bench crowded by sun-drenched sagebrush, views stretch across the canyon to the south. A few steps later you'll cut across the edge of a grassy plateau, then reach a multiple-trail junction at 1 mile. Continue straight on Franciscan Trail. Climb a bit to a junction at 1.3 miles, and turn left onto Ridgeview Loop, following the SCENIC OVERLOOK sign.

Traffic noise from nearby I-280 is steady, but tree cover blocks any vehicular views as the trail climbs. When you step out into chaparral, there's a break in the vegetation where you can get a peek at the Santa Cruz Mountains to the west (this is the extent of the "scenic overlook"). A thicket of chamise lines the trail near Edgewood's highest point, but soon you'll descend through some pretty coast live oaks to a junction at 1.6 miles. Turn left onto Live Oak Trail.

After a brief descent, turn right onto Serpentine Loop, 1.7 miles into the hike. Fences protect habitat as the trail enters serpentine grassland, where incredible displays of wildflowers carpet the sides of the trail in spring. Serpentine Loop reaches a junction at 1.9 miles. This is the turnaround point for the hike, but in wildflower season you might explore more in the area. Whatever you choose, retrace your steps back to the junction with Live Oak Trail.

Instead of returning uphill on Live Oak, continue straight on Serpentine Loop. A few zigzags drop the trail down a hillside to a junction at 2.2 miles. Keep going straight, now back on Sylvan Loop Trail.

Initially this part of Sylvan Loop Trail winds downhill through an open forest of oaks, madrone, and patches of grass, but after a pass through some chaparral, the path again settles into coast-live-oak and California bay woods. At 2.7 miles, a wee waterfall appears on the left after rainstorms. There's one last sunny section before Sylvan Loop Trail reenters woods, then meets the other end of the loop at 2.9 miles. Continue straight and retrace your steps back to the parking lot.

41 HENRY COWELL REDWOODS STATE PARK

KEY AT-A-GLANCE INFORMATION

LENGTH: 4.8 miles

CONFIGURATION: Figure-eight

DIFFICULTY: Easy

SCENERY: Woods, chaparral, redwoods, river

EXPOSURE: Mixed

TRAFFIC: Heavy near trailhead, lighter farther afield

TRAIL SURFACE: Dirt fire roads and trails; one paved trail

HIKING TIME: 2.5 hours

SEASON: Summer is often very hot— late winter and spring are best.

ACCESS: Pay a $10 fee at the entrance kiosk.

MAPS: At the entrance kiosk and tinyurl.com/cowellmap

FACILITIES: Restrooms and water at trailhead

SPECIAL COMMENTS: Dogs are permitted on a few park trails but not on every trail in this hike. Expect horses on most trails.

CONTACTS: 831-335-4598, tinyurl.com/cowellsp

DRIVING DISTANCE: 69 miles from the I-280/CA 1 merge at the San Francisco– Daly City border

GPS INFORMATION

N37° 2.403' W122° 3.801'

101 N. Big Trees Park Rd.
Felton, CA 95018

IN BRIEF

Visitors pour into Henry Cowell State Park, drawn to the park's magnificent redwoods, but beyond a short popular loop through the groves of giant *Sequoia sempervirens*, you'll find a vast and varied park that's lightly traveled, except by locals. This hike is a soup-to-nuts tour through redwoods, sun-baked chaparral, even ponderosa pines. You might also get a glimpse of a narrow-gauge train that passes through the park.

DESCRIPTION

Henry Cowell was a successful Gold Rush–era entrepreneur who once owned 6,500 acres of prime Santa Cruz County real estate. His heirs donated more than 1,600 acres of land abutting a county park founded to preserve one of the area's loveliest redwood groves, and the two properties became a state park in 1954.

Start from the parking lot and follow the big sign toward the redwood grove. This paved, level boulevard, suitable for wheelchairs and

----

Directions

Drive south from San Francisco on I-280 and use the CA 1/19th Avenue merge as your mileage starting point. Drive south about 36 miles on I-280, then take Exit 12 onto CA 85 South. After 7.5 miles, take Exit 11A onto CA 17 South. Drive south about 17 miles on CA 17, then take Exit 3 onto Mount Hermon Road. Turn right and follow Mount Hermon Road about 3.5 miles into Felton. Turn right onto Graham Hill Road, get into the left lane, and turn left onto CA 9. Drive about 0.5 mile south on CA 9, then turn left onto the signed park-entrance road. Drive about 0.5 mile to the entrance kiosk, then continue straight 0.1 mile to the main parking lot, at the end of the road.

Henry Cowell Redwoods State Park

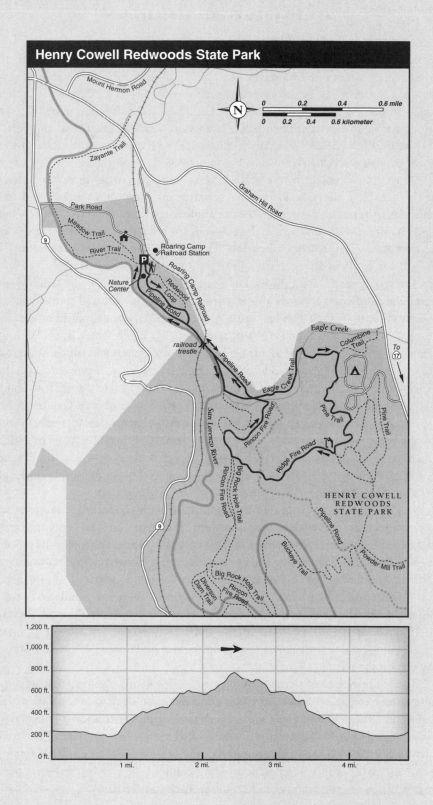

strollers, crosses a fire road near the Nature Center, and then proceeds into the grove, where towering redwoods dwarf a surrounding forest of big-leaf maple, tan oak, and California bay. At the far end of the loop, about 0.4 mile from the parking lot, slip through a gated gap in the trees, then bear right. Running parallel to the railroad tracks, the broad trail ends at a T-junction with Pipeline Road. Turn left.

The trail now descends slightly to the shores of the San Lorenzo River, where big-leaf maples grace the riverbanks. If you happen through this area when a train is either coming or going, you're in for a treat—a trestle crosses directly overhead, and the sight of a chugging locomotive is particularly appealing to kids and train enthusiasts. After a brief descent, Pipeline Trail meets River Trail at 0.6 mile—bear right. The slight trail winds through redwoods, joining a path feeding in from the left; then River Trail reaches a junction. The path to the right leads to Cable Car Beach. River Trail continues straight. Turn left onto Eagle Creek Trail.

The trail ascends along the wall of a canyon above Eagle Creek. Although the surrounding redwood forest is young, these are some mighty tall trees—you can get a good sense of their size by perusing the fallen redwoods that litter the canyon. At 0.9 mile, cross Pipeline Road, remaining on Eagle Creek Trail. With the stream still downslope to the right, Eagle Creek Trail ascends through a forest of redwood, tan oak, madrone, and California bay, with plenty of poison oak, hazelnut, and azalea in the understory. Once across a bridge, Eagle Creek Trail climbs away from the creek through mixed woods of coast live oak and California bay. As the trail surface shifts to white chalky powder, chaparral plants take over— look for pine, manzanita, bush poppy, lizard's-tail, California coffeeberry, sticky monkeyflower, and chamise. At 1.7 miles, under a pocket of woods, you'll reach a junction, with the paths left and straight leading to the campground. Turn right onto Pine Trail.

At a gradual ascent, the thin trail winds through chaparral. The sandy soil seems well suited to native plants, and the sides of the trail are crammed with manzanita, huckleberry, sticky monkeyflower, chinquapin, and ceanothus. Some tan oaks accompany knobcone and ponderosa pines. These two pines are easy to tell apart: knobcones bear closed cones, while towering ponderosas, distinguished by a "jigsaw puzzle" bark pattern, bear open ones. With the ponderosas rising from the stark white soil, you might feel far from the Bay Area; although they are widely distributed through most of the state, ponderosas are very uncommon here. A path heads left to the campground from a junction at 2.1 miles—stay to the right on Pine Trail.

The white ribbon of a trail continues ascending gently through chaparral to a multiple junction at 2.3 miles. An observation deck stands here at the park's highest elevation, offering impressive views north to the ridge surrounding Loma Prieta. This is a good spot for lunch (a picnic table also sits just off the side of the trail), but on a hot day the shade seems miserly. An interpretive sign explains that this part of the park, with its conspicuous white chalky soil, was formerly the ocean floor. When ready to continue, head right on Ridge Fire Road.

The trail does descend off a ridge, but it is no fire road—just a slight path here. Chaparral pea is mixed through manzanita, chamise, sticky monkeyflower, and pines, with some scrubby oaks and young Douglas-fir. A flight of steps drops the trail back into the woods and a junction with Pipeline Road at 2.8 miles. Continue straight on Ridge Fire Road as the trail widens and heads uphill through redwoods. You may hear traffic on CA 9, a short distance to the west but out of sight. Coming to a crest, Ridge Fire Road ends at 3 miles. Turn right onto Rincon Fire Road.

Redwoods rule as the fire road drifts downhill. Ignore two paths breaking off to the left at 3.2 and 3.3 miles. Redwood sorrel, starflower, wild ginger, and iris bloom along the trail in late spring. Rincon Fire Road ends at about 3.6 miles. Turn left on Pipeline Road.

The fire road crosses Eagle Creek, then Eagle Creek Trail. Pipeline Road descends, mostly in the shade of redwoods. You'll pass the junction with River Trail, then enjoy a dead-on view of the railroad trestle as you retrace your route back to the junction with Redwood Grove Loop Trail on the right at 4.4 miles. From the junction just past the trestle, you can walk back through the redwoods to the right, continue straight on Pipeline Road, or veer off to the left on River Trail. Whichever option you choose, it's about 0.4 mile back to the parking lot.

NEARBY ACTIVITIES

The park has a separate area called the **Fall Creek Unit** on Felton Empire Road, northwest of the main park area; call 831-438-2396 for more information. **Roaring Camp Railroads** runs trains through an adjacent redwood forest and seasonally from Felton to Santa Cruz. Call 831-335-4484 or visit **roaringcamp.com**.

42   HENRY W. COE STATE PARK

KEY AT-A-GLANCE INFORMATION

LENGTH: 4.7 miles

CONFIGURATION: Loop

DIFFICULTY: Moderate

SCENERY: Oaks, grassland, ponderosa pines, views of the park

EXPOSURE: First half mostly shaded, second section mostly exposed

TRAFFIC: Light–heavy, depending on the season and day of the week

TRAIL SURFACE: Dirt trails, fire roads

HIKING TIME: 2.5 hours

SEASON: Late winter and spring are pleasant; avoid during heat waves.

ACCESS: Pay $8 fee at visitor center.

MAPS: An excellent park map is available for $5.50 at the visitor center. Additional maps are available at tinyurl.com/coespmaps.

FACILITIES: Drinking water and restrooms at the trailhead; the visitor center, when open, sells a small selection of cold drinks.

SPECIAL COMMENTS: Dogs are permitted in the park only on one short trail, near the park headquarters.

A very good unofficial website, coe park.net, describes the most popular day hikes and details camping options.

CONTACTS: 408-779-2728, tinyurl .com/henrycoesp

DRIVING DISTANCE: 79 miles from the I-280/CA 1 merge at the San Francisco–Daly City border

GPS INFORMATION

N37° 11.180' W121° 32.803'

9000 E. Dunne Ave.
Morgan Hill, CA 95037

IN BRIEF

If you yearn for a real getaway from city life, head to Henry W. Coe State Park. Although Coe is a substantial drive from some parts of the Bay Area, it offers superior day hikes as well as long multiday backpacking treks. This loop is one of Coe's shortest, but it provides an excellent introduction to the park—touring canyons, oak savanna, and a high meadow crowned with towering ponderosa pines. Not to be missed!

DESCRIPTION

Henry Coe is California's second largest state park, and with more than 86,000 acres, it gives you plenty of room to roam through a variety of vegetation and terrific spring-wildflower displays. With so many trails, the choices are a bit mind-boggling, and overzealous visitors can get in over their heads, hiking too far in hot weather while carrying insufficient water. I recommend the loop described here for first-timers. Hiking veterans can expand this trip to a 6.5-mile trek with significantly more elevation change by substituting Fish Trail for Flat Frog, then looping to Hobbs Road via Middle Ridge Trail.

- -

Directions ⟶

Drive south from San Francisco on I-280 and use the CA 1/19th Avenue merge as your mileage starting point. Drive south on I-280 about 36 miles and take Exit 12 onto CA 85 south. Drive south 19 miles, then merge onto southbound US 101 (Exit 1A). Drive south on US 101 about 10 miles to Morgan Hill, then take Exit 366 onto East Dunne Avenue. Drive east 13 miles to the park headquarters and visitor center.

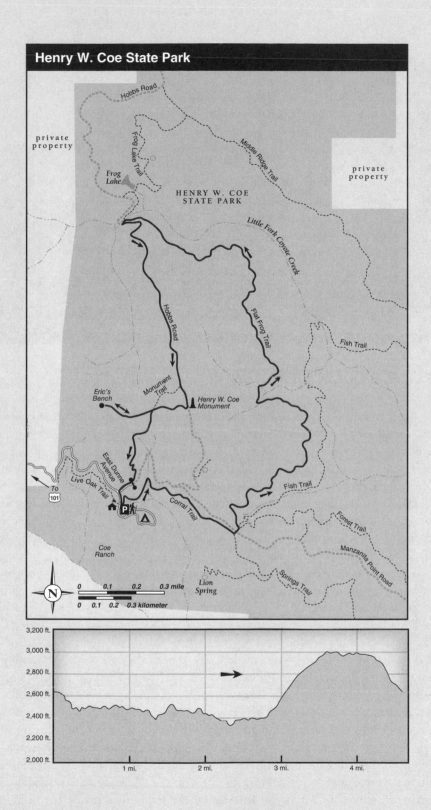

Henry W. Coe State Park

private
property

Hobbs Road

Frog Lake Trail

Frog
Lake

HENRY W. COE
STATE PARK

Middle Ridge Trail

private
property

Little Fork Coyote Creek

Hobbs Road

Flat Frog Trail

Fish Trail

Eric's
Bench

Monument Trail

Henry W. Coe
Monument

East Dunne Avenue

Live Oak Trail

To
101

Corral Trail

Fish Trail

Forest Trail

Manzanita Point Road

Coe
Ranch

Lion
Spring

Springs Trail

N

| 0 | 0.1 | 0.2 | 0.3 mile |

| 0 | 0.1 | 0.2 | 0.3 kilometer |

3,200 ft.

3,000 ft.

2,800 ft.

2,600 ft.

2,400 ft.

2,200 ft.

2,000 ft.

1 mi.   2 mi.   3 mi.   4 mi.

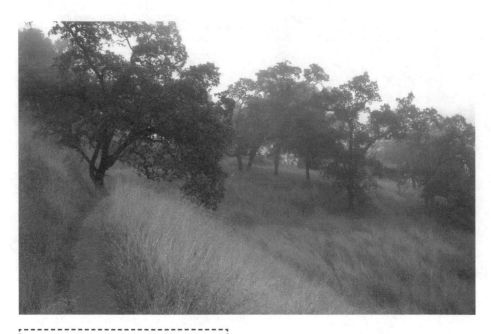

Begin from the park headquarters on the well-signed Corral Trail, which sets off at the edge of the parking lot, across from the visitor center. The narrow trail descends to cross a damp area on a wooden bridge, then begins a level journey on a ledge above a wooded gulch. On the morning of one hike, cobwebs strung through trailside vegetation glistened with dew, like strands of sparking jewels. Buckeye, California bay, and live oak shade the trail most of the way, but in a few pockets, chaparral shrubs including chamise, manzanita, and toyon bask on exposed hillsides. Like many of Coe's shaded paths, Corral Trail hosts lovely displays of fairy lanterns in spring.

The trail finally leaves the woods for good and enters oak savanna, where on a June hike thick fog obscured the landscape and massive valley oaks standing in grassland were reduced to ghostly figures looming in the distance. Up close, disturbed vegetation under the oaks is an obvious sign of the wild-pig population inside the park: Pigs dig up the ground beneath oaks while rooting for acorns. At 0.5 mile, you'll reach a signed three-prong junction. The trail to the right leads to Manzanita Point via Spring Trail, and the path straight ahead to Manzanita Point Road. Veer left toward Flat Frog and Fish Trails. After a few feet, the path crosses Manzanita Point Road and reaches a junction with Flat Frog and Fish Trails. Bear left onto Flat Frog.

After hiking less than 30 minutes, there is virtually no noise from the outside world—except for occasional airplanes traveling overhead, the soundscape is made up of birdsong, quails chirping unseen in the brush, squirrels scampering from tree to tree, and leaves whispering in the breeze. Keeping an easy grade, this slight path follows a contour on the side of the hill with a ravine to the right, winding through a sparse woodland of pines, California bay, manzanita, and a variety of deciduous and evergreen oaks. By mid-June, flowers on fairy lanterns are gone, leaving dangling seedpods, while great washes of elegant clarkia stain the drying grass pink. Occasionally, the trail bisects little huddles of chaparral, as well as increasing amounts of poison oak and creambush, but overall the vegetation is dominated by trees, including some big-leaf maple and madrone. With displays of pink flowers, coyote mint is common in late spring.

As the ravine begins to open out, there are views across the canyon to another ridge, and ceanothus, scrub oak, cercocarpus, and toyon make appearances. Thickets of snowberry crowd Flat Frog Trail, which bends left to follow a creek just before the trail ends at a multiple junction at 2.9 miles. Hobbs Road heads uphill both to the left and right, and Frog Lake Trail sets off for its namesake, sharply to the right. Turn left onto Hobbs Road.

Ascending narrow Pine Ridge, a climb begins, moderate at first but then increasingly sharp. Along the fire road, some California coffeeberry, pines, madrones, and oaks stake their claim above a grassy understory where you might see milkweed and pink-tinted clay mariposa lilies in early June. If you pause to look back downhill, Mount Hamilton's Lick Observatory dome is prominent in the distance to the north. In a little dip, Monument Trail departs to the right at 3.6 miles. Continue straight on Hobbs Road, which soon crests at the flat ridgetop.

Just as the fire road begins to descend, turn left across from a junction with the Ponderosa Trail at 3.7 miles. A short path leads to the Henry Coe monument, a small, headstonelike memorial with Coe's birth and death dates, as well as the following inscription: MAY THESE QUIET HILLS BRING PEACE TO THE SOULS OF THOSE WHO ARE SEEKING. Coe and his family ranched this land until his death in 1943. Shortly thereafter the land was sold, but Coe's daughter Sada repurchased the property, then donated the 12,230-acre parcel to Santa Clara County in 1953. Turn back to the fire road, then cross it onto Ponderosa Trail. This slight path can be hard to follow when the grass is tall, but the obscure section is short. Ponderosa winds slightly uphill through blue oaks and pine, then descends to a junction with Monument Trail at 3.9 miles. Continue straight, following the sign to the vista point.

The path rises gently, then levels out in a broad, grassy plateau, topped with a few mature ponderosa pines, blue oaks, and young madrones. At 4.1 miles, the paths split around Eric's Bench (they eventually rejoin at the park boundary). If you proceed a bit farther down the left fork, you'll come to a graceful blue oak. When you're ready, return to the junction with Monument Trail and turn right.

Descending steadily, the small footpath sweeps through grassland, then switchbacks through a pocket of California bay and ends at 4.5 miles. Turn right onto Manzanita Point Road, where a gate stretches across the fire road and dirt turns to pavement near a house. Manzanita Point Road descends gently toward park headquarters, then ends at 4.6 miles. Veer left onto the park road, and walk the remaining 100 feet back to the parking area.

43 JOSEPH D. GRANT COUNTY PARK

KEY AT-A-GLANCE INFORMATION

LENGTH: 7.4 miles

CONFIGURATION: Balloon

DIFFICULTY: Moderate

SCENERY: Grassland, views

EXPOSURE: Almost entirely unshaded

TRAFFIC: Light

TRAIL SURFACE: Dirt fire roads and trails

HIKING TIME: 4 hours

SEASON: Daily, 8 a.m.–sunset. Best in spring—not a summer destination unless you favor dehydration. Trails are often muddy, but this is an awesome winter hike.

ACCESS: Pay the $6 fee at the park entrance (self-register if kiosk is unattended).

MAPS: At the park entrance and tinyurl.com/jdgrantmap. There's also an information signboard at the trailhead.

FACILITIES: Restrooms and drinking water at trailhead

SPECIAL COMMENTS: Leashed dogs are permitted on some park trails but not on every trail in this hike. Watch out for wild pigs throughout the park.

CONTACTS: 408-274-6121, tinyurl.com/jdgrantcountypark

DRIVING DISTANCE: 56 miles from the US 101/I-280 split in San Francisco

GPS INFORMATION

N37° 20.204' W121° 42.890'

IN BRIEF

On the high slopes of Mount Hamilton, Joseph D. Grant County Park sprawls over 9,000 acres of oak-dotted grassland, less than 15 miles from downtown San Jose. Even though the park is bisected by Mount Hamilton Road, it has an isolated feel to it—I've hiked for hours here and seen only birds, cows, and wild pigs. This hike begins near an old ranch compound, skirts Grant Lake, and then climbs through an oak savanna to the ridgeline. After a sustained jaunt along the grassy ridge, you'll drop through grassland peppered with oaks, then retrace your steps back to the parking lot.

DESCRIPTION

Begin on the signed Hotel Trail at the edge of the parking lot. The first steps are paved, but when the pavement swings right, continue straight, passing the pretty old ranch buildings on the left. After 500 feet, you'll reach a T-junction. Turn left, following the sign toward Mount Hamilton Road.

Directions

Depart San Francisco southbound on US 101 and use the I-280/US 101 split as your mileage starting point. Drive south on US 101 about 44 miles, then take Exit 386A at Santa Clara Street/Alum Rock Avenue (just north of the I-280/I-680 junction). Drive east on Alum Rock Avenue about 4 miles, then turn right onto Mount Hamilton Road. Drive about 8 miles southeast on this narrow, winding road to the park entrance on the right side of the road. Once past the entry kiosk, go straight past the first parking area on the left, then turn left where the road splits and park near the gated entrance to the Hotel Trail.

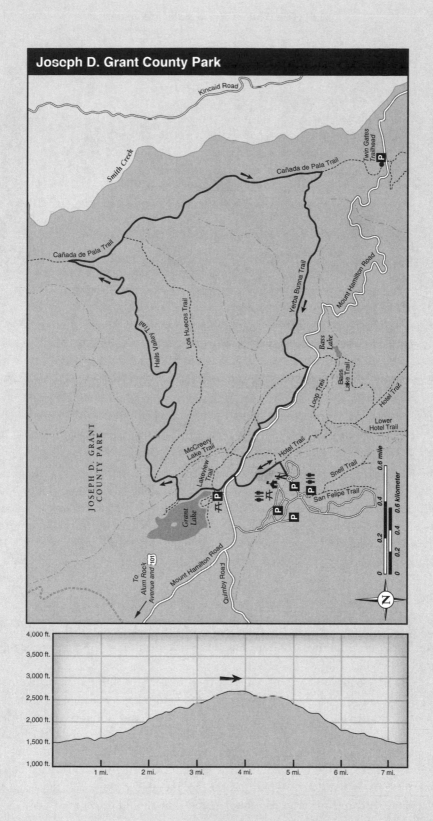

Joseph D. Grant County Park

Kincaid Road

Smith Creek

Cañada de Pala Trail

Twin Gates Trailhead

Cañada de Pala Trail

Mount Hamilton Road

Yerba Buena Trail

Halls Valley Trail

Los Huecos Trail

Bass Lake

Bass Lake Trail

Loop Trail

Hotel Trail

Lower Hotel Trail

McCreery Lake Trail

Hotel Trail

Snell Trail

JOSEPH D. GRANT COUNTY PARK

Lakeview Trail

San Felipe Trail

Grant Lake

0.6 mile

0.4

0.6 kilometer

0.2   0.4

0   0.2

To Alum Rock Avenue and 101

Mount Hamilton Road

Quimby Road

N

4,000 ft.
3,500 ft.
3,000 ft.
2,500 ft.
2,000 ft.
1,500 ft.
1,000 ft.

1 mi.   2 mi.   3 mi.   4 mi.   5 mi.   6 mi.   7 mi.

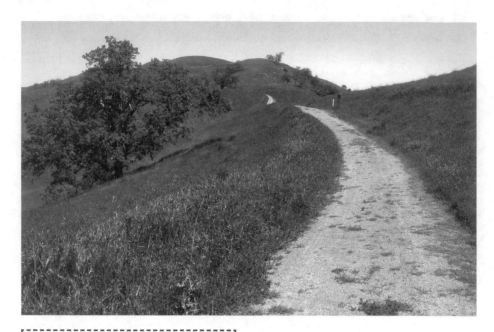

Halls Valley Trail slices through the grassland.

A few steps down the trail, a hard-to-spot path, Loop Trail, departs on the right. Continue on Hotel Trail, here a wide dirt path. Ascending easily, the trail is lined with young coast live oak and coyote brush, and in spring the sloping grassy hillside on the right hosts big patches of rose clover, along with smatterings of blue-eyed grass, vetch, fiddle-necks, and California poppy. A few cottonwoods and alders thrive on the left on the edge of a damp creek basin where I've seen some of the park's marauding wild-pig population. At 0.4 mile, the trail approaches Mount Hamilton Road. Carefully cross the street, then turn left onto Yerba Buena Trail.

The trail approaches, then swings to the right of a small staging area and reaches a junction at 0.6 mile. Turn right toward Halls Valley Trail. Lakeview Trail breaks off to the right, looping back to Yerba Buena Trail. Continue straight. Coyote brush forms thickets on the right, and just off the left side of the trail ducks totter about on the shore of Grant Lake. From a junction at 0.8 mile, turn right onto Halls Valley Trail.

The fire road dips to cross a creek, then rises again through coast live oak, valley oak, eucalyptus, and coyote brush. On one hike, I heard the distinctive *whoof* grunts of wild pigs, concealed from view in a dense clump of coyote brush just off-trail to the right. I didn't linger, since these wild pigs (descendants of game animals and escaped domesticated pigs) can run faster than I can and some of them wield tusks. Should you come across pigs, be sure to give them a wide berth. Their eyesight and hearing are poor, so they might not see you—give them a good holler and raise up your arms to look big, and they should be on their way.

Canal Trail begins on the right at 1 mile, another blink-and-you'll-miss-it trail. Continue another 0.1 mile, then stay to the left at a junction with Los Huecos Trail. At an easy grade, Halls Valley Trail begins to ascend, through coyote brush, California coffeeberry, poison oak, and black, valley, and coast live oaks. Look for yarrow, Ithuriel's spear, and checkerbloom along the trail in late April, when I once saw a long dense swath of orange scarlet pimpernel at the edge of the trail. As the grade picks up slightly, you may notice California bay and a few big-leaf maples; their shade fosters a pretty display of shooting stars, blue larkspur, buttercups, and woodland star in spring. Halls Valley Trail passes through a gate, crosses a creek, and then begins to climb at a steady, moderate grade. On the right in early May, California gilia blooms in a cluster of sagebrush and sticky monkey-flower. The landscape shifts to oak savanna, with lovely blue and valley oaks standing in grassland along the trail, many of them dangling massive clumps of mistletoe, a poisonous, parasitic plant.

Weaving through a landscape of oaks and grassland, the trail permits views north to the highest hills of the park, near Antler Point. In autumn, when the grass is sunbaked blonde, your gaze may be drawn to bright-red patches of poison oak on distant hillsides. On a hot day, every little bit of shade along the trail provides a brief but welcome respite from the sun. With the ridgeline in sight, Halls Valley Trail begins a drop to another creek. Buckeyes blend through California bays on the left—look for fairy lanterns on the right slope in April. The trail makes one last push uphill to the ridge, reaching a junction with Cañada de Pala Trail at 3.1 miles. If you'd like to add 4.5 miles to this hike, you can turn left here and loop to Antler Point; at just under 3,000 feet, it's the highest point in the park. Turn right on Cañada de Pala Trail.

At the peak of wildflower season, the slopes are filled with a variety of common flowers: Look for blue-eyed grass, popcorn flower, johnny-jump-ups, fiddlenecks, California poppy, checkerbloom, blue and white lupine, and blue-dicks. On an early-May hike, I enjoyed one of the best wildflower displays I've ever witnessed in the Bay Area, with heavily concentrated blooms all around. It's a far different scene in summer and autumn, when only oaks interrupt the one-dimensional expanse of golden grassland.

Cañada de Pala, the name of this rancho's original grant, rises gently, then reaches a junction with Los Huecos Trail at 3.5 miles. Continue straight. Across a valley to the east, the domes of Lick Observatory are visible, near the highest elevation on Mount Hamilton, 4,373-foot Copernicus Peak. Cañada de Pala Trail crosses through a gate into cattle range, where cows are present in spring and summer. In April and May, the transition is abrupt—say goodbye to wildflowers and hello to trim, bare grassland and big sections of muddy trail.

As you follow an easy, rolling course, look for a bench on trail-right, a good spot from which to gaze at the long views extending downhill to Grant Lake and beyond to downtown San Jose on clear days. The fire road drops away from this hike's highest elevation, about 2,700 feet, and you should be able to see past the rolling hills along the trail to the ridge forming Grant's southwestern boundary. At 4.8 miles, Yerba Buena Trail begins on the right. If you'd like to stretch this hike to 9.5 miles, you can continue straight here, cross Mount Hamilton Road, pick up San Felipe Trail, and then turn right onto Hotel Trail, which returns to the trailhead through the southern part of Halls Valley. To stick to this 7.4-mile hike, turn right onto Yerba Buena Trail.

The trail begins a moderate descent through cattle range. Even when the cows are in the area, some wildflowers escape them, including owl's clover, woodland star, and blue and white lupine. Poison oak is common, growing here in shrub form. Valley oaks keep a distance from the trail, so there is little shade. Bass Lake is briefly visible downhill to the left. One short uphill precedes a steady descent past a few black oaks on the right, through grassland where mule ear sunflowers, goldfields, johnny-tuck, blue-eyed grass, Ithuriel's spear, California poppy, and buttercups bloom in spring.

At 6.2 miles, Yerba Buena Trail nears the side of Mount Hamilton Road—the gate to the road is locked, but there's a step-over bench. A path to Bass Lake sets off directly across the street, but a locked gate has blocked access every time I've visited. If you can find a way over the fence, a trip to Bass Lake would make an excellent return loop to the trailhead, via the Bass Lake and Hotel Trails. Continue on Yerba Buena Trail, which runs along Mount Hamilton Road, finally leaving the cattle range at a gate at 6.7 miles. The trail here shrinks to a narrower path and keeps to an easy, mostly downhill grade. Look for a big gooseberry bush growing around a rock formation on the left.

A trail to McCreery Lake departs on the right at 6.9 miles. Continue on Yerba Buena Tail to the next junction at 7 miles. Turn left, cross the road, and retrace your steps back to the trailhead.

NEARBY ACTIVITIES

This large park offers many hiking possibilities. For mellow, easy loops, pick trails through Halls Valley, such as Lower Hotel and San Felipe. View a map at **tinyurl .com/jdgrantmap.**

MONTARA MOUNTAIN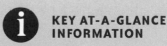

IN BRIEF

Just 10 miles south of San Francisco, coastal scrub–cloaked Montara Mountain rises from the ocean at Pacifica, offering quick and easy access for hikes with incredible views, interesting vegetation, and frequent animal sightings.

DESCRIPTION

This is a two-for-one hike through attached parks to the highest peaks of a small, rugged coastal range. McNee Ranch State Park offers fine views attained via steep fire roads. By starting at San Pedro Valley County Park you can take advantage of the county park's well-graded trails, cutting the difficulty of the climb considerably and reducing the overall distance to just under 7 miles. Combining the two also permits a peek at Brooks Falls, which drops off the north slope of Montara Mountain.

Montara Mountain has a healthy wildlife population—bobcats are sighted so often that *Lynx rufus* has become the mascot of San Pedro Valley County Park, appearing on sweatshirts sold at the park store. Why are there so many animal sightings in these two attached parks on the outskirts of residential Pacifica? Perhaps because San Pedro Valley Park and McNee Ranch State Park abut the San Francisco Watershed, a massive hunk of land stretching across

KEY AT-A-GLANCE INFORMATION

LENGTH: 6.9 miles

CONFIGURATION: Balloon

DIFFICULTY: Moderate

SCENERY: Woods, coastal scrub, waterfall, views

EXPOSURE: Some shade in the first mile, then almost completely exposed until the last mile

TRAFFIC: Light weekdays, moderate weekends

TRAIL SURFACE: Dirt trails, fire roads

HIKING TIME: 4 hours

SEASON: Opens daily at 8 a.m.; closing hours vary (see Contacts, below). Especially good in January and February for manzanitas in bloom, but nice year-round.

ACCESS: Pay $6 fee at entrance kiosk (self-register if kiosk is unstaffed).

MAPS: At the entrance kiosk, at tinyurl.com/sanpedroparkmap, and at a signboard at the trailhead

FACILITIES: Restrooms and water at the trailhead

SPECIAL COMMENTS: No dogs. Bikes aren't allowed on the trail that connects to McNee Ranch but are allowed on the state park's fire roads.

CONTACTS: 408-274-6121, tinyurl.com/sanpedropark

DRIVING DISTANCE: 11 miles from the I-280/CA 1 merge at the San Francisco–Daly City border

Directions ———————————→

Drive south from San Francisco on I-280 and use the CA 1/19th Avenue merge as your mileage starting point. After 1.7 miles, take Exit 47B onto CA 1 South. Drive 7 miles south into Pacifica, turn left onto Linda Mar Boulevard, and drive 2 miles east to the end of the road. Turn right onto Oddstad Boulevard and, almost immediately, make the first left into San Pedro Valley County Park.

GPS INFORMATION

N37° 34.690' W122° 28.531'

600 Oddstad Blvd.
Pacifica, CA 94044

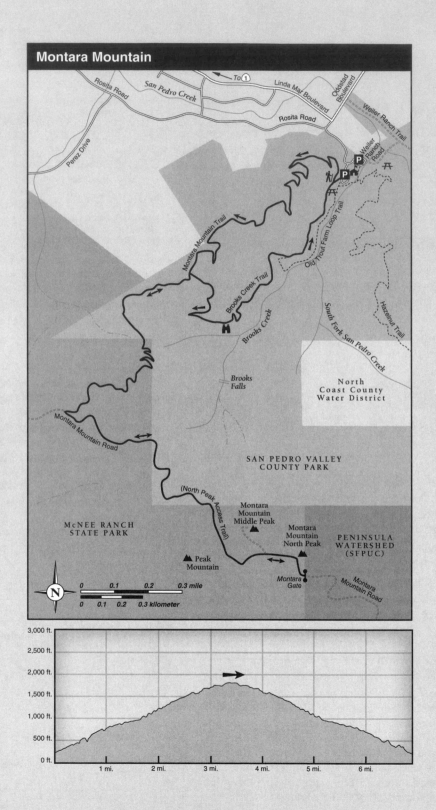

Montara Mountain

To ①

Linda Mar Boulevard

Oddstad Boulevard

Rosita Road

San Pedro Creek

Weiler Ranch Trail

Rosita Road

Perez Drive

Weiler Ranch Road

Montara Mountain Trail

Old Trout Farm Loop Trail

Brooks Creek Trail

Brooks Creek

South Fork San Pedro Creek

Hazelnut Trail

Brooks Falls

North Coast County Water District

Montara Mountain Road

SAN PEDRO VALLEY COUNTY PARK

(North Peak Access Trail)

Montara Mountain Middle Peak

Montara Mountain North Peak

PENINSULA WATERSHED (SFPUC)

McNEE RANCH STATE PARK

Peak Mountain

Montara Gate

Montara Mountain Road

N

| 0 | 0.1 | 0.2 | 0.3 mile |
| 0 | 0.1 | 0.2 | 0.3 kilometer |

3,000 ft.
2,500 ft.
2,000 ft.
1,500 ft.
1,000 ft.
500 ft.
0 ft.

1 mi.   2 mi.   3 mi.   4 mi.   5 mi.   6 mi.

the southern flanks of the mountain range. Although the watershed is mostly closed to public use, plenty of animals enjoy the wildlife corridor, which stretches from Pacifica all the way south to CA 92.

Begin near the restrooms on signed Montara Mountain Trail. The path ascends about 130 feet, then reaches a T-junction where you'll turn right onto Montara Mountain Trail. The trail crosses a service road and begins to climb through a eucalyptus forest. Zigzagging up a hillside, the sounds of residential Pacifica, at first quite loud, begin to fade.

Although in some parts of this forest eucalyptus chokes out all companion plants, there are patches of understory chock-full of natives, including California coffeeberry, hazelnut, toyon, poison oak, creambush, sticky monkeyflower, thimbleberry, currant, ceanothus, and coyote brush. This part of the mountain is not a spring-wildflower hot spot, but a few iris, hound's tongue, and starflower bloom in spring. When the trail leaves the eucalyptus forest, coffeeberry, ceanothus, and coyote brush linger, bridging the gap between woods and coastal scrub. Yerba santa is common, and chinquapin and huckleberry appear in a damp shaded spot. A few manzanitas mix in and then completely overtake the sides of the trail. Different varieties of this evergreen native bloom in stages during winter—I've seen pure pink blossoms on Montara Mountain manzanita in late November, and waves of more common white flowers around Christmas. Others bloom even later, with flowers persisting into early April. When the manzanitas are in full flower the scent is intoxicating, like honeyed perfume—just ask the hummingbirds.

At 1.2 miles, Brooks Falls Trail departs on the left. This is the return leg of the hike; before you continue straight, take a moment to enjoy the ocean view on the right. At an easy ascent, the narrow path squeezes through a dense collection of coastal scrub. A bench on the left side of the trail is a favorite of mine—I often pause to drink some water and gauge the visibility for the rest of the hike. Although the elevation here is less than 1,000 feet, on clear days you can see north to both Golden Gate Bridge towers, Mount Tamalpais, and the entire Point Reyes peninsula.

Continuing uphill, you'll pass a solitary cypress. Manzanita, while still present along the trail, no longer dominates. Silk-tassel shrubs are conspicuous in winter when they dangle curious catkinlike flowers. In spring, when blueblossom ceanothus is in full bloom, bees swarm about, giddy from the abundance of sweet-smelling flowers.

The trail sweeps uphill just off the rounded ridgeline, then begins an ascent up the face of the mountain. Switchbacks ease the climb, but the trail is eroded and rocky, and the plants along this stretch of Montara Mountain Trail are stunted and windswept. At 1.9 miles, with the switchbacking over, you'll pass from the county park into the state park. Just to the right of the transitory sign, walk a few steps out onto a rounded knoll. Views north are awesome, though not as extensive as from the top. You'll likely have this spot completely to yourself.

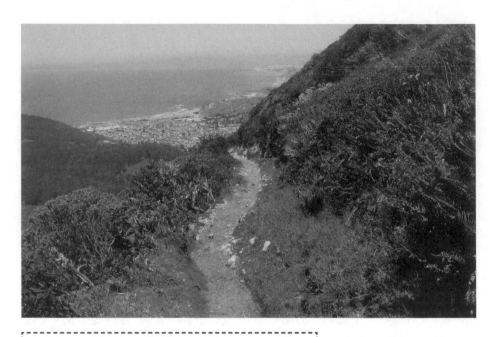

Montara Mountain Trail clings to the hillside high above Pacifica.

When I don't feel like continuing to the summit, I consider this "Far Enough Point." I once watched a chipmunk scampering over the dwarfed vegetation that grows on this granite knoll, and it's also a good vantage point to observe ravens frolicking through the skies, making their odd vocalizations and *wonk-wonk* calls. Return to Montara Mountain Trail; from here it's only 0.3 mile to the fire road, and the trail ascends at a moderate pace, clinging to the steep hillside. At 2.3 miles, Montara Mountain Trail ends, and you'll turn left onto North Peak Access Fire Road, where you should be alert for cyclists descending rapidly.

At first, the ascent doesn't seem so bad, as the wide fire road climbs through a mix of coastal scrub over bare swaths of granite. The first hill is reasonable, but the second is one steep climb. Luckily, it's a short section, whereafter the fire road adopts a more moderate grade, even throwing in one short downhill. In late winter and early spring, currant shrubs bloom along the trail, presenting dazzling pink flowers to contrast the wide-open blue sky. You also might see California poppy, paintbrush, and purple bush lupine. San Francisco wallflower, a yellow-blossomed plant in the mustard family, is so common in April that you might assume it's just another ordinary plant, but this variety of wallflower is rare.

Where the fire road crests and levels considerably, the area off to the right is scarred with paths and an old crashed car (one of several on the mountain). On the left and straight ahead, coyote brush–coated hillsides ascend to radio towers atop the two tallest points on Montara Mountain. From the top of the mountain there are new vistas, including the ocean and coastline to the west and Mount

Diablo to the east. Goldfields blaze yellow patches through the grass along the trail in spring.

When the fire road forks, if you want to climb as high as possible, you can walk uphill on the road to the left. Off to the right, North Peak is fenced and inaccessible. If you continue on the fire road to the right, you'll reach the end of the line and the watershed boundary at 3.5 miles. A fence and locked gate fail to screen views south to fire roads traveling across the spine of the ridge. You'll probably want to revel at the summit before heading back downhill, unless it's a windy day; you'll find plenty of spots suitable for a lunch break. When you're ready, retrace your steps back to the junction with Brooks Falls Trail (sometimes known as Brooks Creek Trail) at 5.8 miles, and turn right.

Along this trail, you might see rabbits nibbling on the trailside vegetation, which includes coyote brush, yerba santa, poison oak, California coffeeberry, creambush, ceanothus, blackberry, and currant. The initial path is nearly level, and then Brooks Falls Trail begins to drop into a canyon. In one damp corner, cow parsnip and forget-me-nots bloom in spring. There are views back up to the ridge, but you'll want to pay attention to the trail, which has some rocks and roots that are easy to trip over.

Manzanitas return, flourishing in a swale of red soil. A bench on the left is perfect for one last rest stop. When Brooks Falls is running, this is the best viewpoint to the three-tier falls. In all the years I've been hiking at San Pedro, I've never seen a gush to write home about, even when the sound of running water downhill in San Pedro Creek is audible. Most of the time Brooks Falls is just three little trickles, but it's still a scenic and quiet spot, and a good place to watch hummingbirds.

As the trail continues downhill, manzanita, huckleberry, chinquapin, and silk-tassel yield to eucalyptus again. At 6.5 miles, a trail doubles back to the right, dropping to follow San Pedro Creek through the remains of an old trout farm on the way back to the trailhead. Either trail is an option, but I usually continue straight on Brooks Falls Trail, which descends through a mix of coast live oak, redwood, pine, Douglas-fir, and dogwood. A picnic area is visible on the right; then the trail ends back at the hike's first junction. Turn right and return to the parking lot.

Note: Fog is very common along this part of the coast; Pacifica can be fogged in while the tip of Montara Mountain is above the fog, or vice versa. I've enjoyed this hike in fog so thick I could see only a few feet, but if you're counting on great views, pick a day with clear, stable weather.

NEARBY ACTIVITIES

San Pedro Valley Park hosts two other loop trails and one wheelchair-accessible interpretive trail that runs along San Pedro Creek. The visitor center features exhibits about Montara Mountain flora and fauna, and hosts a small store with maps and books.

45 MONTE BELLO OPEN SPACE PRESERVE

KEY AT-A-GLANCE INFORMATION

LENGTH: 6.7 miles

CONFIGURATION: Loop

DIFFICULTY: Moderate

SCENERY: Grassland, woods, creek views

EXPOSURE: Mixed

TRAFFIC: Light–moderate

TRAIL SURFACE: Dirt fire roads and trails

HIKING TIME: 3.5 hours

SEASON: Summer is often very hot; late winter and spring are best.

ACCESS: Free

MAPS: At the trailhead's information signboard and at tinyurl.com/monte bellomap

FACILITIES: Pit toilets at trailhead

SPECIAL COMMENTS: No dogs allowed

CONTACTS: 650-691-1200, openspace.org/preserves/pr_monte _bello.asp

DRIVING DISTANCE: 37.2 miles from the I-280/CA 1 merge at the San Francisco–Daly City border

GPS INFORMATION

N37° 19.544' W122° 10.743'

IN BRIEF

With a 2,800-foot elevation, Black Mountain boasts outstanding 360-degree views. Want to look down at the Santa Clara Valley? You got it. Prefer views of the forested Santa Cruz Mountains? No problem—just turn around! This hike descends to cool, quiet Stevens Creek, then ascends out of a canyon to Black Mountain's summit. The return route is all downhill, through an old walnut orchard and grasslands where flowers riot in spring.

DESCRIPTION

Oddly enough, in a preserve where everything seems supersized, I find myself particularly drawn to Monte Bello's most subtle charms. In this open-space preserve the trails, views, and hikes are long, but I get lost in the little things: new oak leaves unfolding, hillsides covered with miniature flowers, and water trickling down a tiny waterfall. It's the perfect place for a solo hike-as-meditation.

From the parking lot, walk to the signed trailhead, then turn right onto White Oak Trail. The narrow trail, which used to begin near Page Mill Road, now follows the edge of grassland along the shoulder of the wooded canyon. Initially there are views south to Black Mountain, but trees soon shade the path and

----

Directions

Depart from San Francisco on southbound I-280 and use the CA 1/19th Avenue merge as your mileage starting point. Drive south on I-280 about 29 miles, then take Exit 20 onto Page Mill Road. Drive west on Page Mill Road about 8 miles, and turn left into the preserve parking lot.

Monte Bello Open Space Preserve

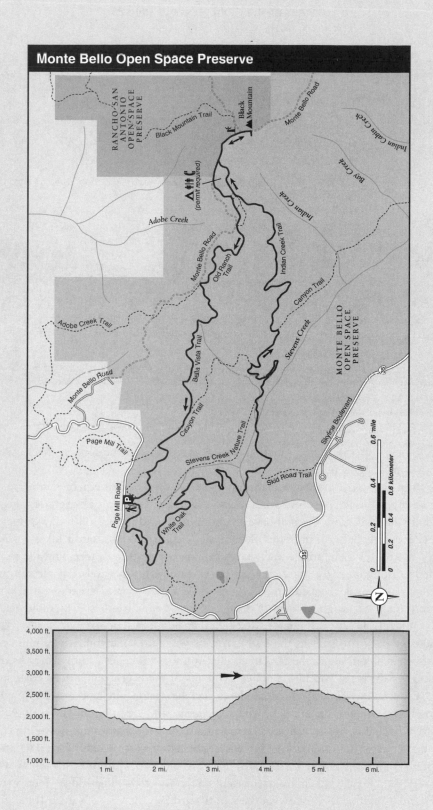

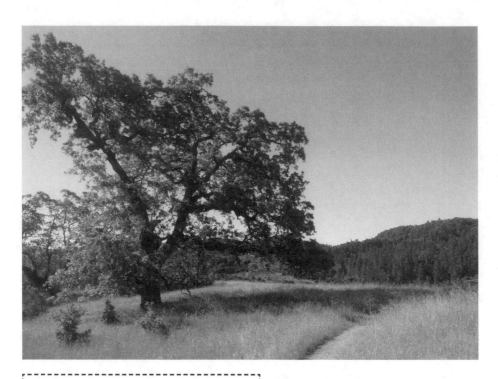

An old white oak stands in grassland at Monte Bello.

block views. At the signed junction, at 0.6 mile, stay to the left on White Oak Trail, which begins to descend.

The trail passes through madrone and oak woods, then emerges into grassland peppered with huge old white oaks. Valley and Oregon oak are both classified as white oaks, but Oregon oaks are an unusual find in the South Bay. Some of these gorgeous oaks on the sides of the trail are Oregon oaks, but it takes a practiced eye to tell them apart—oak leaves can vary from tree to tree, and the most telltale distinguishing feature, the acorn, is around for perusal only in autumn (valley oak acorns are slender and long, while Oregon oaks' are short and fat). Even though it's tough to identify them, it's easy to admire these venerable oaks.

White Oak Trail continues to descend, then adopts a series of switchbacks. The landscape begins to shift as the trail makes its way into a canyon, where mule ear sunflowers bloom along the trail in spring, in the last patches of grassland. As the tree cover thickens, you might notice two oaks of the evergreen variety, coast live and canyon live. Other common plants include California bay, big-leaf maple, gooseberry, Douglas-fir, tan oak, wild rose, ferns, and creambush. The springtime flowers, including western heart's ease, trillium, coltsfoot, and pink-flowering currant, are typical to moist dark woods and creek beds. In the dead of winter, the trail is often completely covered with fallen leaves. White Oak Trail rises to a junction at 2 miles. Skid Road Trail climbs to the right on the way to Skyline Ridge Open Space Preserve. Continue left, following the sign toward Stevens Creek Nature Trail.

This wide trail descends through a forest of Douglas-fir, tan oak, and California bay. At 2.3 miles, Stevens Creek Nature Trail heads back toward the trailhead on the left. Continue to the right, toward Canyon Trail. The trail crosses, then follows Stevens Creek. At a second bridge, a tributary drops into the creek from the left, creating a small cascade in the wettest months. Thimbleberry, blackberry, and blue elderberry thrive in the damp canyon beneath Douglas-fir and California bay, and honeysuckle vines drip from live oaks. Fairy lanterns bloom here in spring. The trail begins to ascend, then makes a sharp turn left, away from the creek. At 2.9 miles, the trail ends at a junction with Canyon Trail. Turn right.

Baby blue-eyes freckle a small, grassy meadow in spring. The fire road sweeps uphill through a pocket of woods, then reemerges into grassland and descends to a junction at 3.1 miles. Turn left onto Indian Creek Trail.

The wide fire road begins to ascend at a sustained, moderate grade. On one August hike, I caught a glimpse of a young coyote sitting in a patch of sloping grassland near the edge of woods on the right. Gradually, the accompanying vegetation shifts from madrone, oaks, and California bay to a chaparral blend of poison oak, sticky monkeyflower, chamise, toyon, California coffeeberry, ceanothus, and yerba santa. You may also notice clematis, a vine with pretty white flowers in spring and puffy seed clusters in autumn.

As the trail ascends, grassland begins to dominate, and graceful displays of popcorn flower, johnny-jump-up, chia, owl's clover, fiddle-neck, blue-dicks, and California poppy appear in spring. At 4.1 miles, a path veers off to the left. Continue straight, following the sign toward Black Mountain. The climb continues until Indian Creek Trail ends at a T-junction at 4.3 miles. Turn right onto Monte Bello Road.

As if to compensate for the climb, the last stretch to the summit, on a broad fire road, is easy. A tangle of California coffeeberry, live oaks, ceanothus, madrone, and pitcher sage blocks views to the east, but just past some communication structures, where a trail begins on the left and descends at an extremely steep grade into Rancho San Antonio Open Space Preserve, the trees and shrubs yield to grassland. Continue a little farther on Monte Bello Road to the top of Black Mountain at 2,800 feet—more of a plateau than an apex. Here, savor views east and south, including Mission Peak and Mount Hamilton. Look for a small boulder field on the right, and follow the unsigned but obvious path into this area. The treeless summit offers exceptional views, particularly of Mount Umunhum to the south and a forested ridge running to the west, much of which is preserved open space. This is a wonderfully scenic spot for a lunch break. When you're ready, return to the junction with Indian Creek Trail, then continue straight on Monte Bello Road.

The fire road descends easily, bordered by woods where you might see mournful duskywing butterflies in summer. When the road forks, stay to the left, following the sign for BACKPACK CAMP. On the right, the wide fire road passes Black Mountain Backpack Camp, a small, no-frills camp requiring advance reservations. Continue through the camp to a junction at 5.1 miles, and bear left onto Old Ranch Trail.

Almost right away, head to the right on a slight path, marked with NO BIKES, NOT A THROUGH TRAIL signs. The path climbs through grassland, then ends at a hilltop with the preserve's best views north, extending past San Francisco to Mount Tamalpais on clear days. In spring, johnny-jump-ups, fiddle-necks, and popcorn flower bloom with abandon through the surrounding grass. Descend back to Old Ranch Trail, then turn right.

The trail descends downslope from the ridgeline, through grassland dotted with coyote brush. The high reaches of a wooded ravine on the left are packed with poison oak, but thankfully Old Ranch Trail keeps its distance. You might see buttercups, owl's clover, California poppy, and blue and white lupine peeking out from spring's lush green grass. Russian Ridge is visible to the northwest, and in the foreground Bella Vista Trail is conspicuous. At 5.6 miles, you'll reach a junction with two paths on the right leading to Monte Bello Road. Stay to the left, now on Bella Vista Trail.

Beautiful views? Yes, indeed, particularly to the north and west. Bella Vista initially sticks to grassland, but as it descends, trailside vegetation becomes more varied and includes small clusters of creambush, California bay, buckeye, live oaks, and big-leaf maple nestled in creases of the hillside. Painted lady butterflies are commonly glimpsed along the trail in summer. After a steady, moderate descent, Bella Vista Trail ends at 6.4 miles. Turn right, onto Canyon Trail.

Coyote brush, buckeye, willow, and toyon mix it up along the trail. Activity along the San Andreas Fault, which runs parallel to the fire road, created the little sag pond on the right. Canyon Trail, keeping to a mostly level grade, passes a spur path on the left, then reaches a junction at 6.6 miles. Turn left, following the sign to Monte Bello parking lot.

The little trail weaves through an old walnut orchard, then sweeps right and ascends slightly. On these grassy slopes high above Stevens Creek, grassland fosters good wildflower displays in spring; on one late April visit, an entire hillside on the left was covered with pink owl's clover. At 6.9 miles, Stevens Creek Nature Trail enters from the left near a rustic stone bench. Before continuing on the trail heading right, take a moment to gaze south, enjoying one last look at Black Mountain and Mount Umunhum. The final stretch to the parking lot is short and level.

NEARBY ACTIVITIES

Los Trancos Open Space Preserve, just across Page Mill Road from the Monte Bello parking lot, offers a self-guided nature tour, with an emphasis on earthquakes and geology—the San Andreas Fault runs through both preserves. For more information, call 650-691-1200 or visit **openspace.org/preserves/pr_los_trancos.asp.**

PORTOLA REDWOODS STATE PARK

IN BRIEF

Portola Redwoods is packed with wooded canyons and rushing creeks, and you could easily spend a three-day camping holiday here and still not hike every trail. This 7.4-mile hike hits many of Portola's high points: Pescadero Creek, Tiptoe Falls, and quiet redwood forests. The last segment is an out-and-back trip to an old-growth redwood. If you're worried that this hike is too tough, you can easily break it into two loops and traverse them separately.

DESCRIPTION

Portola Redwoods State Park is a perfect tree-lover's park, with forests of mostly second-growth redwoods, mature tan oaks, madrones, and Douglas-fir extending as far as the eye can see. Tucked in canyons in the Santa Cruz Mountains' western slope, this remote and sheltered location is a haven for hikers and

----

Directions ———————————→

Depart San Francisco on southbound I-280 and use the CA 1/19th Avenue merge as your mileage starting point. Drive about 29 miles south on I-280, then take Exit 20 onto Page Mill Road. Drive west on Page Mill Road about 9 miles to the junction with Alpine Road and CA 35/Skyline Boulevard. Continue straight through the intersection onto Alpine Road and drive west about 3 miles on this narrow road (be especially careful for bicycle and motor-cycle traffic on weekends). Turn left onto Por-tola State Park Road, and drive on the tiny and winding road the remaining 3 miles to the entrance kiosk. Continue another 0.4 mile to the parking areas near the ranger station. If possible, park in the Madrone lot (to the left, just before the ranger station) or in the spots past the ranger station and across the bridge, on the right side of the road.

KEY AT-A-GLANCE INFORMATION

LENGTH: 7.4 miles

CONFIGURATION: Loop with 2 short out-and-back segments

DIFFICULTY: Moderate

SCENERY: Redwoods, creek

EXPOSURE: Mostly shaded

TRAFFIC: Autumn–spring: moderate weekends, quiet weekdays; summer: moderate–heavy

TRAIL SURFACE: Dirt fire roads and trails

HIKING TIME: 3.5 hours

SEASON: Daily, 6 a.m.–sunset. In winter, park staff remove bridges crossing Pescadero Creek, restricting access to a few trails; summer is the best season.

ACCESS: Pay $10 fee inside the ranger station, or self-register out front if it's unstaffed.

MAPS: At the ranger station and tinyurl.com/portolamap

FACILITIES: Restrooms and drinking water at trailhead

SPECIAL COMMENTS: No dogs allowed

CONTACTS: 650-948-9098, tinyurl.com/portolasp

DRIVING DISTANCE: 45.6 miles from the I-280/CA 1 merge at the San Francisco–Daly City border

GPS INFORMATION

N37° 15.136' W122° 13.086'

Portola Redwoods State Park

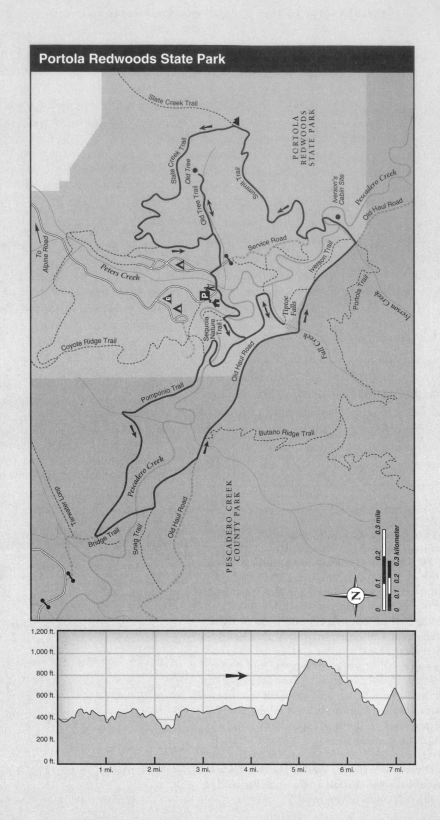

campers who seek refuge from noisy city living and summer heat. Portola Redwoods abuts two other parks, Pescadero Creek County Park and Long Ridge Open Space Preserve. Hikers have the opportunity to start at Portola and hike for miles, but many visitors are content to make short treks on two popular park trails: a short loop near Pescadero Creek and an out-and-back path to an old-growth redwood.

Begin from the side of the ranger station, on signed Sequoia Nature Trail. The path descends slightly through redwood, tan oak, and huckleberry, then bends right and drops to the banks of Pescadero Creek. Use the bridge to cross the creek, then walk along the bank until the trail ascends a few steps and soon reaches a junction at 0.2 mile. Bear left, following the sign toward Iverson Trail. Where the other leg of Sequoia Nature Trail feeds in from the right, stay to the left. The trail rises a bit to a T-junction with Iverson Trail at 0.3 mile. Turn left onto Iverson to begin the first of the hike's two out-and-back segments, ascending through a forest of redwood, tan oak, madrone, and huckleberry. The hillside drops sharply off to the left where the trail runs high above Pescadero Creek, so step carefully.

At 0.5 mile, where a path heads off to the left and down to the creek, stay to the right. This area can be bogged down by winter rains, and somewhat over-grown in summer. Iverson Trail steps over a stream, then reaches a junction at 0.6 mile, where you'll turn right and climb briefly and easily to Tiptoe Falls. Although the falls cascade only a few feet before spilling into a pool, Tiptoe Falls is a pretty and calm place that can relax and rejuvenate you in the way that only rushing water can. When you're ready, retrace your steps back to the junction with Iverson Trail and the connector to Sequoia Nature Trail at 0.9 mile. Continue straight, remaining on Iverson Trail.

The trail descends gently to wander along the forest floor. Some wildflowers that bloom here throughout spring include starflower, redwood sorrel, milkmaids, and trillium. The trail drops to the shores of Pescadero Creek, and once again you'll cross on a bridge. On the other side, the trail ascends a bit on some steps, then reaches a junction at 1.2 miles. Turn left onto Pomponio Trail. At a nearly flat grade, Pomponio follows the general course of Pescadero Creek, although the distance precludes views of the water. The forest understory is particularly dense here, with huckleberry thickets squeezing the trail in areas. Huckleberry is an evergreen shrub common to redwood canyons. Its fruit, which somewhat resembles blueberries, rip-ens in some parts of the Bay Area by late summer. Along this trail, they aren't usu-ally edible until October—the seasons seem to arrive late at Portola.

With a transition marked by signs facing both directions, Pomponio Trail leaves the state park and enters Pescadero Creek County Park. In summer, you might see fairy lanterns along the trail, and by autumn, honeysuckle berries dangle from vines twined through trees and shrubs. Madrone, California bay, creambush, toyon, ceanothus, and wild rose succeed huckleberry as the trail widens and passes through a slightly sunnier area. Where there are breaks in the forest, you can actu-ally see the surrounding forest of Douglas-fir and redwood towering above the trail. At 2.2 miles, Pomponio Trail ends at a junction with Bridge Trail. The path straight across leads to Tarwater Trail Camp.

Turn left onto a broad fire road that is level until it drops a short distance to cross Pescadero Creek. Tan oak, redwood, Douglas-fir, and big-leaf maple line the trail, which begins a moderate climb. At 2.5 miles, pass Snag Trail on the right and continue straight on Bridge Trail. Now nearly level again, Bridge Trail passes a damp, tree-lined meadow on the right, then ends at 2.8 miles. Continue left, now on Old Haul Road. Almost right away, Ridge Trail begins on the right. The trail climbs about 1,500 feet in a little more than 2 miles, then leaves the county park and heads toward Big Basin Redwoods State Park via an easement trail connection. For now, keep an easy pace straight ahead on Old Haul Road. On the high south bank of Pescadero Creek, Old Haul Road passes through redwood, huckleberry, creambush, Douglas-fir, and tan oak. In winter months, you'll likely hear water rushing as feeder creeks flow downhill on the way to Pescadero Creek. The largest of these streams, Fall Creek, tumbles into Tiptoe Falls a short distance off to the left but is inaccessible from the fire road.

At 4.1 miles, Portola Trail and Iverson Creek drop to the fire road from the right and a service road descends on the left—turn left onto the service road. Now back in the state park, you'll begin a somewhat steep descent. Iverson Trail begins on the left, but this segment of the trail has been perennially plagued with landslides. Slightly downhill from the junction with Iverson sit the remains of the cabin belonging to that trail's namesake: Christian Iverson, a Danish immigrant who was the first recorded European settler in the area. This little redwood structure was built in the 1860s and remained intact until the 1989 earthquake toppled it.

The service road winds downhill to a junction at 4.5 miles. If you're already tired, this is your opportunity to bail on the remaining hike: Simply follow the service road back to the trailhead. Otherwise, turn right onto Summit Trail. Initially, Summit Trail is a broad fire road, but once past a pair of water tanks, the trail shrinks to a footpath. At a moderate grade, the trail ascends through an assortment that by now should be familiar: Douglas-fir, redwood, tan oak, madrone, and huckleberry. If you arrive in late winter hoping for wildflowers, you'll probably be disappointed; instead look for a variety of colorful mushrooms. Wild rose is really the only understory plant here besides huckleberry to make a statement.

Curve left with Summit Trail as it travels across the sloping walls of a canyon. At one point, the trail crosses over the top of a tiny ridge, then continues to contour across the hillside. A pretty wooded knoll extends off to the right. What's marked on the map as the "summit," the highest point on this loop, doesn't quite live up to its name. You'll know you're there when you spot a handful of chamise and manzanita shrubs. There are no views, and this tiny hilltop has barely enough room for a group of three to sit. However, it's a peaceful spot to pause and listen to the wind sweep through the trees. Summit Trail descends, curves left, then levels out on a ridge and ends at 5.3 miles. At this junction, bear left onto Slate Creek Trail, which leads back to the ranger station trailhead. An easy descent commences. In some places, redwood needles and tan oak leaves cover the trail in a cushy carpet. Many of the tree trunks here are charred from a long-ago fire. Yellow banana slugs, if you

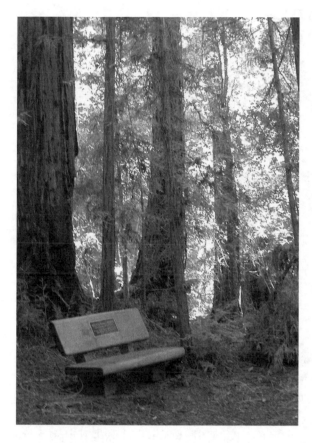

happen to encounter them, really stand out in this forest of brown and green.

Continuing a loop around the canyon, Slate Creek Trail weaves through a quiet forest where bird-calls filter through the air. Just past a memorial grove sign, look on the right for a bench nestled in the middle of a redwood fairy ring— an excellent lunch stop. Soon after, at 6.2 miles, a path to the campground departs on the right. Continue to the left on Slate Creek Trail, traverse a short, steep downhill section on some stairs, and then return to a gentle grade. Moss-covered tree stumps and evergreen plants create an incredibly lush atmosphere. Slate Creek Trail passes through a massive fallen redwood, then reaches a junction at 6.6 miles, where you'll turn left onto Old Tree Trail for a short out-and-back. Passing a huge fallen tree lying on the right, Old Tree Trail makes its way into the heart of the canyon at an easy incline, following along a seasonal creek. Western wood anemone bloom here in late winter.

At 6.9 miles, you'll reach the end of the trail and its namesake, an old tree. Cradled in a deep canyon, this redwood has a circumference of more than 12 feet and seems to scrape the sky. When you're ready, walk back to the junction with Slate Creek Trail, then continue straight. The wide path descends gently, then ends at 7.3 miles at the park road. Turn right and walk the remaining 0.1 mile along the road to the ranger station.

Note: The park is sometimes closed after heavy storms, so during winter check trail conditions with park staff before leaving home (see Contacts, page 219). From October to the end of the rainy season, bridges are removed from trails that cross Pescadero Creek. If the bridges are out and the creek is high, start your hike on Iverson Trail, across from Madrone Picnic Area parking lot, and omit the trip to Tiptoe Falls.

47 PULGAS RIDGE OPEN SPACE PRESERVE

KEY AT-A-GLANCE INFORMATION

LENGTH: 2.5 miles

CONFIGURATION: Loop

DIFFICULTY: Easy

SCENERY: Woods and chaparral

EXPOSURE: Mostly shaded

TRAFFIC: Moderate–heavy

TRAIL SURFACE: Dirt trails

HIKING TIME: 1 hour

SEASON: Good year-round

ACCESS: Free

MAPS: At the trailhead and tinyurl
.com/pulgasmap

FACILITIES: Vault toilet at the
trailhead

SPECIAL COMMENTS: Dogs are
permitted on-leash on the trails and
off-leash in a designated area.

CONTACTS: 650-691-1200,
openspace.org/preserves/pr_pulgas
_ridge.asp

DRIVING DISTANCE: 21.8 miles from the
I-280/CA 1 merge at the San Francisco–
Daly City border

GPS INFORMATION

N37° 28.504' W122° 16.969'

IN BRIEF

This hike is an easy loop through woods and chaparral at a preserve for dogs and hikers who love them (or at least don't mind them).

DESCRIPTION

Pulgas Ridge is a small preserve on the outskirts of San Carlos and Redwood City, literally just across a canyon from Edgewood County Park and Natural Preserve (see Hike 40). Both parks share a similar landscape of mixed woods, grassland, and chaparral. Both are right off I-280—a mixed blessing/curse of fast access and highway noise. The biggest difference between the two parks has four legs and a wagging tail: dogs are prohibited at Edgewood but welcome at Pulgas.

From 1926 to 1972, Pulgas Ridge housed a City of San Francisco tuberculosis sanatorium. After the hospital closed, the property was purchased by the Midpeninsula Regional Open Space District (MROSD), and the buildings were torn down in the 1980s. When I first hiked here in 2000, a motley collection of plants growing along the old paved roads was the last relic of the sanatorium era. District staff and volunteers have gradually removed cacti, oleander, rockrose, broom,

Directions

Drive south from San Francisco on I-280 and use the CA 1/19th Avenue merge as your mileage starting point. Drive south on I-280 about 20 miles and take Exit 29 onto Edgewood Road. Turn left and drive east on Edgewood about 1 mile, then turn left onto Crestview Road. Almost immediately, turn left onto Edmonds Road. Continue about 0.2 mile to the signed preserve parking lot, on the right.

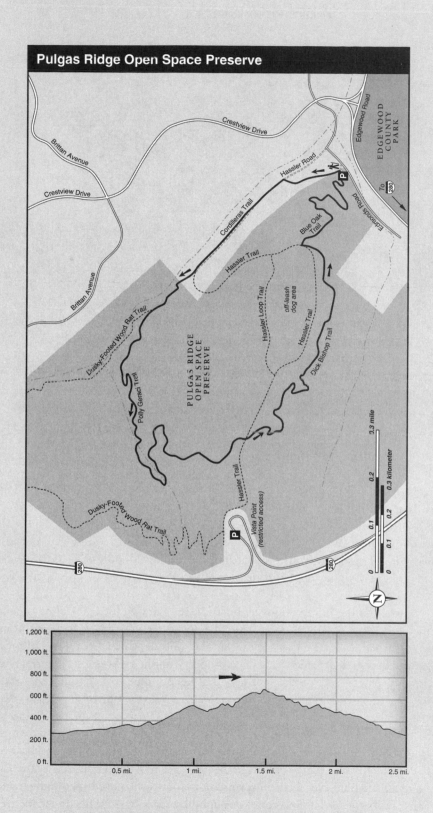

Pulgas Ridge Open Space Preserve

Crestview Drive

Brittan Avenue

Crestview Drive

Brittan Avenue

Hassler Road

Edgewood Road

EDGEWOOD COUNTY PARK

To 280

Edmonds Road

Cordilleras Trail

Hassler Trail

Blue Oak Trail

Dusky-Footed Wood Rat Trail

Polly Geraci Trail

Hassler Loop Trail

off-leash dog area

Hassler Trail

Dick Bishop Trail

PULGAS RIDGE OPEN SPACE PRESERVE

Hassler Trail

Vista Point (restricted access)

Dusky-Footed Wood Rat Trail

P

280

280

0.3 mile

0.2

0.1

0.3 kilometer

0.2

0.1

0

N

1,200 ft.					
1,000 ft.					
800 ft.					
600 ft.					
400 ft.					
200 ft.					
0 ft.					
	0.5 mi.	1 mi.	1.5 mi.	2 mi.	2.5 mi.

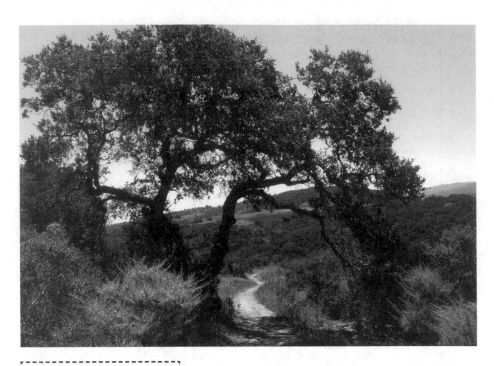

A shady spot on Dick Bishop Trail

and other nonnative specimens, replanting oaks in their stead. Only the crumbling old roads remain.

In 2006, MROSD added a parking lot and two new trails at Pulgas Ridge, greatly increasing loop possibilities. The off-leash dog area is still the preserve's hot spot for hikers with canine companions—Dick Bishop (formerly Sagebrush) Trail allows hikers to skip this area altogether. Dusky-Footed Wood Rat Trail combined with Hassler and Polly Geraci Trails is another loop option. Regardless of your hiking proximity to the off-leash area, come prepared to cross paths with dogs at Pulgas.

Start from the information signboard at the parking lot and follow the trail signed TO POLLY GERACI TRAIL. The path accompanies a string of power lines to the left, as it traverses a gently sloping hillside. Coast live oaks, California bays, and buckeyes provide shade. The property on the right is a substance-abuse-treatment center—stay on the trail here and keep it quiet. After some easy undulating, the trail bends right, passes through a narrow, tree-dotted meadow, crosses a road, and meets Cordilleras Trail at a T-junction. Turn left. Now parallel to the road, the trail borders water-district lands; stay on the trail (don't walk on the road). Not too much to look at along the flat trail, mostly poison oak shrubs, nonnative broom plants, some coast live oaks, and acacias. You might see a few Ithuriel's spear and blue-eyed grass in spring. At 0.4 mile, the paved road (here named Hassler Trail) sweeps left and continues uphill. A gated trail heads under the trees to the right. Turn right, enter the preserve, and, after a few feet, turn left onto Polly Geraci Trail.

The narrow path crosses a creek and begins an easy ascent through buckeye, madrone, coast live oak, and California bay woods. At 0.5 mile, Dusky-Footed Wood Rat Trail breaks off to the right (this is a great option for a longer hike with more substantial elevation change). Continue straight.

The wildflower display begins here in February, with red Indian warrior, blue hound's tongue, white milkmaids, and big displays of fetid adder's tongue. This plant is easy to miss until you see one, and then you'll likely see it everywhere you look—the smooth green leaves are mottled with brown spots, and the flowers are streaky brown and white. Polly Geraci Trail is one of the best locations in the Bay Area to spot this member of the lily family.

The trail switchbacks uphill, climbing out of the shaded canyon to a sun-drenched, sandy chaparral plateau. Traffic noise from I-280 is audible, and there is one stretch where the freeway is briefly visible, off to the right. Chamise and manzanitas dominate this landscape, where you also might notice sticky monkey-flower, blue elderberry, yerba santa, ceanothus, pitcher sage, and toyon. At 1.5 miles, Polly Geraci Trail ends at a signed junction. Hassler Trail, to the right, runs uphill along the ridgeline, connecting to the Dusky-Footed Wood Rat Trail near a Caltrans vista point. To the left, Hassler leads downhill to the off-leash dog area. Continue straight, now on Dick Bishop Trail.

As the trail begins an easy descent, there are sweeping views south to the forested slopes of the Santa Cruz Mountains and, even closer, of Edgewood County Park and Natural Preserve. Sagebrush and coyote brush line the trail initially, but after a while pockets of coast live oaks provide occasional shade. At 2.1 miles, Dick Bishop Trail ends at Blue Oak Trail. Turn right.

Under a mix of blue and coast live oak, madrone, and California bay, the narrow trail winds downhill. This is another good stretch for wildflower-hunting in spring, with delicate ivory-hued fairy lanterns appearing in May and golden brodiaea blooming reliably every June. Blue oaks are uncommon on the peninsula—these deciduous native oaks are more at home in southern Santa Clara, Contra Costa, Marin, and Sonoma Counties. Edgewood County Park, less than a quarter-mile to the south, has plenty of oaks, but no blues. Blue Oak Trail ends at 2.5 miles, just above the trailhead and Edmonds Road. Bear left to the parking lot.

NEARBY ACTIVITIES

If you and your dogs prefer a sunnier Peninsula destination, check out **Pearson-Arastradero Preserve** (1530 Arastradero Rd., Palo Alto), about 10 miles south of Pulgas Ridge between Page Mill and Alpine Roads. Arastradero's trails roam gently rolling grassy hills, and dogs are welcome on-leash. For more information, call 650-329-2423 or visit **tinyurl.com/arastradero.**

48   PURISIMA CREEK REDWOODS OPEN SPACE PRESERVE

KEY AT-A-GLANCE INFORMATION

LENGTH: 7 miles

CONFIGURATION: Loop with a very short out-and-back segment

DIFFICULTY: Moderate

SCENERY: Redwoods, creek, chaparral

EXPOSURE: Nearly equal parts shade and sun

TRAFFIC: Moderate weekends, quiet weekdays

TRAIL SURFACE: Dirt fire roads and trails

HIKING TIME: 3.5 hours

SEASON: Good year-round; cool in summer if you get an early start.

ACCESS: Free

MAPS: At information kiosk a short distance from the parking lot; tinyurl.com/purisimamap

FACILITIES: Pit toilets near trailhead

SPECIAL COMMENTS: No dogs allowed

CONTACTS: 650-691-1200; openspace.org/preserves/pr_purisima.asp

DRIVING DISTANCE: 26.5 miles from the I-280/CA 1 merge at the San Francisco–Daly City border

GPS INFORMATION

N37° 26.253' W122° 22.237'

IN BRIEF

This loop follows Purisima Creek upstream into a canyon, then breaks off through wooded Soda Gulch. You'll wind uphill through chaparral, then descend rapidly on a moderately steep fire road, which returns to the creek, redwoods, and trailhead.

DESCRIPTION

Large-scale logging was commonplace in the Santa Cruz Mountains, with redwood lumber widely used as building material for San Francisco structures. By the early 1900s, most of the redwood giants had been cut and hauled out of the canyons and steep hillsides. Although some small virgin groves of redwoods still stand throughout the Santa Cruz Mountains, usually tucked in hard-to-reach canyons, most of the redwood forests are second-growth woods. Purisima Creek Redwoods is no exception, although when wooded canyons are this gorgeous, I find myself transfixed by the trees rather than by the stumps.

Life along Purisima Creek and the surrounding canyons changes with the seasons. In early winter, redwood needles pad the trails, and after rainstorms, newts can be spotted

---

Directions

Drive south from San Francisco on I-280 and use the CA 1/19th Avenue merge as your mileage starting point. Drive 14 miles south on I-280, take Exit 34 onto CA 92 west, and drive 8 miles to the junction with CA 1. Turn south (left) onto CA 1 and drive about 1 mile; then turn left onto Higgins–Purisima Road (a.k.a. Higgins Canyon Road). Drive on this narrow, winding road about 4.5 miles to the trailhead, on the left side of the road just past the tiny white bridge.

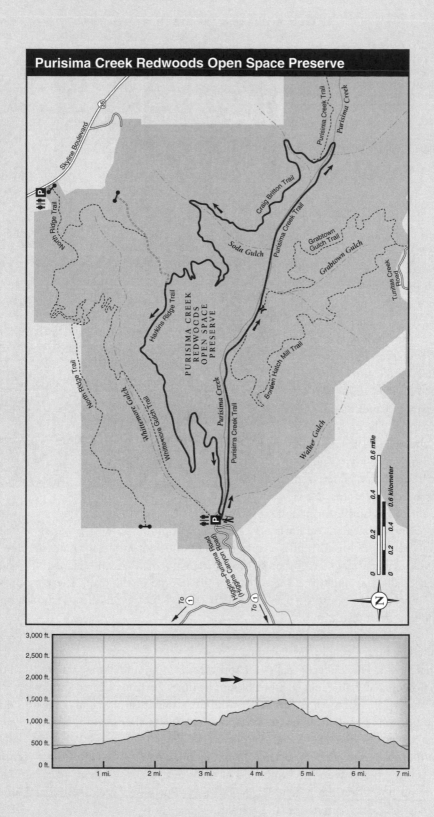

Purisima Creek Redwoods Open Space Preserve

35

Skyline Boulevard

North Ridge Trail

Purisima Creek Trail

Purisima Creek

Purisima Creek

Craig Britton Trail

Soda Gulch

Grabtown Gulch Trail

Grabtown Gulch

Tunitas Creek Road

Harkins Ridge Trail

PURISIMA CREEK
REDWOODS
OPEN SPACE
PRESERVE

North Ridge Trail

Whittemore Gulch

Whittemore Gulch Trail

Purisima Creek

Purisima Creek Trail

Borden Hatch Mill Trail

Walker Gulch

0.6 mile

0.4

0.6 kilometer

0.2

0.4

0.2

0.4

0

0

Higgins–Purisima Road
(Higgins Canyon Road)

To ①

To ①

N

3,000 ft.

2,500 ft.

2,000 ft.

1,500 ft.

1,000 ft.

500 ft.

0 ft.

1 mi.   2 mi.   3 mi.   4 mi.   5 mi.   6 mi.   7 mi.

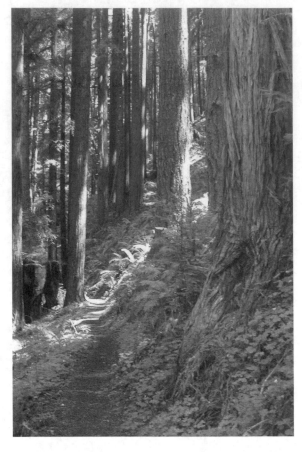

Craig Britton Trail weaves through a forest of redwood, with fern and redwood sorrel in the understory.

making their way to the creek to breed. Late winter and spring bring wildflowers to brighten the floors of the darkest canyons. Summer's abundant daylight encourages daylong hikes through chaparral spiced with the aroma of blooming native shrubs.

As you make your way from the parking lot into the preserve, almost immediately you can feel and see the cooling influence of Purisima Creek and the redwoods. The canyon wall on the right is a tangle of such moisture-loving plants as thimbleberry, alder, red elderberry, and ferns. Near the pit toilets and information signboard, Whittemore Gulch Trail departs to the left. Continue straight on Purisima Creek Trail. Running above the banks of Purisima Creek, the broad trail is nearly flat and almost completely shaded by redwoods. Banana slugs are often sighted curled up on logs and plants, although occasionally you might see one or two in the middle of the trail. These mollusks are important composters, chewing fallen leaves, needles, and mushrooms, and expelling fresh fertile soil.

After 1 mile of easy walking, you'll reach a junction with Borden Hatch Mill Trail. Continue straight on Purisima Creek Trail. The grade picks up a bit but remains easy. Huckleberry makes an appearance in an understory where trillium, starflower, and California larkspur bloom in June. Purisima Creek Trail meets the junction with Grabtown Gulch Trail; continue straight on Purisima Creek Trail.

Purisima Creek Trail presses on uphill, delving farther into the redwood canyon. A little bridge marks the confluence of Soda Gulch and Purisima Creek. You'll cross Soda Gulch again later on in this hike. After one more bridge routing the trail back across to the south side of the creek, the trail begins to climb with more purpose. At a sharp bend left, you'll leave Purisima Creek behind and, after one last hill, reach a junction at 2.3 miles.

Purisima Creek Trail continues uphill toward Skyline Boulevard. Turn left onto Craig Britton Trail (formerly Soda Gulch Trail). Continuing the journey through the darkest part of the canyon, this Bay Area Ridge Trail segment is a stunner. The narrow path winds through redwoods, angling across steeply sloped hillsides. Ferns sprawl through the understory and nestle on the shores of a little creek crossed by a small wooden bridge. Winter storms uproot trees pretty much every year, forcing temporary reroutes or short scrambles over or around the fallen giants. There's a "wow" around nearly every corner, including a surprising grassy spot where a few coast live oaks and ceanothus shrubs permit views west.

Craig Britton Trail crosses Soda Gulch on another pretty little bridge. The sound of water is supremely refreshing on a hot summer day. Finally, as the trail begins to climb, you'll slalom through a very dark patch of redwoods and then emerge on the sun-drenched slopes of the mountain, blinking in the sudden sunlight. Views here stretch to the ocean.

Switchbacks route the trail through ceanothus, coyote brush, toyon, coffeeberry, and lizard's-tail. Paintbrush, sticky monkeyflower, and cow parsnip are just a few of the wildflowers that linger into summer, thriving under a coastal influence that keeps the hillsides here green when inland parks' wildflowers are already dry and brown. A few madrones and coast live oaks shade the trail occasionally, which you'll likely appreciate around noon on a sunny day. At 4.9 miles, where Craig Britton Trail ends at a junction with Harkins Ridge Trail, turn left.

The contrast between Harkins Ridge Trail, a wide steep fire road, and the intimacy of hiking-only Craig Britton Trail is illuminated immediately. Harkins Ridge sets off downhill like it means business, through towering Douglas-fir and an understory of creambush, hazelnut, huckleberry, yellow bush lupine, and coyote brush. Watch out for cyclists zipping down the steepest sections, where the sharp grade might give hikers with unstable knees a pause. Because views have been mostly obscured by the redwoods until this part of the hike, the trail compensates for the steep descent with lots of stunning vistas. To the right you can see North Ridge and the high eastern flanks of Montara Mountain. Dead ahead to the west, hills undulate all the way to the ocean.

The trail soon veers left and begins a series of broad switchbacks, heading down into the canyon. As redwoods exert their influence, look also for hazelnut and currant. Harkins Ridge Trail ends at a junction with Whittemore Gulch Trail at 7 miles. Turn left, cross Purisima Creek for the last time, turn right, and retrace your steps back to the parking lot.

NEARBY ACTIVITIES

You can also begin a Purisima hike from the preserve's main trailhead on CA 35, 4 miles south of CA 92.

49 RANCHO SAN ANTONIO OPEN SPACE PRESERVE

KEY AT-A-GLANCE INFORMATION

LENGTH: 6.4 miles

CONFIGURATION: Figure-eight

DIFFICULTY: Easy–moderate

SCENERY: Grassland, woods, creek

EXPOSURE: Nearly equal parts shaded and exposed

TRAFFIC: Busy, busy, busy— 365 days a year

TRAIL SURFACE: Dirt fire roads and trails

HIKING TIME: 2.5 hours

SEASON: Good anytime

ACCESS: Free

MAPS: At information signboard 0.3 mile inside the park; tinyurl.com /rsamap

FACILITIES: Restrooms and water at the trailhead

SPECIAL COMMENTS: No dogs allowed. Arrive early on weekends for parking.
   The eastern hunk of this vast preserve is actually a Santa Clara County park but is managed by the Midpeninsula Regional Open Space District. Trail signs can be a bit confusing near the trailhead, and maps aren't up for grabs until you get into the open-space part of the complex.

CONTACTS: 650-691-1200, openspace.org/preserves/pr _rancho_san_antonio.asp

DRIVING DISTANCE: 38.3 miles from the I-280/CA 1 merge at the San Francisco– Daly City border

GPS INFORMATION

N37° 19.973' W122° 5.271'

IN BRIEF

After a mile of gentle strolling, you'll leave the crowds behind and climb through oaks and grassland to a vista point. Press on uphill, through chaparral where coyotes have been spotted, then descend to a shaded canyon and follow a creek back toward the farm. A bypass route skirts the area and returns to the trailhead through woods and grassland.

DESCRIPTION

Once you've nailed down a parking space, you'll start this hike with the masses, walking to Deer Hollow Farm. Begin from the parking lot near the restrooms and cross Permanente Creek on a footbridge (not the sturdy vehicular bridge on the other end of the parking lot). On the far side of the bridge, turn right onto Permanente Creek Trail, following the sign toward Deer Hollow Farm. This broad dirt trail runs along the creek through a flat grassy area.

Once past a massive California bay and some tennis courts, the trail ends at a multiple junction. Turn left, cross a paved path and the road, and you'll arrive at the boundary with the open-space preserve. Pick up a map from the signboard and continue on Lower Meadow Trail, a wide dirt path through a pretty swatch of grass dotted with coast live oaks and

Directions

Drive south from San Francisco on I-280 and use the CA 1/19th Avenue merge as your mileage starting point. Drive south on I-280 about 36 miles, then take Exit 13 at Foothill Expressway. Turn right, drive south on Foothill Boulevard, and take the first right onto Cristo Rey Drive. Drive about 1 mile and turn left into the park.

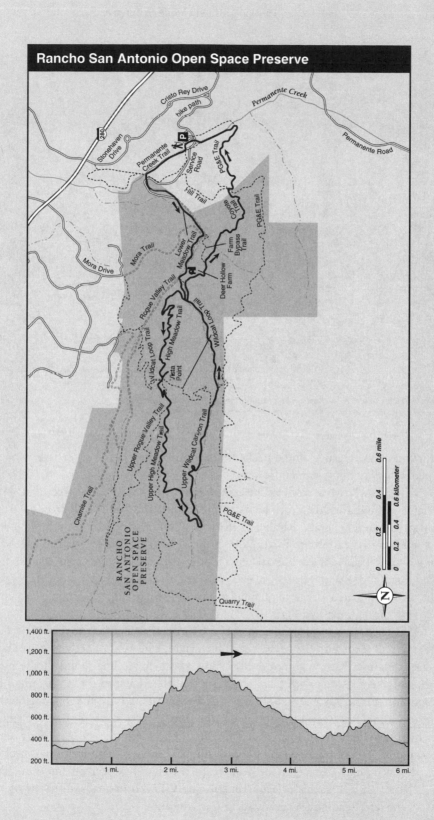

Rancho San Antonio Open Space Preserve

Cristo Rey Drive

hike path

Permanente Creek

Permanente Road

280

Stonehaven Drive

P

Permanente Creek Trail

Service Road

PG&E Trail

Hill Trail

Coyote Trail

PG&E Trail

Mora Trail

Mora Drive

Lower Meadow Trail

Farm Bypass Trail

Deer Hollow Farm

Rogue Valley Trail

High Meadow Trail

Wildcat Loop Trail

Wildcat Loop Trail

Vista Point

Upper Rogue Valley Trail

Upper High Meadow Trail

Upper Wildcat Canyon Trail

Chamise Trail

PG&E Trail

RANCHO SAN ANTONIO OPEN SPACE PRESERVE

Quarry Trail

0.6 mile

0.6 kilometer

0.2   0.4

0   0.2   0.4

0

N

1,400 ft.

1,200 ft.

1,000 ft.

800 ft.

600 ft.

400 ft.

200 ft.

1 mi.   2 mi.   3 mi.   4 mi.   5 mi.   6 mi.

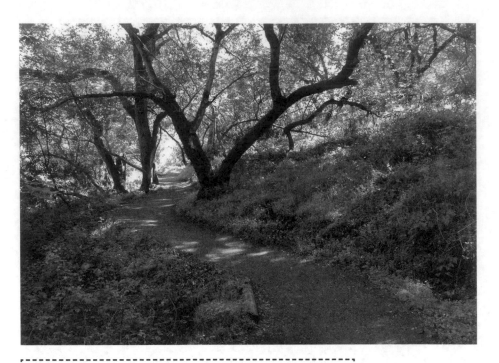

Coyote Trail is one of many Rancho San Antonio trails favored by runners.

California bays. Orange fiddle-necks bloom along the trail here in late winter, preceding yellow mule-ear sunflowers.

When Lower Meadow Trail meets the paved road, cross the street and skirt a permit parking area, then pick up a continuation of the trail. You'll cross a creek, then walk on a level grade parallel to the park road. At 0.8 mile, a multiple junction sends trails scattering in every direction. Across the paved road to the left, Farm Bypass Trail loops around Deer Hollow Farm. The other two routes, the paved road and a path straight ahead, proceed to the farm. Mora Trail, to the right, avoids the area altogether, climbing up to a grassy ridge. Continue straight, following the sign marked FOOT TRAFFIC.

This little path rolls gently up and down on the edge of grassland. At 0.9 mile, the trail feeds into the paved road. Turn right. The buzz of activity surrounding Deer Hollow Farm includes excited kids, vocalizing animals, and the hum of farm equipment. Along with farm buildings that date back to the 1850s, mature persimmon, pomegranate, and other fruit trees create an old-time, bucolic atmosphere. Although the farm is not open to the public every day, you can still enjoy watching goats and cows from the trail side of the fence and peer into a pretty garden of flowers and vegetables. Wild animals seem ridiculously comfortable near the farm, and you might see deer or quail only a few feet off the trail. Just past a barn that wears a historical patina, Rogue Valley Trail heads off to the right. Stay to the left, heading toward Wildcat Canyon Trail.

A few steps past some pit toilets, you'll pass Farm Bypass Trail, which enters from the left. Continue straight through a damp area where willow, big-leaf maple, buckeye, ninebark, and blackberry brambles form a dense wall of vegetation. At 1.2 miles, Wildcat Canyon Trail continues straight, while a path to Coyote Trail sets off to the left. Turn right onto High Meadow Trail.

An assortment of native plants lines this broad trail, including silk-tassel, sagebrush, sticky monkeyflower, poison oak, pitcher sage, coast live oak, buckeye, and toyon. High Meadow Trail curves uphill at a moderate grade, then turns left and begins a series of long switchbacks, which softens the ascent. As the trail meets the lower reaches of a sloping, grassy meadow, blue oaks and coast live oaks appear. Coast live oaks are evergreen and enjoy each other's company, while deciduous blue oaks stand in more-solitary formations here. Blue oaks are easy to pick out in autumn, when their leaves are at their bluest, and in late winter, when they leaf out. Mule ear sunflowers bloom along the trail in abundance as early as March, and if you visit in late May or early June, you might see a few mariposa lilies.

The trail continues uphill on the edge of the sloping grassy hillside, passing coast live oak, toyon, and a few cercocarpus. Look for several venerable valley oaks that grace the grassland to your left.

At 2.1 miles, moving clockwise at a multiple junction, the first path to the left heads to a vista point, Wildcat Loop Trail descends to Wildcat Canyon Trail, High Meadow Trail keeps climbing, and the other segment of Wildcat Loop Trail drops toward Rogue Valley Trail. Turn left for a short out-and-back on the path to the vista point.

The trail ascends quickly, then ends at a belvedere. Straight ahead, the sloping, grassy meadow peppered with oaks descends to the south, framing a view across Silicon Valley to peaks of the Mount Hamilton range. Return downhill to the previous junction, then resume uphill on High Meadow Trail.

After a few steps, the trails split. Either route is an option, but the path on the right is less steep than the fire road, so bear right.

Angling across the hillside, the trail enters a shaded area where California bays mix with coast live oak, sticky monkeyflower, poison oak, and toyon. After a switchback, the path meets and crosses the steep fire road. The difference between the two sides of the hill is remarkable. On these sunny slopes, chamise basks in the sun along with sagebrush and toyon. There are good views to the northwest of Black Mountain, which tops out at 2,800 feet. At 2.5 miles, the two legs of High Meadow Trail rejoin for good at a junction where Upper Rogue Valley Trail drops off the ridge on the right. Continue to the left on High Meadow Trail.

The trail ascends slightly through chaparral and then reaches a junction at 2.8 miles. Upper High Meadow Trail continues uphill straight ahead, presenting a good option for extending this hike 2 miles, on a loop through one of the most remote parts of the preserve, but for today's hike bear left onto Upper Wildcat Canyon Trail.

Descending, Upper Wildcat Canyon Trail winds through madrone, toyon, silk-tassel, chamise, California coffeeberry, pitcher sage, and coast live oak. As the trail drops into Wildcat Canyon, a forest of California bays overtakes the landscape; then the trail bends left and runs along a creek. It's hard to believe that this quiet section of the park is less than 2 miles from the farm area. With steep hills rising up to the right and left, this trail really captures the essence of a canyon, and in the heat of summer, the sound of water and total shade are welcome. In October and November, big-leaf maples create a gorgeous autumnal tableau, releasing their colorful leaves to drift slowly down to the trail and creek. The trail descends gently to a junction at 4.2 miles with Wildcat Loop Trail. Continue to the right, now on Wildcat Canyon Trail.

Creambush, coast live oak, California bay, and blackberries tangle along the trail, accompanying a large colony of western leatherwood. Early wildflowers include trillium, hound's tongue, and milkmaids. A connector to PG&E Trail departs to the right at 4.3 miles, but continue left on Wildcat Canyon Trail.

As you make your way out of the heart of the canyon, the trail crosses the creek on tiny bridges under gracefully arching California bays. At 4.8 miles, you'll reach a familiar junction with High Meadow Trail. Continue straight a few feet, then bear right toward Farm Bypass Trail.

Buckeyes dominate the landscape as the narrow trail ascends easily. You might notice California bay, poison oak, and pitcher sage, as well as trilliums in late winter. Farm Bypass Trail breaks off to the left at 5 miles, but continue to the right on Coyote Trail.

Runners favor this trail for its easy grade and abundant shade. In this fairly open woodland, the limited understory vegetation makes it easy to find wildflowers such as woodland star and mission bells. When the trail enters a sunny area, look for clematis, a trailing vine, draped over shrubs. Gooseberry, ceanothus, sagebrush, poison oak, and sticky monkeyflower are common here. Just past some blue oaks, the trail ends at 5.7 miles. PG&E Trail doubles back to the right, and Hill Trail descends on the left, past a water tank. Make a soft right, following the sign reading TO COUNTY PARK.

Vetch covers much of the hillside on the right, and coast live oak, California bay, buckeye, and blue oak are scattered about. Where the trail descends to a junction near the equestrian parking at 6.1 miles, turn left. The perfectly flat path accompanies Permanente Creek, on the right, screened by willows. At 6.4 miles, you'll reach a junction with a paved bike path and the park road. Turn right and cross the bridge to return to the parking lot.

RUSSIAN RIDGE OPEN SPACE PRESERVE 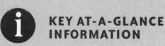 50

IN BRIEF

When spring in all its glory graces the Bay Area, Russian Ridge is one of the top destinations to enjoy swaths of green grass, gentle breezes, and wildflowers. This loop showcases the best of the preserve on an easy circuit through grass-land and clusters of venerable live oaks.

DESCRIPTION

Russian Ridge Open Space Preserve sprawls over one of the Santa Cruz Mountains' rare treeless ridges, so the views are incredible. And because the trailhead is right off CA 35, Russian Ridge is easy to get to and easy to hike—it takes just 10 minutes of walking to reach the ridgeline.

If you're on a wildflower mission, you might go no farther than an out-and-back jaunt along the ridge. Here, usually peaking in early May, a dramatic blossom extravaganza unfolds, with some massive carpets of lupines shading the grass purple and liberal multihued sprinklings from tidytips, owl's clover, California poppy, creamcups, and johnny-jump-ups. Although Russian Ridge is renowned as a wildflower destination, the preserve offers good hike possibilities year-round.

Directions ➞

Depart from San Francisco on southbound I-280 and use the CA 1/19th Avenue merge as your mileage starting point. Drive south on I-280 about 29 miles, then take Exit 20 onto Page Mill Road. Drive west on Page Mill Road about 9 miles to the junction with CA 35/ Skyline Boulevard. Cross Skyline and continue straight onto Alpine Road; then, almost immediately, make the first right into the preserve parking lot.

i KEY AT-A-GLANCE INFORMATION

LENGTH: 3.6 miles

CONFIGURATION: Balloon

DIFFICULTY: Easy

SCENERY: Grassland, oaks, wildflowers

EXPOSURE: Mostly unshaded

TRAFFIC: Moderate weekends, quiet weekdays, busy during wildflower peak

TRAIL SURFACE: Dirt trails and fire roads

HIKING TIME: 2 hours

SEASON: Good anytime; amazing in spring

ACCESS: Free

MAPS: At information signboard in the parking lot; tinyurl.com/russian ridgemap

FACILITIES: Pit toilets at trailhead

SPECIAL COMMENTS: No dogs allowed

CONTACTS: 650-691-1200, openspace.org/preserves/pr _russian_ridge.asp

DRIVING DISTANCE: 38.8 miles from the I-280/CA 1 merge at the San Francisco–Daly City border

GPS INFORMATION

N37° 18.926' W122° 11.316'

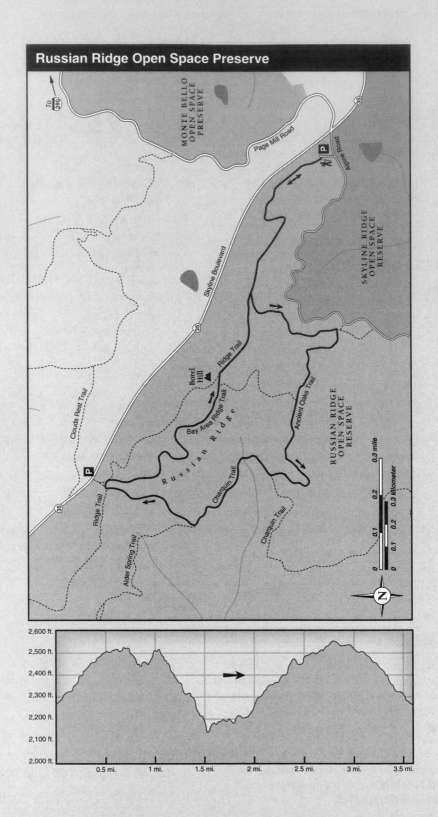

Russian Ridge Open Space Preserve

From the trailhead, begin walking uphill on Ridge Trail. The first stretch runs parallel to CA 35, but soon the trail passes a cluster of buckeye and jogs left, cushioning the noise from the road. The trail turns again and now begins to follow the ridgeline, gaining elevation at an easy pace. Grassland sprawls on both sides of the trail, and as you head northwest, the trail stretches out straight ahead into an inviting ribbon. At 0.6 mile, bear left, following the sign marked TO ANCIENT OAKS TRAIL.

Sweeping south downslope from the ridge, the trail passes through some pockets of California bays and oaks. You'll likely hear vehicles on Alpine Road, partly visible in some places on the left. At 0.9 mile, ignore a spur trail that heads straight, ending shortly at the road, and turn right onto Ancient Oaks Trail.

Pass buckeyes cuddled up in the creases of the hillside on the left, as the narrow trail crosses through grassland and descends slightly. On clear days, there are long views west to the ocean as well as to Mindego Ridge, a volcanic formation. California poppy and blue and white lupine dot the grassland through here in spring. You might see gopher snakes sunning themselves on the trail. Where the trail steps into the woods and reaches a junction at 1.2 miles, continue left, on Ancient Oaks Trail.

Although gorgeous live oaks play a starring roll along the trail, you might also see madrone and Douglas-fir. In the shaded understory, look for hound's tongue in spring. The trail winds downhill, taking a brief foray through grassland before returning to woods again. Creambush and hazelnut mingle with ferns to create a lush atmosphere, particularly in winter after a rainstorm, when you might catch newts crossing the trail. At 1.6, miles Ancient Oaks Trail ends. Turn right onto Charquin Trail (formerly Mindego Ridge Trail) and begin to climb out of the woods, skirting the base of the grassy ridge. In summer, look for painted lady and red admiral butterflies near a wet seep on the right. You'll reach a three-way junction at 1.9 miles—you have an opportunity to extend this hike an additional 1.3 miles, via Alder Spring and Hawk Trails to the left. Bear right, though, on Charquin Trail, toward the vista-point parking.

Ascend easily through quiet grassland. Follow the trail to a crest and junction at 2.2 miles. Continuing straight, the trail ends at Skyline Boulevard, across from a small vista-point parking area. The Bay Area Ridge Trail extends to the left and right. Turn right onto Bay Area Ridge Trail; after a few steps, the path splits (both trails reconnect after about 0.5 mile)—stay to the right.

Small rock outcrops sit off the sides of the trail, which ascends slightly through grassland just off the ridgeline. This is a good segment in which to look for coyotes, active residents of the preserve. Views west are outstanding. Flowers are sprinkled through the grass in spring, a visual snack for the main course still to come. At 2.7 miles, a path connecting to Ancient Oaks Trail departs on the right, but continue straight on Ridge Trail. A few feet farther uphill, the other leg of Ridge Trail feeds in from the left. Stay to the right.

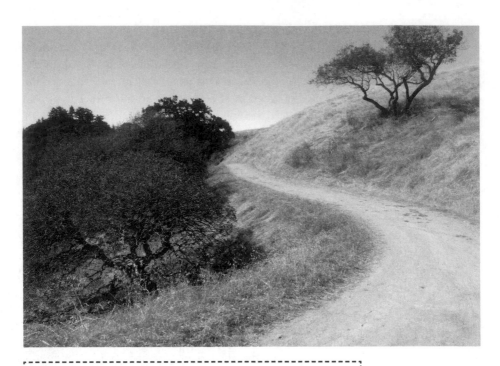

Golden summer grass and dried leaves on a buckeye tree at Russian Ridge

Now hugging the spine of the ridge, the trail enters an area legendary among Bay Area wildflower enthusiasts. During the peak of the season, usually early May, flowers pop (literally and figuratively) out of the lush green grass along the trail. These are "common" wildflowers, including johnny-jump-ups, owl's clover, blue and white lupine, California poppy, tidytips, creamcups, clarkia, and blue-eyed grass, but the display's frequency and urgency are what knock your socks off. Marvel at your leisure, but take care to stay on the trail and, of course, don't pick the flowers! If you follow the change of seasons at Russian Ridge, you'll note that while in spring the grass is short and verdant, by midsummer the hillsides are cloaked in thigh-high grass, and the only flowers still in bloom are usually a few tired-looking tidytips and mule ear sunflowers.

Continuing, Ridge Trail descends gradually, offering views south to the hills of Monte Bello Open Space Preserve, topped by 2,800-foot Black Mountain. When you reach the junction with the path to Ancient Oaks Trail again at 3 miles, continue straight and retrace your steps back to the parking lot.

SAN BRUNO MOUNTAIN STATE AND COUNTY PARK 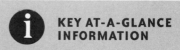 51

IN BRIEF

Sprawling just south of San Francisco, San Bruno Mountain is the perfect park for a quick get-out-of-town hike. This 3.5-mile loop climbs through coastal scrub to a ridge where views include the mountains of Marin and San Mateo Counties. After cresting near the mountain's summit, the hike descends back to the trailhead, offering San Francisco and Mount Diablo views all the way downhill.

DESCRIPTION

One of the Bay Area's most important urban-fringe open spaces, San Bruno Mountain has evaded development plans since the 1960s. One group wanted to shave land off the top of the mountain to fill the bay near San Francisco Airport, and many developers eyed the land for housing tracts. Development plans were firmly squelched in 1976, when the rare Mission Blue butterfly, which lives only on San Bruno Mountain and San Francisco's Twin Peaks, was placed on the U.S. Fish and

---

Directions

From southbound US 101 in San Francisco County, take Exit 429B at Third Street/Cow Palace. Drive south on Bayshore Boulevard about 2 miles, turn right on Guadalupe Canyon Parkway, and drive uphill about 2 miles to the park entrance on the right side of the road. Once past the entrance kiosk, follow the park road under Guadalupe Canyon Parkway to the trailhead, near the native-plant garden on the left.

From northbound US 101, take Exit 426A toward the Cow Palace and drive north on Bayshore Boulevard; then turn left onto Guadalupe Canyon Parkway and follow the remaining directions above.

---

i KEY AT-A-GLANCE INFORMATION

LENGTH: 3.5 miles

CONFIGURATION: Loop

DIFFICULTY: Easy

SCENERY: Coastal scrub, views

EXPOSURE: Nearly all full sun

TRAFFIC: Moderate; the loop is popular in spring.

TRAIL SURFACE: Dirt trails

HIKING TIME: 2 hours

SEASON: Opens daily at 8 a.m.; closing times vary (see Contacts, below). Perfect in spring, but bring a jacket in case it's windy.

ACCESS: Pay $6 day-use fee at the entrance kiosk.

MAPS: At entrance kiosk, trailhead, and tinyurl.com/sanbrunomap

FACILITIES: Restrooms and water near entrance kiosk

SPECIAL COMMENTS: No dogs allowed

CONTACTS: 650-992-6770, tinyurl.com/sanbrunomtnpark

DRIVING DISTANCE: 5.5 miles from the US 101/I-280 split in San Francisco

GPS INFORMATION

N37° 41.710' W122° 26.061'

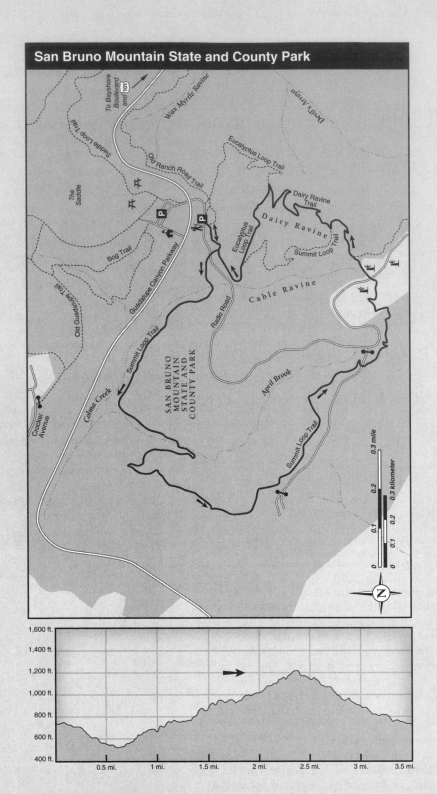

San Bruno Mountain State and County Park

Wildlife Service's endangered-species list. Although houses have crept up the sides of the mountain and communications equipment protrudes from the summit area, more than 2,000 acres of San Bruno Mountain are protected and the mountain, surrounded by densely populated neighborhoods, feels like an island.

Removal of invasive vegetation has been a long-term volunteer project for San Bruno Mountain advocacy groups. Eucalyptus, cotoneaster, ivy, gorse, and broom thrive in some areas. Even with so much nonnative vegetation, a hiker might see plenty of native plants on just one San Bruno Mountain visit. There is an abundance of common flora, but you'll see lots of unusual and some endangered plants as well, including a wallflower, an owl's clover, and a few varieties of manzanita. April and May are the peak times for wildflowers.

The San Bruno Mountain loop begins at a large trail sign in front of the native-plant garden. Follow the arrow pointing right to Summit Loop Trail, and you'll wind through the garden, then reach a signed junction with Eucalyptus Loop Trail. Bear right onto Summit Loop Trail and then, after a few steps, cross the road.

Summit Loop Trail begins a slight descent through an area where eucalyptus, ivy, and cypress thrive near a creek. On the right, a damp bowl-shaped meadow fosters willows. Scorpionweed, blue-eyed grass, checkerbloom, fringe cup, and cow parsnip bloom in spring, tangled through coyote brush, coffeeberry, and lizard's-tail. Guadalupe Canyon Parkway is visible and audible to the north, but the trail soon bends left, crosses April Brook, and then starts climbing south on a few switchbacks.

As you reach the ridgeline, the grade tapers off and plants along the trail seem to hunker down, keeping a low profile against winds that regularly whip across the mountain. Oregon grape nestles in rock outcrops, and annual wildflowers, here sprinkled through sagebrush, include paintbrush, johnny-jump-ups, and varieties of owl's clover.

On clear days, views extend north to the Point Reyes Peninsula and Mount Tamalpais. Summit Loop Trail veers left off the ridgeline and runs downslope. Cottontails can be glimpsed at the edge of the trail, but on approach they dive into thickets of coastal scrub composed of California coffeeberry, coyote brush, lizard's-tail, sticky monkeyflower, twinberry, and poison oak. A cluster of hummingbird sage near a kink in the trail puts forth bold, bright pink flowers in spring.

On the final push toward the summit, the trail crosses a paved service road, then snakes uphill not far from the park road. Nearly ever year here in January, I see San Francisco wallflower blooming. In spring, stands of iris bloom in a community of stunted-looking sagebrush, coyote brush, and lizard's-tail. Tiny-leaved yerba buena trails along the ground, within sight of downtown San Francisco. This plant lent its name to the village that became the city of San Francisco in 1847.

Some shortcuts and one unsigned spur off to the right make the trail a little hard to follow, but just keep heading uphill toward the communications towers. Looking west, the Farallon Islands are often visible if it's not too foggy. At 2.4 miles, Summit Loop Trail crosses a paved road. You'll likely want to hurry through this

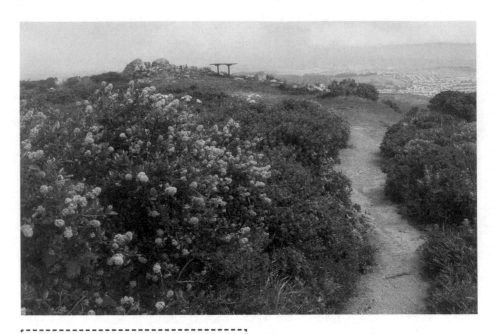

Ceanothus shrubs line the path to a scenic vista.

area, marred with ugly communications buildings, dishes, and towers (but I did experience my first-ever Bay Area coyote sighting near this junction). After a few steps, a gorgeous blend of coastal scrub signals a return to a more natural setting.

Just as the trail begins to descend, East Ridge Trail departs on the right. Continue straight on Summit Loop Trail. At an easy pace, the trail drifts downhill toward a bench off to the right where hikers can gaze north to San Francisco or across the bay to Mount Diablo. In spring, goldfields occupy grassy patches off the trail like an invading army. At 2.6 miles, you'll reach a signed junction. Turn right onto Dairy Ravine Trail.

On long, fluid switchbacks through coastal scrub, Dairy Ravine Trail descends. I've seen wildflowers blooming along the trail here as early as mid-January, and during the peak season you'll likely see plenty of scorpionweed, blue-eyed grass, blue-dicks, seaside daisy, California poppy, and paintbrush. Soon, Dairy Ravine Trail ends at a signed junction at 3 miles. Again, although either trail is an option, bear left onto Eucalyptus Loop Trail.

Following a slight descent, the trail levels as it passes through a stretch of invasives. Three of the park's problem plants—eucalyptus, ivy, and cotoneaster—all grow together in a small colony of exotics. Here, Eucalyptus Loop Trail drops easily back to a junction with Summit Loop Trail at 3.2 miles, where you'll continue straight/right.

The two loops run together downhill, then split at 3.4 miles. Turn right at the split and walk back through the garden to the trailhead.

SIERRA AZUL OPEN SPACE PRESERVE

IN BRIEF

Sierra Azul may be the biggest Bay Area pre-serve you've never heard of. With more than 17,300 acres, the massive preserve sprawls over the flanks of Mount Umunhum, in the Sierra Azul range just southwest of San Jose. This moderate out-and-back hike is a great introduc-tion to Sierra Azul's varied landscapes.

DESCRIPTION

Sierra Azul Open Space Preserve has a long and colorful history. The preserve's highest point, Mount Umunhum, was a sacred peak to the Ohlone Indians, who graced the rugged peak with this melodious name, which trans-lates as "the resting place of the humming-bird." In the 1950s, the U.S. Air Force built a radar station at the top of Umunhum, and until 1979, the facility scanned the coast for potential Soviet threats. When the station closed, the Air Force left behind crumbling buildings, contaminated property, and, at the top of the mountain, a prominent six-story structure, which still stands today. Locals have fond memories of (mostly illegal) excursions

KEY AT-A-GLANCE INFORMATION

LENGTH: 5.4 miles

CONFIGURATION: Out-and-back

DIFFICULTY: Easy

SCENERY: Chaparral, grassland, views

EXPOSURE: Mostly shaded, with some full sun

TRAFFIC: Moderate

TRAIL SURFACE: Dirt fire road

HIKING TIME: 2.5 hours

SEASON: Good anytime but very hot in summer

ACCESS: Free

MAPS: At the trailhead and tinyurl.com/sierraazulmap

FACILITIES: Vault toilets at trailhead

SPECIAL COMMENTS: Dogs are permit-ted on some preserve trails, but not on this one.

CONTACTS: 650-691-1200; openspace.org/preserves/pr_sierra_azul.asp

DRIVING DISTANCE: 56 miles from the I-280/CA 1 merge at the San Francisco–Daly City border

---

Directions

Drive south from San Francisco on I-280 and use the CA 1/19th Avenue merge as your mile-age starting point. Drive south about 36 miles on I-280, then take Exit 12 onto CA 85 South. After 10 miles, take Exit 8 at Camden Avenue. Stay in either of the two left lanes, and at the end of the exit ramp, turn left onto Camden. Drive 2 miles, then turn right onto Hicks Road. Drive 6 miles and, at a stop sign, turn right onto (frequently unsigned) Mount Umunhum Road—if you reach Almaden Road, you've gone too far. Almost immediately, turn right into the preserve parking lot.

GPS INFORMATION

N37° 10.520' W121° 51.855'

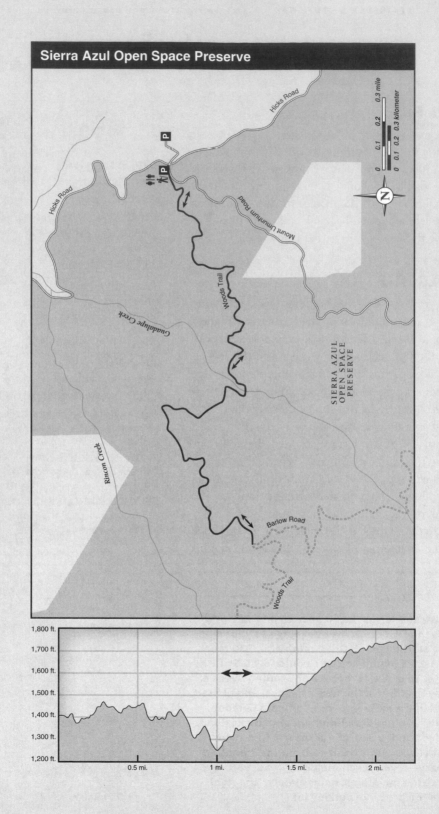

Sierra Azul Open Space Preserve

on the slopes of Mount Umunhum, as well as bittersweet feelings about the sugar cube–shaped mountaintop building that was made inaccessible more than 20 years ago.

The Midpeninsula Regional Open Space District began purchasing Sierra Azul property in the 1980s. Like a jigsaw puzzle in progress, a series of relatively small additions has resulted in one huge but somewhat fragmented preserve. Many areas are still off-limits to the public, while other parcels are surrounded by private inholdings, and the battle to clean up the top of Umunhum has raged for years. The dangerous conditions at the summit are being addressed, and the top will be reopened at some point.

Most of the preserve trails are long fire roads that shoot up and down the hillsides at steep grades, making Sierra Azul a favorite with experienced mountain bikers and equestrians. Hikers can make all-day treks along rolling ridgelines, such as the 11-mile (one-way) trip from Lexington Reservoir to the Jacques Ridge trailhead. Sierra Azul rivals some of the largest state parks in the Bay Area for sheer size and diversity, encompassing chaparral, redwood groves, mixed woodlands, headwaters, and grassy slopes, all just a short drive from San Jose.

Start from the parking lot on the wide fire road, Woods Trail. This trail is used by cyclists and equestrians, so stay alert for traffic throughout your hike. Mount Umunhum's summit, marked by a six-story concrete building, is visible uphill in the distance as the trail makes its way at a nearly level pace into a lightly wooded area. You may hear chickadees chirping from the coast live oak, madrone, and California bay trees, and see Oregon juncos picking through leaf litter along the trail. In late spring, checkerspot, fritillary, and California sister butterflies flutter above poison oak, sticky monkeyflower, coyote brush, and creambush shrubs in the understory.

Woods Trail descends gently and crosses a creek at about the 0.5-mile mark. Big-leaf maples and California buckeyes mix through the other trees here. In the shaded slope on the left side of the trail, look for Chinese houses, fairy lanterns, ribbon clarkia, and pale-lemon-colored Ferdinand's iris in spring. On a May hike, I saw a little ringneck snake basking in a pool of sunlight in the middle of the trail here.

As the trail continues to descend, the sound of rushing water gets ever louder until you reach Guadalupe Creek, just past 1 mile. Woods Trail crosses the waterway, then begins to climb somewhat steeply, passing a few eucalyptus trees. A large Douglas-fir marks its territory along the trail with scattered cones. As the trail ascends into a grassy area dotted with coyote brush, scan the sides of the trail for some of the many flowers that bloom throughout here in spring, including purple ookow, ivory mariposa lilies, blue-eyed grass, white and golden yarrow, and pink clarkia. Where Woods Trail bends left, expansive views unfold from the right side of the trail, stretching past Almaden Quicksilver County Park and the city of San Jose to Mount Hamilton and Mission Peak. If it's not too hot, the pocket of nearly level grassland here is a great stop for a picnic.

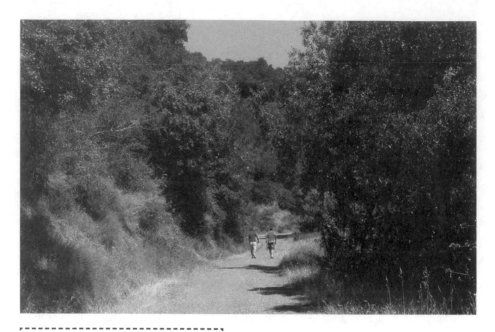

Woods Trail invites easy, leisurely strolling.

Woods Trail passes under power lines, levels out a bit, and reenters partially shaded woods, home to California bay, madrone, live oak, toyon, poison oak, buckeye, chaparral pea, and manzanita. A sunny, open stretch hosts a collection of chaparral plants including yerba santa, chamise, pitcher sage, mountain mahogany, and sticky monkeyflower.

Swallowtail butterflies are commonly spotted along the trail in late spring— these large butterflies, cream or yellow with black accents, flap and glide more like a bird than flutter like a typical butterfly. Anise swallowtails are the most common Bay Area swallowtail, but on a May hike here, I saw pale swallowtails, no doubt drawn to host plants coffeeberry and creambush, both found in abundance on the slopes of Mount Umunhum. The two swallowtails have similar yellow-and-black markings, but anise swallowtails have a stronger yellow hue and large patches of black on the middle tops (shoulders) of both wings.

More great views unfold uphill to the summit before Woods Trail reenters shaded woodland again, where a rare oak hybrid called oracle or Shreve oak graces the right side of the trail. This deciduous oak, a cross between a black oak and an interior live oak, is most conspicuous in autumn, when the leaves turn a beautiful orange color. In this final shaded segment, where wild rose, columbine, and western heart's ease (tiny white violets) bloom in spring, the trail ascends slightly to a signed junction with Barlow Road at 2.7 miles. Woods Trail continues uphill straight ahead, and Barlow Road climbs to Mount Umunhum Road to the left. Retrace your steps back to the parking lot.

SKYLINE RIDGE OPEN SPACE PRESERVE

IN BRIEF

If you enjoy the tranquility of little mountain lakes, I recommend this short but stunning Skyline Ridge hike. This loop skirts Horseshoe Lake, climbs to a chaparral-covered ridge, then descends through grassland to Alpine Pond. The return route ascends to the ridge, then drops through woods and grassland back to the trailhead.

DESCRIPTION

There are quite a few open-space preserves and parks sprawled on the crest of the Santa Cruz Mountains, but Skyline Ridge is a favorite. The preserve is home to two small man-made lakes that were created to ensure a steady supply of water for former ranches. Horseshoe Lake is partly rimmed with Douglas fir and Christmas-tree-farm escapees, while Alpine Pond, tucked in the far northern corner of the preserve, hosts Skyline Ridge's nature center. Stretched between the two ponds is a ridge composed of grassland and chaparral, where views extend far to the west, south, and east. This is a good hike for families with kids because it's fairly short and there's good wildlife-viewing at the ponds. You will likely see plenty of waterfowl here,

KEY AT-A-GLANCE INFORMATION

LENGTH: 4.1 miles

CONFIGURATION: Loop with a short out-and-back segment

DIFFICULTY: Easy

SCENERY: Ponds, grassland, chaparral, ridge views

EXPOSURE: A few pockets of shade, otherwise full sun

TRAFFIC: Moderate

TRAIL SURFACE: Dirt fire road and trails

HIKING TIME: 2 hours, plus any additional time spent lollygagging around the ponds

SEASON: Good all year—nice wildflowers in spring

ACCESS: Free

MAPS: At the trailhead and tinyurl .com/skylineridgemap

FACILITIES: Vault toilet at trailhead, another one near Alpine Pond

SPECIAL COMMENTS: No dogs allowed

CONTACTS: 650-691-1200, openspace.org/preserves/pr _skyline_ridge.asp

DRIVING DISTANCE: 39.7 miles from the CA 1/I-280 merge at the San Francisco–Daly City border

Directions

Depart from San Francisco on southbound I-280 and use the CA 1/19th Avenue merge as your mileage starting point. Drive south about 29 miles on I-280, then take Exit 20 onto Page Mill Road. Drive west on Page Mill about 9 miles to the junction with CA 35/Skyline Boulevard. Turn left onto Skyline Boulevard and drive south about 0.8 mile; then turn right into the preserve. Stay to the right and follow the park road to the northern parking lot.

GPS INFORMATION

N37° 18.736' W122° 10.616'

Skyline Ridge Open Space Preserve

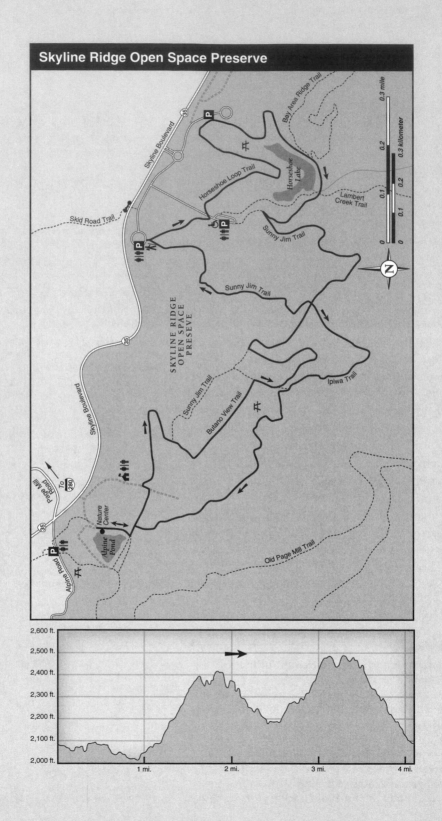

but less commonly spotted animals visit the ponds as well—on one hike, I came within 10 feet of a bobcat completely engrossed in a shoreline hunt.

From the trailhead's information signboard a few feet off the parking lot, bear left, following Sunny Jim Trail toward Horseshoe Lake. This narrow, nearly level path bisects a damp, sloping meadow where coyote brush is mixed through a few yellow bush lupine shrubs. At 0.1 mile, the path reaches a parking lot reserved for handicapped visitors. Turn left, walk up the access road a few feet, and then bear right onto a slim path, Horseshoe Lake Trail.

The trail ascends slightly, leaving coyote brush for a grassland dotted with Douglas-fir, coast live oak, and a few other conifers—a Christmas-tree farm is a short distance off to the south. In spring, look for blue and white lupine, California poppy, blue larkspur, clarkia, and Ithuriel's spear. You'll get a peek at Horseshoe Lake's northern arm, downhill to the right.

The trail crests in the midst of a coast-live-oak and California bay grove, where two picnic tables on opposite sides of the trail provide secluded spots for lunch. Horseshoe Lake Trail descends, crosses a culvert, and reaches a junction at 0.6 mile. Turn right and pass through a damp area where willows huddle on the right. After a few steps, a second trail heads uphill to the left; like the previous trail, this one leads to the equestrian parking lot. Continue to the right, as Horseshoe Lake Trail passes through a lush area, with poison oak, blackberry, thimbleberry, and buckeye dominating. The south arm of the lake sits just off to the right.

Once across a tiny footbridge, the trail curves right, leveling in woods where columbine blooms in spring. At 0.8 mile, you'll reach a junction. Stay to the right on Horseshoe Loop Trail to reach the shore of the lake. From here, you'll have nice views; if you want to spend more time on the shoreline, there's a bench on the right. At 0.9 mile, Horseshoe Loop Trail bends right. Continue straight and, after a few feet, stay to the right at a junction with Lambert Creek Trail. Horseshoe Loop Trail climbs slightly, through pines and coyote brush, to a junction at 1 mile. Turn sharply left, following the sign toward Alpine Pond.

Sunny Jim Trail, here a broad fire road, climbs moderately, passing a few live oaks, buckeyes, California bays, and madrones on the way into grassland. White brodiaea, clarkia, and yarrow bloom along the trail in early June. When the trail bends right, enjoy views of forested ridges off to the west, including Portola Redwoods State Park. At 1.4 miles, Sunny Jim Trail meets a three-part junction. The path to the right returns to the trailhead—turn left.

A sign warns of entry into an area inhabited by rattlesnakes. I've never seen any rattlesnakes on this trail, but should you encounter one, here's the protocol: If the snake is stretched out on a trail with plenty of real estate surrounding it, you can probably just gingerly walk around it, keeping yourself as far as possible from its head. If the rattlesnake is coiled, that means it's stressed. Back off a good distance and wait for it to chill out, uncoil, and slither away. Gopher snakes, also common in this and all parts of the Bay Area, resemble rattlesnakes but are nonvenomous. Both snakes have a similar cream, tan, and brown pattern, but the easiest

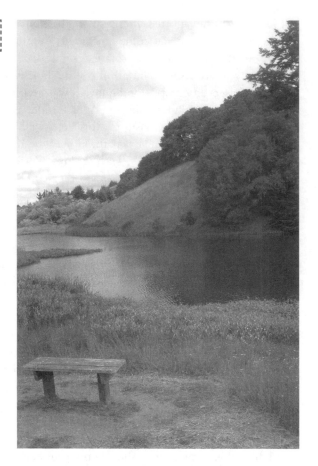

Horseshoe Lake

way to tell them apart (from a safe distance, natch) is by head shape. Gopher snakes have no distinction from their "necks" to their heads, but rattlers have diamond-shaped heads. Both, by the way, make noises to warn off predators, rattlesnakes by shaking their rattles and gopher snakes by vibrating their tails against the ground.

As you climb easily through grassland, the views south and west continue to impress. Although this hillside is infested with invasive yellow star thistle, spring wildflowers are still quite good, with an abundance of owl's clover, clarkia, and California poppy blooming in May. Later, in June, look for yellow mariposa lilies, blended through the tall grass with dandelions. As the trail veers right and runs downslope from the ridge, the trailside vegetation shifts to chaparral, with chamise, manzanita, ceanothus, and yerba santa common, as well as a few shrubs of silk-tassel and pitcher sage. A pocket of coast live oak provides some unexpected shade. At 1.8 miles, Ipiwa Trail squeezes past a boulder on the right, then reaches a junction with an unnamed trail heading right to the top of the ridge. Continue straight.

The next section is dominated in late spring by orange-blossomed sticky monkeyflower shrubs, overshadowing neighboring sagebrush and lizard's-tail. Descending easily, Ipiwa Trail offers views to the grassy shoulders of Russian Ridge to the north. The trail leaves grassland and enters woods, where California bays are dwarfed by some positively massive old live oaks. Now nearly level, Ipiwa Trail reaches a junction at 2.3 miles with a still-somewhat-paved trail. Cross the pavement and continue on Ipiwa Trail, winding through Douglas-fir, pine, California bay, and buckeye to the south shore of Alpine Pond at 2.4 miles.

The Daniels Nature Center (open weekends) features exhibits about the preserve's history and wildlife, but even when the center is closed, you can enjoy the pond's shoreline, where I've seen crawfish meandering through mud in the driest months of the year. A wheelchair-accessible pond-viewing station is set up on the side of the building. When you're ready, return to the previous junction with the paved trail and turn left. (You can also loop around the lake, but the trail's proximity to Skyline Boulevard and Alpine Road makes the walk a bit noisy.)

The sides of wide and paved but crumbling Sunny Jim Trail host good displays of Chinese houses and fairy lanterns in spring. Ignore a path breaking off to the right, signed NOT A THROUGH TRAIL, and continue easily uphill to a T-junction with a paved road at 2.5 miles. Turn left and, after a few feet, just before the ranger-station compound, turn right, following the sign toward Horseshoe Lake.

White poplars, nonnative trees with silvery leaves, are conspicuous on the right. The broad trail passes an old tennis court, then sweeps sharply right and begins to climb, bordering a forest of interior live oak, Douglas-fir, and tan oak on the left. At 2.8 miles, Sunny Jim Trail heads left while Butano View Trail continues straight. Both trails converge eventually (consider Sunny Jim if it's hot)—continue straight on Butano View Trail.

The wide trail climbs, passes a water tank, and then bends left. As you ascend along a grassy ridge, savor great views west. At 3.1 miles, a connector heads off to the left—continue to the right, soon reaching a second junction with a path leading to Ipiwa Trail. Proceed to the left, climbing past tall oaks to a hilltop and the high point of the hike. Butano View Trail begins to descend, then ends at a junction with Sunny Jim Trail at 3.4 miles. Turn right.

A short and somewhat steep descent reaches the junction with Ipiwa Trail once again. This time, turn left.

The trail steps into woods composed of big-leaf maple, live oak, Douglas-fir, California bay, and hazelnut. Descending past a cluster of buckeye, you'll reemerge in grassland, where elegant brodiaea, yellow mariposa lilies, and clarkia bloom in early June. At 4.1 miles, the trail ends back at the trailhead.

NEARBY ACTIVITIES

At Skyline Ridge's neighboring preserve, **Long Ridge**, you can hike through woods to a grassy hilltop where a stone bench memorializes Wallace Stegner, an author and preservationist who lived the last years of his life in nearby Portola Valley. More info: 650-691-1200, **openspace.org/preserves/pr_long_ridge.asp**.

54 SWEENEY RIDGE

KEY AT-A-GLANCE INFORMATION

LENGTH: 5.6 miles

CONFIGURATION: Out-and-back

DIFFICULTY: Easy–moderate

SCENERY: Coastal scrub, views

EXPOSURE: Exposed except for a few tiny pockets of shade

TRAFFIC: Heavy on the Sneath Lane Trail, lighter farther afield

TRAIL SURFACE: Paved fire road, dirt fire road

HIKING TIME: 3 hours

SEASON: Daily, 8 a.m.–sunset. Good all year; best late winter–spring. Stay away on a foggy day . . . unless you like that kind of thing.

ACCESS: Free

MAPS: None at the trailhead. A good map to the area is Pease Press's *Trails of the Coastside & Northern Peninsula* ($6.95; peasepress.com). For an online option, visit the website below.

FACILITIES: There's a vault toilet up on the ridge, but no facilities at the trailhead.

SPECIAL COMMENTS: Leashed dogs welcome. Get up-to-date information about the Bay Area Ridge Trail segment through water-district lands at ridgetrail.org.

CONTACTS: 415-561-4323, www.parksconservancy.org/visit /park-sites/sweeney-ridge.html

DRIVING DISTANCE: 7.8 miles from the CA 1/I-280 merge at the San Francisco–Daly City border

GPS INFORMATION

N37° 37.159' W122° 27.246'

IN BRIEF

Although the Sweeney Ridge trailhead is just minutes from San Francisco and begins at the edge of a residential neighborhood, a climb of less than an hour on a paved fire road through coastal scrub leads to a quiet ridge with sweeping views. Once at the ridge, this hike meanders past the Portola Discovery site to a turnaround point at the boundary with water-district lands, where you'll retrace your steps back to the trailhead.

DESCRIPTION

In many ways, Sweeney Ridge exemplifies the past, present, and future of Bay Area open space. In 1769, Spanish explorer Gaspar de Portolà got his first glimpse of San Francisco Bay from the ridge. From 1956 to 1974, Sweeney Ridge was home to a Nike missile site, the remains of which are still visible. Currently, Sweeney Ridge is the gateway to Peninsula Watershed property that stretches from the edge of the ridge across Montara Mountain to CA 92. The Bay Area Ridge Trail Council has worked for years to allow public access into the water-district lands, and in 2003 docents started leading hikes through the watershed, beginning at Portola Gate (the southern terminus of the Sweeney Ridge Trail).

Directions

Depart San Francisco on southbound I-280 and use the CA 1/19th Avenue merge as your mileage starting point. Drive about 5.5 miles south on I-280, then take Exit 43B onto Sneath Lane (just before the I-380 exit). Turn left onto Sneath Lane and drive west 2 miles to the trailhead, at the end of the road.

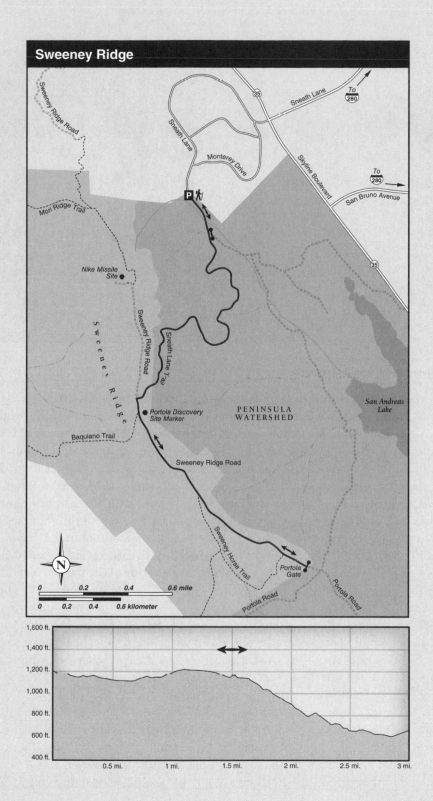

Sweeney Ridge

Sweeney Ridge Road

Sneath Lane

Sneath Lane

Monterey Drive

35

To
280

Sneath Lane

Skyline Boulevard

To
280

San Bruno Avenue

35

Mori Ridge Trail

Nike Missile
Site

Sweeney Ridge

Sweeney Ridge Road

Sneath Lane Trail

Portola Discovery
Site Marker

Baquiano Trail

PENINSULA
WATERSHED

San Andreas
Lake

Sweeney Ridge Road

Sweeney Horse Trail

Portola
Gate

Portola Road

Portola Road

N

| 0 | 0.2 | 0.4 | 0.6 mile |
| 0 | 0.2 | 0.4 | 0.6 kilometer |

1,600 ft.

1,400 ft.

1,200 ft.

1,000 ft.

800 ft.

600 ft.

400 ft.

0.5 mi. 1 mi. 1.5 mi. 2 mi. 2.5 mi. 3 mi.

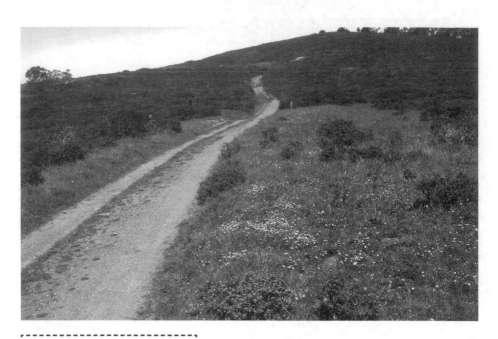

Sweeney Ridge Trail ascends gently.

Begin from the parking area at the end of Sneath Lane and squeeze through the V-shaped stile onto Sneath Lane Trail. This old paved road descends slightly through a damp area where dogwood, coyote brush, twinberry, California coffeeberry, and toyon tangle together. In late spring, blooming mustard, wild radish, and fennel are common. Just past a junction with a gated water-district fire road on the left, the trail passes through a cluster of eucalyptus and begins to climb at a modest grade. The sides of Sneath Lane Trail are lined with coastal scrub plants, most notably coyote brush, ceanothus, creambush, poison oak, sagebrush, lizard's-tail, and sticky monkeyflower. Shrubby willows soak up moisture in the draws of the hillsides, accompanied by currant and gooseberry. In early spring, I often make this part of the hike at a near-crawl, scanning the right side of the trail for a variety of wildflowers, including milkmaids, fringe cups, iris, hound's tongue, and woodland star. Even in early summer you're likely to see a multitude of paintbrush in bloom, as well as California poppy, California larkspur, and the last lingering fairy lantern blossoms. Three edible favorites fruit along the trail in June: strawberry, thimbleberry, and blackberry. And if you hike quietly, you might see cottontail rabbits browsing on trailside vegetation. Many locals use Sneath Lane Trail as a daily exercise route, so expect traffic from cyclists, joggers, and walkers.

As the trail winds up the hillside, a yellow fog line joins the journey. This line down the middle of the trail is unnecessary on a clear day, but when thick, wet, fiercely blowing fog descends on the ridge, creating whiteout visibility, the line assists hikers and cyclists on the journey back toward the trailhead. Just beyond the start of the fog line, the trail curves right and ascends moderately steeply. At the end of this stretch, you may want to stop at a bench on the right and enjoy the views north and east, which encompass San Francisco, Mount Tamalpais, San Bruno Mountain, and San Francisco Bay.

Traffic (and noise) from planes is steady. The grade slackens back to moderate and continues to taper off as the trail presses on uphill, through the upper reaches of a eucalyptus grove. Look downhill to the left for a good view of San Andreas Lake, one of the reservoirs that make up the Peninsula Watershed. At 1.7 miles, the trail crests at a junction with Sweeney Ridge Road, a Bay Area Ridge Trail segment. Turn left.

About 100 feet down the dirt fire road, bear left toward the discovery site. The path cuts through coastal scrub, then reaches the Portola Discovery site, marked by a small monument. Adjacent to the marker, there's a "mountain finder," with the prominent landforms visible from Sweeney Ridge etched onto a granite cylinder. On clear days you might be able to make out Mount Hamilton to the southeast, but even in the smog of summer, views include Montara Mountain and the Pacifica coastline to the west. From this clearing, walk a few steps to the right, returning to the fire road at the junction with Baquiano Trail, which travels west to the park boundary. Turn left and resume hiking south on Sweeney Ridge Road.

The fire road descends easily through dense shrubs of coyote brush, lizard's-tail, and California coffeeberry. Here, a knoll on the left blocks noise from the east, and birdsong fills the void quite nicely. Iris, buttercup, mission bells, and blue-eyed grass, all early-spring flowers, bloom through the coastal scrub, and goldfields commonly flower clustered together in pockets of grassland, forming bright yellow patches. In early June, look for annual lupines, checkerbloom, paintbrush, and yarrow in bloom.

At 2.2 miles, Sweeney Horse Trail departs to the right, but continue straight. In a saddle, traffic noise from I-280 drifts up to the ridge, where twinberry, ceanothus, and a few huckleberry shrubs mingle through the scrub. Views west to Montara Mountain continue to impress.

Sweeney Ridge Road ascends slightly, and the Portola Gate comes into view. At 2.8 miles, the other end of Sweeney Horse Trail feeds in from the right; then Sweeney Ridge Road ends at Portola Gate. This is the trailhead for watershed hikes. Retrace your steps back to the trailhead.

NEARBY ACTIVITIES

Explore the northern part of Sweeney Ridge from the trailhead at Skyline College: From Skyline Boulevard, turn west onto College Drive (less than 1 mile north of Sneath Lane). Turn left at the college entrance, then park in Lot 2. From the Skyline College trailhead, Sweeney Ridge Road extends 2.3 miles south, past the old Nike missile site area, to the junction with Sneath Lane Trail. You can extend this hike on an out-and-back excursion west along Mori Ridge Trail, but to avoid a steep uphill return, turn back before the last sharp drop to Shelldance Nursery.

55 UVAS CANYON COUNTY PARK

KEY AT-A-GLANCE INFORMATION

LENGTH: 4 miles

CONFIGURATION: Balloon with 2 very short spurs

DIFFICULTY: Easy

SCENERY: Woods, waterfalls, chaparral

EXPOSURE: Mostly shaded

TRAFFIC: Light except in summer, when campers increase trail traffic

TRAIL SURFACE: Dirt trails and fire roads, with some rocky stretches along Swanson Creek

HIKING TIME: 2 hours

SEASON: Daily, 8 a.m.–sunset; best in winter for waterfalls

ACCESS: Pay the $6 fee at the entrance station.

MAPS: At entrance station, start of Waterfall Loop, and tinyurl.com /uvascanyonmap

FACILITIES: Restrooms and drinking water at trailhead

SPECIAL COMMENTS: Dogs welcome

CONTACTS: 408-779-9232, tinyurl .com/uvascanyoncountypark

DRIVING DISTANCE: 69.7 miles from the CA 1/I-280 merge at the San Francisco– Daly City border

GPS INFORMATION

N37° 5.049' W121° 47.566'

8515 Croy Rd.
Morgan Hill, CA 95037

IN BRIEF

Uvas Canyon Park has a premium waterfall-to-mileage quotient. Most Bay Area waterfalls require substantial hikes, but that's not the case at Uvas, where three of the falls can be reached with very little effort. The fourth requires a bit more grunt but is still an easy trek. With four waterfalls on four different creeks, you can visit them all on this 4-mile hike on a tour through the canyon's woods and chaparral.

DESCRIPTION

Uvas hikes are all about waterfalls. It's no wonder, given the park's location, tucked back in a canyon. Steep hillsides channel runoff to a series of creeks that flow with the greatest intensity after sequential winter rainstorms. However, if you enjoy autumn foliage (such as it is in the Bay Area), you might make a special trip to Uvas in October or November, when

- -

Directions

Drive south from San Francisco on I-280 and use the CA 1/19th Avenue merge as your mileage starting point. Drive south about 36 miles on I-280, then take Exit 12 onto CA 85 South. After about 12 miles, take Exit 6 at Almaden Expressway. Turn south onto Almaden, drive about 5 miles to the end of the expressway, and turn right onto Harry Road. Almost immediately, turn left onto McKean Road. Drive south on McKean, which turns into Uvas Road after about 6.5 miles. Continue on Uvas another 3.7 miles, then turn right onto Croy Road (look for a brown county-park sign before the turnoff). Drive about 3.8 miles to the park entrance, at the end of the road. *Note:* The last stretch of Croy passes through the Swedish-American private community of Sveadal. Drive slowly.

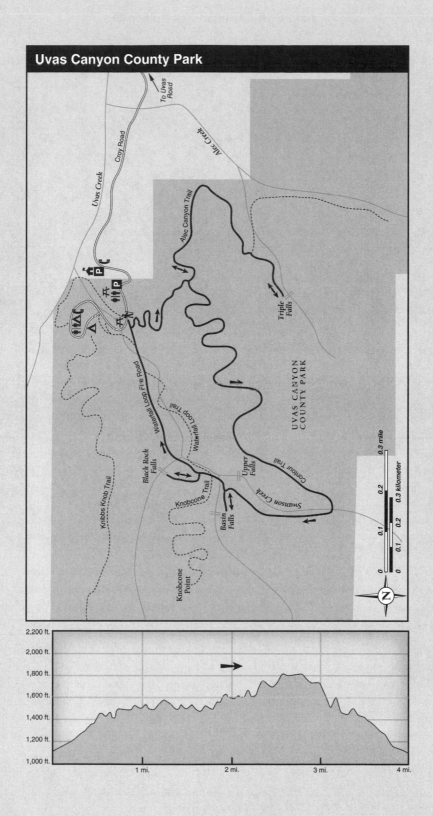

Uvas Canyon County Park

To Uvas Road

Alec Creek

Croy Road

Uvas Creek

Alec Canyon Trail

Triple Falls

UVAS CANYON COUNTY PARK

Waterfall Loop Fire Road

Waterfall Loop Trail

Black Rock Falls

Knibbs Knob Trail

Upper Falls

Swanson Creek

Contour Trail

Knobcone Trail

Basin Falls

Knobcone Point

0.3 mile

0.1   0.2   0.3 kilometer

0   0.1   0.2

N

2,200 ft.
2,000 ft.
1,800 ft.
1,600 ft.
1,400 ft.
1,200 ft.
1,000 ft.

1 mi.   2 mi.   3 mi.   4 mi.

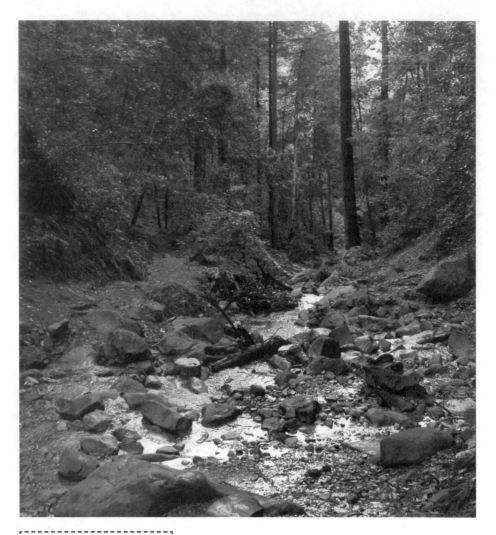

Swanson Creek in Uvas Canyon

the leaves on the park's many big-leaf maple trees flush orange and drift slowly down onto the creek beds and trails.

Part of Uvas's charm is that the journey to the park is such a pleasant prelude to a day hike. Once you get off the highway, back roads travel through bucolic country, a landscape of rolling hills studded with oaks. This part of Santa Clara County has largely escaped the era of the tech boom, when developers dug up orchards and installed acres of tilt-up buildings. There are few megamansions, but still lots of old horse ranches and lonely stretches where you might see wildlife. On one visit to Uvas, I spotted a huge bobcat along the side of McKean Road, ambling through the far reaches of a golf course.

The trailhead for this hike is at the end of the Black Oak Group Area, a reservable picnic spot. Leave the parking spaces adjacent to that area for picnickers, and park instead in the day-use lot just uphill and around the corner from the park entrance and the ranger station. From the lot, ascend a flight of steps toward the restrooms, then walk up the park road and, where it forks, bear left, following signage for Waterfall Loop. Begin hiking at the gated start of a dirt fire road, about 0.1 mile from the day-use parking lot. Check the wooden box on the right for the self-guided nature trail brochure and a map. After a short easy stretch, Waterfall Loop begins on the right. Continue straight on Alec Canyon Trail.

The fire road winds uphill on a series of broad switchbacks, through a forest of California bay, madrone, tan oak, and Douglas-fir. The grade fluctuates between easy and moderate. A bench on the side of the trail is a good spot for a rest, as there's a break in the vegetation that permits good views east. Just uphill from the bench, Alec Canyon Trail meets Contour Trail at 0.5 mile. You'll return to Contour Trail, but for now continue straight on Alec Canyon Trail.

The trail ascends gently out of the woods and through a stretch of chaparral. In February, when toyon shrubs still are weighted down with clusters of red berries, you might see buckbrush in bloom. At about 0.7 mile, Alec Canyon Trail crests and reaches Manzanita Point. Silk-tassel, toyon, and manzanita sprawl on the hillside downslope from a rest bench. More sweeping views stretch east out of the canyon. On a steady but easy descent, the trail passes through a chaparral-plant community dominated by chamise, where you might also see coyote mint and hollyleaf cherry. Buckeyes mark a transition into a damper area, and then California bays and redwoods come into view along the steep banks of a creek.

Look for a sign pointing right and uphill to Triple Falls at about 1 mile, following the narrow path along the creek bed to the falls. It's not far, only 0.2 mile, but the trail is pretty steep, and damp leaves on the path can make the ascent a bit slippery. California nutmeg makes an appearance along the trail. This native tree with evergreen needles can be confused with a young redwood or Douglas-fir, until you touch the tip of a needle. Redwood and Douglas-fir needles are rounded, but nutmeg needles are quite sharp! Native Americans are said to have used these needles for tattooing.

At the end of the spur you'll reach Triple Falls, the most remote of Uvas's waterfalls. This little redwood canyon is a quiet place, where the burble of the creek competes with the steady rush of the fall, a three-stage procession of water dropping about 35 feet in total. With the first waterfall visited, return to the junction with Alec Canyon and Contour trails at about 1.8 miles. Turn left onto Contour Trail.

The narrow path cuts across a steeply walled canyon, mostly under the shade of madrone, Douglas-fir, coast live oak, tan oak, and California bay. There's a fair bit of elevation wobble, but only in short stretches. Two nooks and crannies are crossed with the aid of a plank and a little wooden bridge. Sunlight rarely punctuates the dark creases of the canyon, but the parts of the mountain that jut out get enough sunshine to sustain manzanita and toyon shrubs. The sound of rushing water grows ever louder, until the trail drops to the banks of Swanson Creek at about 3 miles. Except for two very short spurs to visit waterfalls, it's all downhill from here, as you follow the creek back toward the trailhead. The flow rate can seem a bit tame this far up the canyon, but a low water level permits the trail to cross over to the opposite bank here. Use caution descending and crossing the creek, especially when the rocks are wet. The ground is less rocky on the other side, and the descent is easy through Douglas-fir, California bay, and big-leaf maple.

You may notice a little path ascending on the left, heading to an old hothouse site. Along the trail, tiny facets of broken glass twinkle on the hillsides surrounding a length of pipe. On a short set of steps, the trail descends through an area prone to landslides, then reaches Upper Falls, Swanson's Creek's largest drop. Just past Upper Falls, the path to Basin Falls departs at about 3.3 miles. Turn left.

It's an easy and brief ascent to the falls, a 15-foot cascade that creates a charming pool before continuing down the canyon to join Swanson Creek. Return to the main trail and continue downhill. In a little flat area, two other trails head off—Knobcone Trail to the left and Waterfall Loop Trail to the right. You'll also find a few picnic tables with good creek views. The ground cover that pervades the area is vinca, a nonnative. Continue straight on Waterfall Loop Fire Road. Less than 0.1 mile down the trail, veer left onto the path to Black Rock Falls.

The path ascends slightly, then curves left into a steeply walled canyon. This waterfall, a little taller than Basin Falls, may be my favorite at Uvas. It's an incredibly lush setting, where moss covers big-leaf maple trunks and giant boulders with abandon. Milkmaids bloom here and there in winter. When you return to Waterfall Loop Fire Road, if you've brought along the nature trail guide, now's the time to fish it out and follow along. Buckeye, big-leaf maple, sycamore, canyon live oak, and California bay may be spotted and identified with the aid of the guide.

The trail descends at a moderate grade. In winter, you might see scores of ladybugs hibernating on the trailside vegetation. This curious natural phenomenon is one of the benefits of Bay Area winter hiking, as this is only time of year these beetles can be seen in such concentrated colonies. Waterfall Loop Trail rejoins the fire road, and the two run together, crossing the creek one last time just downstream from what's left of an old retaining pond.

Stay to the right as a trail veers off toward the campground, and at about 4 miles you'll return to the junction with Alec Canyon Trail. Turn left and walk back to the parking lot.

WINDY HILL OPEN SPACE PRESERVE

IN BRIEF

Windy Hill showcases the micro and macro sides of nature. From the highest reaches of this preserve, there are excellent views from ocean to East Bay; on narrow, winding paths that climb through quiet woods, there are spectacular displays of wildflowers and autumn foliage. At Windy Hill, you can see the woods for the trees, and then some.

This loop begins at the edge of Portola Valley, then ascends through woods to the top of Windy Hill. The return leg is a fast descent on a fire road with a quick detour around Sausal Pond.

DESCRIPTION

I've enjoyed many magical hikes at Windy Hill over the years, in every season. In summer the woods are cool; spring brings tons of flowers; in autumn, maple leaves blaze with color; and winter is lonely with starkly naked oaks and nearly deserted trails. The preserve has two major trailheads at the top and bottom of the mountain. I like to start in Portola Valley, get the climbing out of the way first, and cruise downhill back to the trailhead. If, however, you prefer to face the ascent on the return, begin at the CA 35 trailhead, but note that Spring Ridge Trail is significantly steeper than Hamms Gulch Trail.

Directions ———————————➤

Drive south from San Francisco on I-280 and use the CA 1/19th Avenue merge as your mileage starting point. Drive south about 27 miles on I-280, then take Exit 22, Alpine Road. Head west on Alpine about 3 miles, then turn right onto Portola Road. Drive about 1 mile and turn left into the preserve parking lot.

KEY AT-A-GLANCE INFORMATION

LENGTH: 7.4 miles

CONFIGURATION: Loop

DIFFICULTY: Moderate

SCENERY: Grassland, woods, pond

EXPOSURE: Nearly equally shaded and exposed

TRAFFIC: Moderate

TRAIL SURFACE: Dirt fire roads and trails

HIKING TIME: 3.5 hours

SEASON: Good anytime, although Spring Ridge Trail is very hot in summer.

ACCESS: Free

MAPS: At the trailhead's information signboard and tinyurl.com/windyhillospmap

FACILITIES: Pit toilets at the Portola Valley trailhead and the CA 35 trailhead

SPECIAL COMMENTS: Leashed dogs are permitted on this hike but not on all Windy Hill trails.

CONTACTS: 650-691-1200, tinyurl.com/windyhillosp

DRIVING DISTANCE: 31.6 miles from the CA 1/I-280 merge at the San Francisco–Daly City border

GPS INFORMATION

N37° 22.517' W122° 13.408'

Windy Hill Open Space Preserve

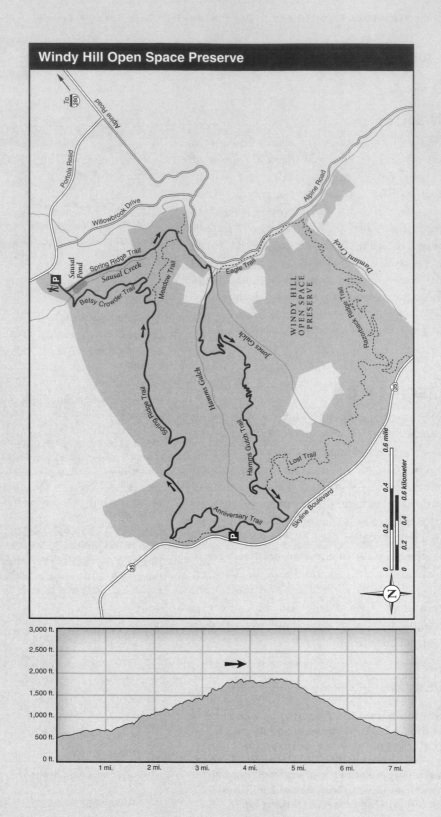

The lower trailhead, just off Portola Road, is a parking lot next to The Sequoias, a retirement community. Begin on a connector trail that winds through oak, buckeye, poison oak, and coyote brush. After about 300 feet, you'll reach a junction near Sausal Pond. Turn left onto Spring Ridge Trail.

At a level grade, the broad trail creeps along the preserve boundary. As they grow, young planted native shrubs, including currant and toyon, should help to block the noise from the Sequoias complex, visible on the left. Sausal Pond sits off to the right behind tangles of blackberry, poison oak, and young coast live oak. Spring Ridge Trail begins to ascend a bit, passing huge old valley oaks. You may see or hear red-winged blackbirds and quail in this area. At 0.6 mile, Spring Ridge Trail curves right and heads uphill, and a path leaves the preserve on the left. Continue straight, following the sign toward Alpine Road.

Madrone, California bay, big-leaf maple, and coast live, black, and valley oaks shade the level trail, where hound's tongue and buttercups bloom in late spring. In autumn, you might notice shrubs with marble-sized white berries—the aptly named snowberry plant. Quite a few hawthorn shrubs blend into the vegetation on the right. Hawthorn is not a plant commonly spotted in natural areas in these parts, and it's easy to pick out in autumn, when its red berries dangle from tooth-leaved branches.

You'll reach an important junction at about 0.8 mile: First the trail crosses a paved private road; then a trail leads left to Alpine Road. Continue straight onto Hamms Gulch Trail. A few steps later, the connector to Spring Ridge Trail, named Meadow Trail, departs to the right. Continue straight.

In the grassy understory beneath gorgeous black and valley oaks, blue-dicks and blue-eyed grass bloom in early spring. Watch out for poison oak, which is common along this slim path. Hamms Gulch Trail enters the woods. A creek runs slightly downslope to the left, and this riparian microclimate hosts plants that prefer a damp environment, including currant, California bay, and buckeye, plus trilliums and milkmaids in late winter.

The trail dips to cross a creek, then reaches a junction with Eagle Trail at 1.2 miles. Stay to the right on Hamms Gulch Trail, which abandons the waterway and begins to climb. In early March, hound's tongue is usually very prolific, blooming in giant colonies along the length of the trail, but you'll also likely see many other wildflowers, including shooting stars, trilliums, and milkmaids. The forest is a pretty mix of madrone, oaks, California bay, and some maple, redwood, and Douglas-fir. Hazelnut, creambush, poison oak, currant, and gooseberry compose the bulk of the understory.

Hamms Gulch Trail is well graded with many switchbacks and, except for a few short steeper sections, makes for an easy climb. Occasional breaks in the forest reveal views across the gulch to Spring Ridge Trail. In a sunny patch of chaparral, nearly hidden in thick stands of coyote brush, look for western leatherwood, an extremely rare shrub that is easiest to spot when yellow blossoms appear in late winter.

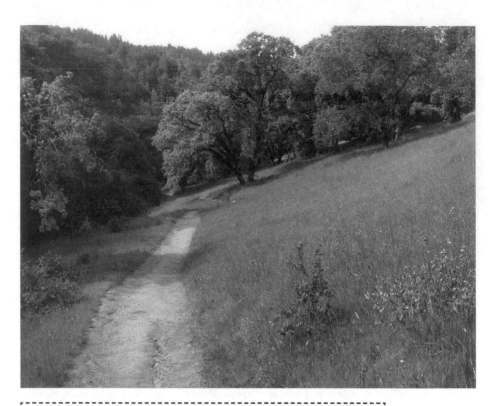

Majestic oaks pepper the grassland along the lower portion of Hamms Gulch Trail.

After another foray through the woods, Hamms Gulch Trail skirts the edge of a sloping, grassy meadow—the only significant grassland on the trail. Benches placed here and there along the trail are a welcome sight for weary hikers. The trail just keeps climbing, and you may begin to notice some incredibly large Douglas-firs mixed through tan oak, big-leaf maple, oaks, and madrone. At 3.8 miles, Hamms Gulch Trail ends at a T-junction. Turn right onto Lost Trail.

Lost Trail makes its way out of the forest, then runs along the edge of the woods, allowing good close-up views of those giant Douglas-firs. On the left side of the trail coyote brush dominates, with some currant mixed in. This level stretch is a nice intermission between the ascent of Hamms Gulch and the descent of Spring Ridge.

Within audible range of CA 35 on the left, Lost Trail cuts across grassland on the high flanks of Windy Hill. Blue-eyed grass, mule ear sunflowers, fiddle-necks, and California poppy are common in early spring. Views east extend to Mount Diablo. At 4.2 miles, you'll reach a picnic area on the left, near the CA 35 trailhead. More than once I've seen hikers sprawled on top of the picnic tables, resting at either the midpoint or end of their journeys. Continue straight past the trailhead, now on Anniversary Trail, built and named to commemorate the 10th anniversary of Windy Hill's preservation.

The trail parallels CA 35, then veers right and makes the brief ascent to the hilltop. There are no formal trails to the actual top, but you can easily pick one of the paths that rise a few feet to the crest. If you've been wondering why the preserve is named Windy Hill, visit on a breezy day and the mystery will be revealed—air rushes unimpeded east from the ocean to this prominent Santa Cruz Mountains hilltop. A 360-degree panorama encompasses the Santa Clara Valley, Mounts Hamilton and Diablo, and soft grassy hills descending to the ocean. Once past the crest at 4.9 miles, the trail drops through coyote brush to a junction near a roadside parking area and CA 35. Turn right onto Spring Ridge Trail.

The broad fire road descends somewhat steeply through grassland. Look for blue-eyed grass, California poppy, lupines, and popcorn flower blooming in early spring. In the first stages of the descent, little huddles of coast live oak provide the only shade, but as Spring Ridge Trail heads downhill, woods begin a gradual squeeze toward the trail. Meadow Trail, the connector to Hamms Gulch Trail, sets off on the right at 6.5 miles. In April, blue and white lupines put on a good show in the grass on both sides of the trail at this junction. Continue to the left on Spring Ridge Trail. The grade thankfully eases to moderate as the trail winds through madrone, coast live oak, California bay, toyon, buckeye, and poison oak. California coffeeberry dangles red and black berries in late autumn to the delight of Windy Hill's bird and coyote population. Spring Ridge Trail emerges in an area dominated by coyote brush and offers some views east. The quad-aching descent finally ends at 6.8 miles at a junction with Betsy Crowder Trail. Turn left.

This gentle grade is welcome after Spring Ridge's descent. The trail is named in honor of Betsy Crowder, a guidebook author and Midpeninsula Regional Open Space District board member who died in 2000. In her 70s at the time of her death, Betsy was a vibrant and strong woman who worked tirelessly on preservation issues. Whenever I saw her at outdoor volunteer projects, I was amazed at her youthful spirit. Her namesake trail drifts through a grassy meadow favored by deer, then drops into a forest of California bay, madrone, buckeye, hazelnut, coffeeberry, and coast live oak. Sausal Pond is barely visible. In early spring, look for the dregs of blooming hound's tongue, plus trilliums and blue-dicks. The path curves right around a few massive eucalyptus and draws near a road outside the park boundary. Vinca, a nonnative ground cover, sprawls through the understory. If you peer through the trees on the right, you may notice a tall, level berm, which contains the north side of Sausal Pond.

At 7.4 miles, Betsy Crowder Trail ends. Turn left and return to the trailhead on the connector trail.

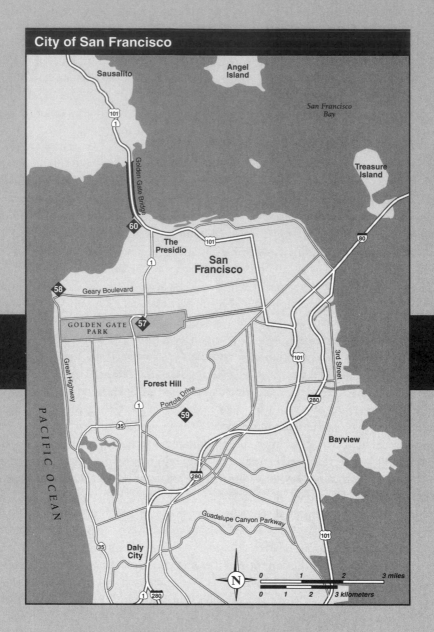

City of San Francisco

Sausalito

Angel Island

San Francisco Bay

101

1

Treasure Island

Golden Gate Bridge

60

The Presidio

101

San Francisco

1

80

58

Geary Boulevard

57

GOLDEN GATE PARK

3rd Street

Great Highway

Forest Hill

Portola Drive

101

59

1

280

35

Bayview

280

PACIFIC OCEAN

35

Daly City

Guadalupe Canyon Parkway

101

1 280

N

0   1   2   3 miles

0   1   2   3 kilometers

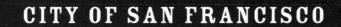

CITY OF SAN FRANCISCO

57 GOLDEN GATE PARK: STOW LAKE

KEY AT-A-GLANCE INFORMATION

LENGTH: 2.2 miles

CONFIGURATION: Spiral

DIFFICULTY: Easy

SCENERY: Pond, woods

EXPOSURE: Mix of shade and sun

TRAFFIC: Heavy

TRAIL SURFACE: Paved path and dirt trails

HIKING TIME: 1 hour

SEASON: Good anytime

ACCESS: Free

MAPS: None at the trailhead. *The Walker's Map of San Francisco*, published by Pease Press, is a good option ($7.95; peasepress.com). PDF and interactive maps available at golden-gate-park.com/category /maps.

FACILITIES: Restrooms, water, and food at the boathouse

SPECIAL COMMENTS: Dogs welcome if leashed or under voice control

CONTACTS: 415-831-2700, sfrecpark.org/destination/golden -gate-park

DRIVING DISTANCE: 4 miles from the San Francisco Civic Center

GPS INFORMATION

N37° 46.175' W122° 28.476'

IN BRIEF

Somewhere between a walk and a hike (a wake? a hilk?), this little jaunt spirals around Stow Lake and up to the top of Strawberry Hill.

DESCRIPTION

Beautiful Golden Gate Park is a manufactured masterpiece, transformed in the late 1800s from a sand-blown landscape of dunes. Over time, the land has been planted, shaped, and tweaked a million ways, and today GGP's more than 1,000 acres host an incredible assortment of activities: There are grassy meadows for picnics, museums, sports fields, ponds, and playgrounds.

The park's paths range from wide and paved to narrow and dirt, but there is little actual hiking to be found. Many areas of the park offer lovely strolls, and if that's what you're after, consider the Arboretum or North Lake. Park visitors can get a sense of our native landscape in the oak-woodlands section (just north of the Conservatory of Flowers), but the trails in that part of GGP are short and can feel a bit seedy.

Directions ———————————➤

From northbound 19th Avenue in San Francisco, just as you enter Golden Gate Park, turn right onto Martin Luther King Jr. Drive. After 0.2 mile, turn left onto Stow Lake Drive. Follow the road around the lake and past the boathouse, and where the road splits, stay to the right. Park near the yellow gate on the right.

From southbound 19th Avenue in San Francisco, in Golden Gate Park, turn right onto Crossover Drive. After 0.1 mile, turn left onto Transverse Drive, then left again onto John F. Kennedy Drive. After 0.4 mile, turn right onto Stow Lake Drive; where the road splits, stay to the left. Park near the yellow gate on the right.

Golden Gate Park: Stow Lake

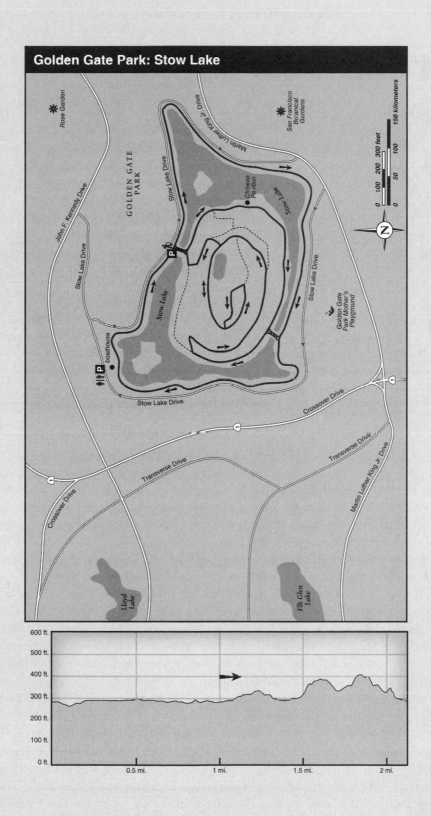

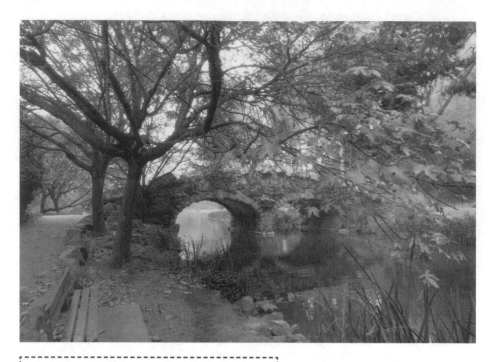

Scenic old stone bridge and colorful maples at Stow Lake

My favorite GGP destination for hybrid walk/hikes is Strawberry Hill, which is perhaps better known for its surrounding artificial moat, Stow Lake. A flat, paved trail rings the lake, and dirt paths and stairs wind up and down the hill, allowing walkers to create a variety of exercise routes. The hill and lake offer excellent city bird-watching with frequent surprises, like glimpses of great horned owls, red-tailed hawks, and great blue herons.

Start at the yellow-gated bridge on the lake's north side. For a quicker walk, you can head right over the bridge, but to get the most out of your excursion, begin walking east on the paved trail, following in the same direction as the one-way park road. The trail is a popular route for walkers and stroller-pushers. Look to the right for a view to one of the lake's small tree-dotted islands. Common waterfowl, including American coots and mallards, are year-round natives around the lake. You'll also likely see (and hear) Canada geese, Brewer's blackbirds, pigeons, and crows. I was surprised once to come across a soft-shell turtle along the trail—must have been dumped here, as is the fate of some Muscovy ducks who have been "retired" at the lake.

The paved trail curves around the east edge of the lake, offering great views across the water to man-made Huntington Falls and the Chinese Pavilion. On the south shore, at 0.58 mile, you'll pass one of GGP's treasures, Rustic Bridge, constructed in 1893. This pretty little bridge crosses the lake and connects to Strawberry Hill, but our route continues straight around the lake on the paved path.

Traffic noise from Transverse Drive (out of sight to the west) is heavy here as the path bends north and heads towards the boathouse area. Look right to the lake's largest island, where great blue herons commonly nest in spring. Pass the boathouse (or stop here for a bathroom break, food and drink, or a boat rental) and now follow the path east. At 1 mile, you'll reach the walk's starting point, at the yellow gate. Turn right across the bridge.

At the end of the bridge, turn left onto the dirt trail. For now ignore the stairs and paths that head uphill to the right, continuing on the flat trail as it crosses the bottom of Huntington Falls, a popular destination for wedding photos, then passes through a grove of planted redwoods. Once past the Chinese Pavilion, the path bends right. You'll typically encounter tons of squirrel beggars along the trail here. At 1.35 miles, pass the other side of the stone bridge and continue on the dirt path, which sweeps slightly uphill to the right and reaches an unsigned junction at 1.45 miles. Turn right, then, after a few steps uphill, right again.

The wide dirt trail climbs gently through some Monterey pines, which block most of the views south. At 1.7 miles, the trail flattens at a junction. Steps head back downhill to the right. A wide trail doubles back toward the left, heading to the hilltop, but continue straight on the trail that runs along a tiny fenced reservoir.

Lucky, sharp-eyed hikers might get a glimpse of great-horned owls which often nest in the trees in this part of Golden Gate Park. I seem to be blind to them, but many more-skilled birders spot them during nesting season and sometimes after the birds have fledged. The trail is level along the reservoir but then climbs again, passing a grove of toyon and coast live oak on the left. At 1.83 miles, pass a set of steps on the left and continue straight.

As you make the final push to the hilltop, notice surprisingly tall and sturdy pines and cypress trees along the trail. At 1.9 miles, the trail reaches the flattened top of Strawberry Hill. An interpretive panel prompts visitors to look for butterflies here, and sure enough, there are commonly swallowtails, admirals, and ladies fluttering about in warm, sunny weather. Turn left to admire a partial view north to the Golden Gate Bridge and Marin Headlands. The rocky rubble on the east side of the hilltop is the remains of an observatory that was destroyed by the 1906 earthquake.

When ready, follow a sandy path west along the crest of the hill. The path descends through a cluster of native shrubs, including lizard's-tail, coyote brush, lupine, and native blackberry. Buckwheat blooms here in summer. Old stone steps drop to a junction with the fire road, at 1.97 miles. Turn right.

Retrace your steps past the reservoir back to the junction at 2.08 miles. Turn left onto a trail (with a green handrail) that quickly descends and forks. Bear left and descend more steps to a junction, at lake level, at 2.17 miles. Retrace your steps back across the bridge to the trailhead.

58 LANDS END

KEY AT-A-GLANCE INFORMATION

LENGTH: 2.8 miles

CONFIGURATION: Out-and-back

DIFFICULTY: Easy

SCENERY: Coastline

EXPOSURE: Mix of shade and sun

TRAFFIC: Heavy

TRAIL SURFACE: Dirt fire road and trail with many steps

HIKING TIME: 2 hours

SEASON: Good anytime

ACCESS: Free

MAPS: Trail map (under glass) at the trailhead's information signboard and at the website in Contacts, below. *The Walker's Map of San Francisco*, published by Pease Press, shows all trails in the area ($7.95; peasepress.com).

FACILITIES: Restrooms, water, and food at the visitor center

SPECIAL COMMENTS: Dogs welcome if leashed or under voice control. Be mindful of the additional dog regulations posted along the trails.

CONTACTS: 415-426-5240, parksconservancy.org/visit /park-sites/lands-end.html

DRIVING DISTANCE: 5.5 miles from the San Francisco Civic Center

GPS INFORMATION

N37° 46.856' W122° 30.702'

IN BRIEF

Lands End is a rugged bit of coastline in the northwest corner of San Francisco, around the bend from the historic Cliff House and the flat expanse of Ocean Beach. Locals come here to jog or walk the trails, while tourists enjoy the views of the Golden Gate Bridge.

DESCRIPTION

Coastal Trail is the "main street" at Lands End, popular with local runners, dog-walkers, stroller-pushing parents, and folks from out of town. Camino del Mar Trail runs along the bluff above Coastal Trail, departing from the War Memorial parking lot and ending near the Palace of the Legion of Honor. You can make a loop of both trails, but I don't recommend it, as this loop entails walking down the middle of a street dedicated to museum parking as well as a sidewalk past the museum and golf course.

In addition to trekking out and back on Coastal Trail, hikers can explore spur paths leading to the Sutro Bath ruins and Lands End proper. Veteran hikers will likely find Coastal Trail lovely but tame. The round trip to Eagle's Point is less than 3 miles, and the elevation change (albeit for two sets of steps) is slight. It's a good choice for beginners because it's an out-and-back hike—simply head back to the trailhead when you've had enough.

Directions

Lands End is in northwest San Francisco. Drive west on Geary Boulevard, which, past 39th Avenue westbound, becomes Point Lobos Avenue. Continue west on Point Lobos, cross 48th Avenue, and turn right into the parking lot, on the right side of the street—if you reach the Cliff House, you've gone too far.

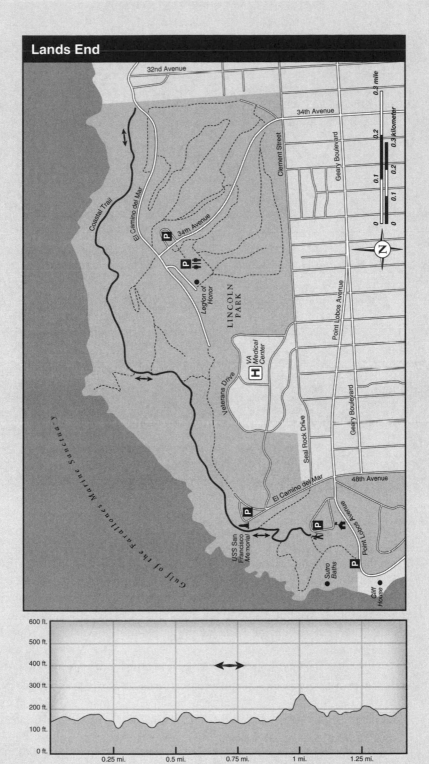

Lands End

32nd Avenue

34th Avenue

Clement Street

Geary Boulevard

0.3 mile

0.2

0.1

0

0.3 kilometer

0.2

0.1

0

El Camino del Mar

Coastal Trail

34th Avenue

P

P

Legion of Honor

LINCOLN PARK

Point Lobos Avenue

VA Medical Center
H

Veterans Drive

Seal Rock Drive

Geary Boulevard

48th Avenue

El Camino del Mar

P

P

P

USS San Francisco Memorial

Point Lobos Avenue

Sutro Baths

Cliff House

Gulf of the Farallones Marine Sanctuary

600 ft.

500 ft.

400 ft.

300 ft.

200 ft.

100 ft.

0 ft.

0.25 mi.   0.5 mi.   0.75 mi.   1 mi.   1.25 mi.

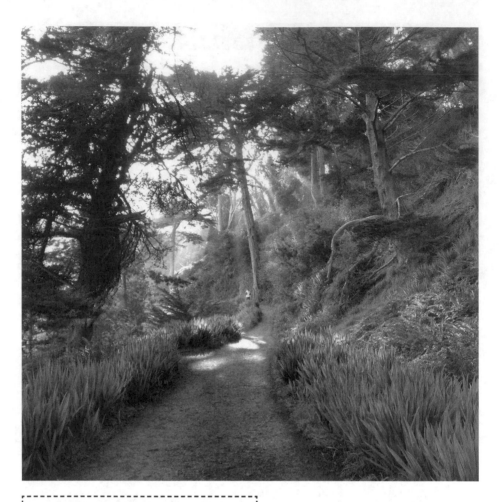

Sun filters through Monterey pines on Coastal Trail.

If you're new to San Francisco, or to hiking, do use caution at Lands End: Stay back from the steep, unprotected drop-offs along some stretches of the trail, stay on the trails, and learn to recognize and avoid poison oak. I would not normally issue these cautions, but it's not uncommon for folks to get lost or stranded at Lands End, particularly on the rocks at the coastline. Don't wreck your day with a helicopter rescue!

Begin from the parking lot at Merrie Way. A big, pleasant parking lot and an information display greet you. A visitor center hosts interpretive displays, restrooms, and a cafe. Ascend a few stairs to a kiosk with a map and information about Lands End; then begin hiking on Coastal Trail. Tall Monterey pines tower over a restored area with a lovely assortment of native plants, including buckwheat, bush lupines, coyote brush, monkeyflower, lizard's-tail, and yarrow. Just before the wide paved trail sweeps back to the right, a signed trail descends left to the Sutro Bath area. Continue straight on Coastal Trail.

A second gentle curve swings the trail north again, climbing slightly. Where a second paved trail enters from the right, bear left. Soon you'll reach the first interpretive panel—although Lands End appears relatively untouched by civilization, a railroad ran along the coast here in the 1880s, and in the 1900s ships wrecked on the rocks (some sharp-eyed hikers can spot the wrecks during low tide). Visit on a foggy day and get an earful of the foghorns described on one panel—each horn has a different tone to assist ships navigating through our local pea soup.

At 0.3 mile, Coastal Trail reaches a signed junction and overlook. On a clear day, views sweep north across the water to the Marin Headlands and the Golden Gate Bridge. A set of steps leads up the War Memorial area, but our route straight, continues on Coastal Trail.

A retaining wall on the right holds up a hillside dotted with Monterey pines. At a second overlook, the trail shifts to dirt but remains nearly flat—if you're visiting with a stroller or in a wheelchair, you'll most likely want to turn around here. Beware a massive hedge of poison oak on the left shortly before Coastal Trail passes an unmarked path heading uphill on the right. Continue straight. The trail rolls up and down a bit over loose, sandy soil. Another trail, this one signed, breaks off to the right. Again, continue straight on Coastal Trail.

Thickets of willow and cypress crowd the trail. Cheerful orange-colored nasturtiums drape over the trailside shrubs; you might also see poison hemlock, with white, lacy flowers and purple-blotched stems. At 0.8 mile, a paved trail enters from the right, leading up through the Lincoln Park golf course to the Palace of the Legion of Honor. Continue left on Coastal Trail.

Shortly past the junction, a signed trail near the emergency call box heads downhill to the left, leading to the actual Lands End—a nice side trip to a rocky beach (not described here), but note that the climb back up is rough.

On Coastal Trail, a set of ascending steps brings the easy section of this hike to an end. Look for native strawberry and yerba buena plants on the grassy hill to the right. The trail crests and almost immediately begins to drop, again on steps. Eucalyptus and cypress trees shade the trail and screen most of the view, but as the trail sweeps downhill a dramatic vista north across the Golden Gate opens up.

The trail hugs the coast, then turns slightly inland near Deadman's Point, passing through more eucalyptus before emerging with sweet coastal views, now including the posh Sea Cliff neighborhood slightly to the northeast. You may see or hear some common Bay Area birds here, including chickadees and a variety of sparrows. At 1.4 miles, the golf course is visible on the right and Coastal Trail reaches Eagle's Point on the left.

The trail ends here, at 32nd Avenue and Camino del Mar. After soaking in the views, retrace your steps back to the trailhead.

59 MOUNT DAVIDSON

i KEY AT-A-GLANCE INFORMATION

LENGTH: 1 mile

CONFIGURATION: Balloon

DIFFICULTY: Easy

SCENERY: Grassland and woods, city views

EXPOSURE: Mix of shade and sun

TRAFFIC: Light

TRAIL SURFACE: Dirt trails

HIKING TIME: 1 hour or less

SEASON: Good anytime

ACCESS: Free

MAPS: None at the trailhead. *The Walker's Map of San Francisco,* published by Pease Press, is a good option ($7.95; peasepress.com). Website below links to Google Maps.

FACILITIES: None

SPECIAL COMMENTS: Dogs welcome if leashed or under voice control

CONTACTS: sfrecpark.org/destination /mt-davidson-park

DRIVING DISTANCE: 4.6 miles from the San Francisco Civic Center

GPS INFORMATION

N37° 44.211' W122° 27.234'

IN BRIEF

This easy hike winds through woods and grassland on San Francisco's highest hill.

DESCRIPTION

Mount Davidson, at 938 feet, is the highest natural point in San Francisco but is often overlooked as a hiking destination. Most locals recognize MD as the hill with the cross on top; film buffs remember it from *Dirty Harry.* But as those late-night infomercials say, wait, there's more!

The 40-acre Mount Davidson Park is laced with trails that offer expansive views. It's also enjoyable in the fog, when the swirling mist muffles noise from the surrounding city and sporadic birdsong drifts through the woods.

Although Mount Davidson is a small park completely surrounded by development, the trails are unsigned and it's surprisingly easy to get lost in the woods. Be sure to follow my directions closely and check to make sure

----

Directions ——————————→

From northbound CA 1 (19th Avenue) in San Francisco, bear right onto Junipero Serra Boulevard. Junipero Serra ends at Sloat Boulevard—continue straight/right, now on Portola Drive. After about 0.7 mile, turn right at a traffic light onto Marne Avenue (same junction as Miraloma Drive). Drive one block on Marne and turn right onto Lansdale Avenue. Drive one block and turn left onto Dalewood Way. Drive one block uphill on steep Dalewood to the park entrance, at the junction of Lansdale and Dalewood.

Note: Feel free to consult a map and create your own directions. Many other streets reach the park, but you'll need a map unless you're familiar with the neighborhood.

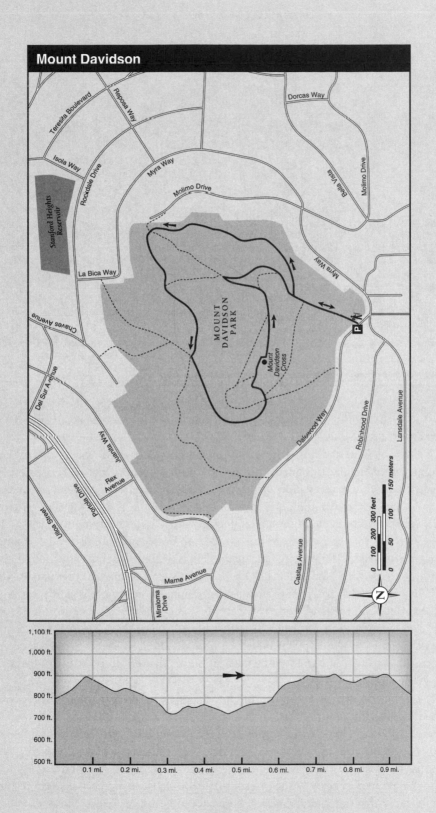

Mount Davidson

Teresita Boulevard
Reposa Way
Dorcas Way
Isola Way
Rockdale Drive
Myra Way
Bella Vista
Molino Drive
Molimo Drive
Stanford Heights Reservoir
La Bica Way
Myra Way
Chaves Avenue
P/R
MOUNT DAVIDSON PARK
Mount Davidson Cross
Del Sur Avenue
Dalewood Way
Robinhood Drive
Lansdale Avenue
Juanita Way
Rex Avenue
Casitas Avenue
Portola Drive
Ulloa Street
Marne Avenue
Miraloma Drive

0 100 200 300 feet
0 50 100 150 meters

N

1,100 ft.
1,000 ft.
900 ft.
800 ft.
700 ft.
600 ft.
500 ft.

0.1 mi. 0.2 mi. 0.3 mi. 0.4 mi. 0.5 mi. 0.6 mi. 0.7 mi. 0.8 mi. 0.9 mi.

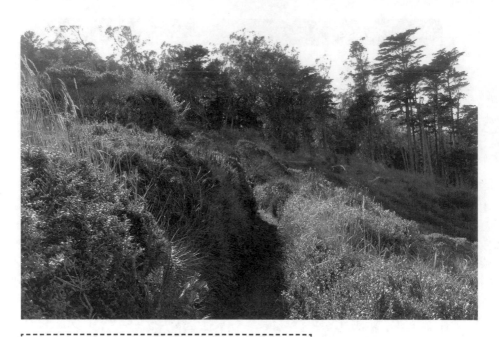

You'll squeeze through huckleberry shrubs on Mount Davidson.

you're on the right track, especially at the junction in the woods at the end of the native-treasures segment.

Starting from the bus stop at the junction of Dalewood Way and Lansdale Avenue, head up the unsigned but obvious trail. Within a few feet, a forest of eucalyptus and Monterey pine shades the broad dirt path. The understory here is mostly blackberry and nonnative plants, including some showy fuchsias. After a brief climb, you'll reach an unsigned junction at 0.1 mile. Bear right.

The trail moves away from the woods into grassland, initially hugging a tall fence on the right. The rocky cut on the left is a good place to spot blue-dicks blooming in spring. Red-tailed hawks are often seen hunting on this part of the hill, and crowned sparrows and phoebes are common. Descending gently, the trail sweeps through grassland dotted with ferns and coyote brush, just upslope from the park boundary on the right. It then rises a bit and crosses a rocky outcrop. Views north to downtown San Francisco unfold. The trail squeezes past a second fence. At 0.3 mile, unsigned paths head uphill to the left and out of the park to the right. Continue straight.

As the trail curves around to the north slope of the mountain, trailside vegetation shifts from grassland to coastal scrub. There are lots of lovely native-plant treasures to enjoy here, including huckleberry, creambush, monkeyflower, coyote brush, currant, and snowberry. A few feet before the trail heads back into the woods, at about 0.39 mile, a rough path ascends on the left. Continue straight.

A large serviceberry shrub stands off to the left—to my knowledge, Mount Davidson is the sole San Francisco home for this native shrub. Eucalyptus and

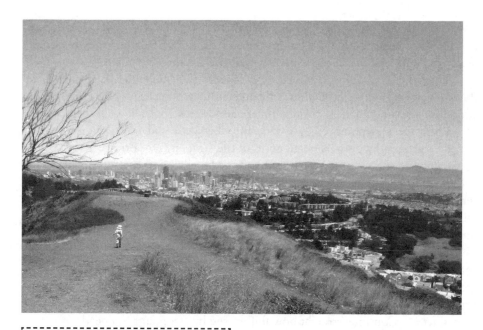

A gorgeous city view from the mountaintop

Monterey pine shade the trail as it keeps to an easy grade. This is a very good stretch of woods for bird-watching—look (or listen) for chickadees, northern flickers, and wrens. Scrub jays are common, but I've seen Steller's jays too, as well as many hummingbirds. Mixed through red elderberry and ferns, the understory blackberry bushes produce tasty fruit during warm summers, but on cold years they fail to thrive. At 0.47 mile, you'll reach an important but unsigned junction—bear left.

The trail ascends through pine and eucalyptus; invasive ivy blocks out nearly every understory plant save blackberry. The trail passes a rock outcrop and bends left. At 0.61 mile, the trail ends at a fire road. Cross the road and continue straight.

Ascend a set of pretty stone steps. Look for yerba buena, a tiny-leaved trailing native plant, growing on the right. Crush a leaf to release its powerful, sweet mint scent. As the stone steps end, continue a few feet more, then turn left and ascend again.

The steps, constructed from wood planks and logs, are steep. Notice that the bunchgrasses crowding the trail remain green year-round. The first time I ascended to the top of Mount Davidson it was socked in, and as I walked, the soft, pale, billowing fog wrapped around me like a fleece blanket. It's so damp on this part of the mountain that ferns grow in the crooks and stumps of some of the eucalyptus, pine, and cypress trees. The steps end at a clearing, to the left. Bear right and ascend the final steps to the mountaintop and the cross.

This flat summit is a broad clearing dominated by the Mount Davidson cross. Constructed in 1934, the cross and lands immediately surrounding it were sold by the city in 1997 to the Council of Armenian American Organizations of Northern

California to commemorate the Armenian genocide of 1915–1923. Throngs of people visit on Easter, but the rest of the year is quite peaceful. After inspecting the cross, walk east along the wide, flat trail toward the viewpoint.

Butterflies love hilltops, and butterfly lovers will be delighted by their colorful fluttering at the mountaintop in summer and autumn. Sometimes I see common red admirals and painted ladies, but often there are dozens of swallowtails here, too.

From the viewpoint, enjoy wonderful views east and north. Unfortunately, the city's geography permits no glimpses of the Golden Gate Bridge. When you're ready, descend the set of steps to the left of the large metal water-department box. This hillside has been seeded with lupines, yarrow, and sagebrush. Look for more serviceberry shrubs here, with conspicuous white flowers in April and May. At 0.8 mile, the trail continues straight to a lower viewpoint (explore it if you like), but our route continues to the right.

The trail passes over rocky ground where I've seen garter snakes (the only snakes I've ever encountered within San Francisco's city limits). In spring, California poppies and buckwheat bloom along the path. After a brief descent—watch for poison oak on the right mixed through blackberry—you'll return to the hike's first junction. Continue straight downhill to the bus stop and trailhead.

THE PRESIDIO:
BATTERIES TO BLUFFS TRAIL

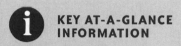

IN BRIEF

Think of a dream San Francisco hike: a path overlooking the ocean, with gorgeous views of the Golden Gate Bridge; a peaceful place where you could sit and watch the waves crash, or get your morning exercise running through a scenic landscape while birds sing and flowers bloom. You don't have to imagine this trail, because it already exists—it's the Batteries to Bluffs Trail in The Presidio.

DESCRIPTION

Batteries to Bluffs Trail runs parallel to and downslope from Lincoln Boulevard and consists mostly of sets of steps and some flat sections of trail. You can hike in either direction, starting from the parking lot at the Golden Gate Overlook, as described here, or from the side-of-the-street parking on Lincoln Boulevard (this is my preferred trailhead, but there isn't much parking).

Begin at the parking area near Golden Gate Overlook. If you want to take in the view

----

Directions

From southbound US 101 in San Francisco, just past the Golden Gate Bridge toll plaza, turn right onto Merchant Road. After about 500 feet, turn right onto Lincoln Boulevard, then almost immediately right again into the parking lot at Golden Gate Overlook, or continue to side-of-the-road parking on Lincoln near Kobbe Avenue.

From northbound 19th Avenue in San Francisco, bear left onto Crossover Drive in Golden Gate Park. Continue, now on 25th Avenue, to the junction with El Camino del Mar. Turn right. Continue, now on Lincoln, into The Presidio, to side-of-the-road parking near the junction with Kobbe Avenue, or to the parking lot at Golden Gate Overlook.

KEY AT-A-GLANCE INFORMATION

LENGTH: 1.9 miles

CONFIGURATION: Out-and-back

DIFFICULTY: Easy

SCENERY: Coastline, beach, Golden Gate Bridge views

EXPOSURE: Almost completely exposed

TRAFFIC: Moderate

TRAIL SURFACE: Dirt fire roads and trail with many steps

HIKING TIME: 1 hour

SEASON: Good anytime

ACCESS: Free

MAPS: At the trailhead's information signboard and nps.gov/goga/plan yourvisit/maps.htm. *The Walker's Map of San Francisco,* **published by Pease Press, is another good option ($7.95; peasepress.com).**

FACILITIES: None

SPECIAL COMMENTS: No dogs allowed

CONTACTS: 415-561-4323, presidio.gov

DRIVING DISTANCE: 5 miles from the San Francisco Civic Center

GPS INFORMATION

N37° 48.207' W122° 28.609'

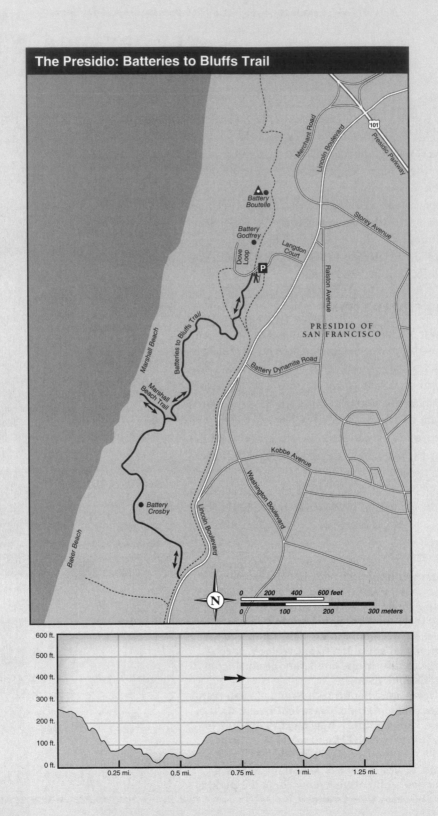

The Presidio: Batteries to Bluffs Trail

Battery Boutelle

Battery Godfrey

Dove Loop

Langdon Court

Merchant Road

Lincoln Boulevard

Storey Avenue

Presidio Parkway

101

Ralston Avenue

PRESIDIO OF SAN FRANCISCO

Battery Dynamite Road

Marshall Beach

Batteries to Bluffs Trail

Marshall Beach Trail

Kobbe Avenue

Washington Boulevard

Battery Crosby

Baker Beach

Lincoln Boulevard

N

0   200   400   600 feet

0   100   200   300 meters

600 ft.

500 ft.

400 ft.

300 ft.

200 ft.

100 ft.

0 ft.

0.25 mi.   0.5 mi.   0.75 mi.   1 mi.   1.25 mi.

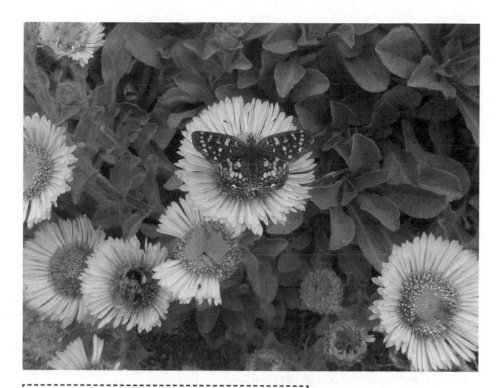

A bee and a butterfly stop to peruse the blooms along the trail.

of the Golden Gate, follow the paved path to the north, then return to the parking lot when ready. Three different paths depart to the south: one edging along Lincoln, the second where a driveway connects two segments of parking lots, and a third on the western edge of the second parking lot. All three join, but for this hike, take the middle path.

The wide dirt trail weaves through a thin forest of Monterey cypress and pine. The understory is mostly invasive ivy. At .07 mile, bear right (the path left leads to the Pacific Overlook on Lincoln). A sign at the top of wooden steps marks the start of Batteries to Bluffs Trail.

And here you'll begin the descent, with the trail already showing off fantastic views south to Lands End. In autumn you may see white-crowned sparrows flitting from ceanothus to coyote brush shrubs. Poison oak is a near-constant companion along the path. In spring look for purple iris in bloom. The steps keep dropping, and the trail passes a bare rocky hillside. At 0.22 mile, note an overlook with a bench on the right—this is an excellent rest stop on the way back uphill. The trail descends again, passing through a clump of willows. At 0.43 mile, turn right at the signed junction with Marshall Beach Trail.

The narrow path descends, then ends at one last set of stairs leading to the beach, at 0.5 mile. Here, you can gaze north to the Golden Gate Bridge and the Marin Headlands. I often see brown pelicans flying in formation overhead, and on

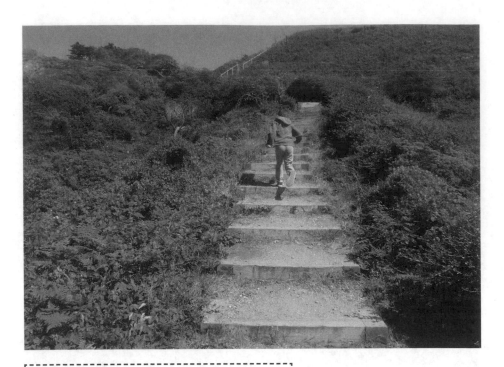

Batteries to Bluffs Trail ascends through lush coastal scrub.

one September visit, I was delighted to watch a pod of porpoises cavorting offshore. Explore the beach if you like; when ready, retrace your steps back to the junction with Batteries to Bluffs Trail, then turn right.

The trail crosses a year-round trickling stream. Toyon, coyote brush, and coffeeberry thrive here. Soon, Batteries to Bluffs Trail begins to climb—yes, more steps! At the top, the trail heads over the top of Battery Crosby; use caution here so you don't fall down to the left. As you enjoy views south to Baker Beach, watch for lizards scampering about. A few more steps head down to join a wide dirt track that leads up to Lincoln Boulevard. You could start back toward the Golden Gate Overlook now, at 0.83 mile, but consider walking up to Lincoln and the official end of the trail. If you do, you'll likely see purple bush lupine as well as San Francisco wallflower, buckwheat, and other lovely wildflowers blooming here in spring. This is also the section of trail where I commonly spot coyote scat.

When you're ready, retrace your steps back to the trailhead.

APPENDIX A:
HIKING CLUBS AND INFORMATION SOURCES

BAY AREA HIKER
bahiker.com

I created this website in 1999 to explore the diverse and wonderful spectrum of hikes in the San Francisco Bay Area. Here you'll find detailed descriptions and photos of more than 200 hikes, along with discussion forums. Bay Area Hiker is also an exceptional resource (if I do say so myself) for identifying local flora and fauna. For the companion Facebook page, go to **tinyurl.com/bahiker.** —*J. H.*

BAY AREA RIDGE TRAIL COUNCIL
ridgetrail.org
1007 General Kennedy Ave., Ste. 3
San Francisco, CA 94129
415-561-2599

BERKELEY HIKING CLUB
berkeleyhikingclub.pair.com
P.O. Box 9762
Berkeley, CA 94709

CALIFORNIA ALPINE CLUB
calalpineclub.org
P.O. Box 2180
Mill Valley, CA 94942-2180

CALIFORNIA DEPARTMENT OF PARKS AND RECREATION
www.parks.ca.gov
1416 9th St.
Sacramento, CA 95814
800-777-0369

CONFUSED OUTDOOR CLUB
confused.org

EAST BAY REGIONAL PARK DISTRICT
ebparks.org
P.O. Box 5381
Oakland, CA 94605-0381
888-327-2757

FRIENDS OF MT TAM
friendsofmttam.org
P.O. Box 7064
Corte Madera, CA 94976
415-258-2410

GREENBELT ALLIANCE
greenbelt.org
631 Howard St., Ste. 510
San Francisco, CA 94105
415-543-6771

INTREPID NORTHERN CALIFORNIA HIKERS (INCH)
rawbw.com/~svw/inch/index.php

MARIN COUNTY OPEN SPACE DISTRICT
marincountyparks.org/depts/pk /divisions/open-space
3501 Civic Center Dr., Room 260
San Rafael, CA 94903
415-499-6387

MIDPENINSULA REGIONAL OPEN SPACE DISTRICT
openspace.org
330 Distel Cir.
Los Altos, CA 94022-1404
650-691-1200

APPENDIX A
(CONTINUED)

**MOUNT DIABLO
INTERPRETIVE ASSOCIATION**
mdia.org
P.O. Box 346
Walnut Creek, CA 94597-0346
925-927-7222

SAN MATEO COUNTY PARKS
www.co.sanmateo.ca.us/portal
/site/parks
555 County Center, 5th Floor
Redwood City, CA 94063-1646
650-363-4020

SANTA CLARA COUNTY PARKS
sccgov.org/portal/site/parks
298 Garden Hill Dr.
Los Gatos, CA 95032
408-355-2200

**SANTA CRUZ MOUNTAIN TRAIL
ASSOCIATION**
scmta-trails.org
P.O. Box 1141
Los Altos, CA 94023

**SIERRA CLUB,
LOMA PRIETA CHAPTER**
lomaprieta.sierraclub.org
3921 E. Bayshore Rd.
Palo Alto, CA 94303
650-390-8411

**SIERRA CLUB,
SAN FRANCISCO CHAPTER**
sanfranciscobay.sierraclub.org/hiking
2530 San Pablo Ave., Ste. I
Berkeley, CA 94702-2000
510-848-0800

TRAIL CENTER
trailcenter.org
3921 E. Bayshore Rd.
Palo Alto, CA 94303
650-968-7065

APPENDIX B:
PLACES TO BUY MAPS

ANY MOUNTAIN
anymountain.net

Berkeley
2777 Shattuck Ave.
Berkeley, CA 94705
510-665-3939

Concord
THE WILLOWS SHOPPING CENTER
1975 Diamond Blvd.
Concord, CA 94520
925-674-0174

Corte Madera
71 Tamal Vista Blvd.
Corte Madera, CA 94925
415-927-0170

Dublin
4906 Dublin Ave.
Dublin, CA 94568
925-875-1115

Fremont
43485 Boscell Rd.
Fremont, CA 94538
510-498-8510

Redwood City
928 Whipple Ave.
Redwood City, CA 94063
650-361-1213

San Jose
1600 Saratoga Ave.
San Jose, CA 95129
408-871-1001

LOMBARDI SPORTS
lombardisports.com
1600 Jackson St.
San Francisco, CA 94109
888-456-6223 or 415-771-0600

PEASE PRESS
peasepress.com
1717 Cabrillo St.
San Francisco, CA 94121
415-387-1437

REI
rei.com

Berkeley
1338 San Pablo Ave.
Berkeley, CA 94702
510-527-4140

Brentwood
2475 Sand Creek Rd.
Brentwood, CA 94513
925-516-3540

Concord
THE WILLOWS SHOPPING CENTER
1975 Diamond Blvd., Ste. B-100
Concord, CA 94520
925-825-9400

Corte Madera
213 Corte Madera Town Center
Corte Madera, CA 94925
415-927-1938

Dublin
7099 Amador Plaza Rd.
Dublin, CA 94568
925-828-9826

Fremont
43962 Fremont Blvd.
Fremont, CA 94538
510-651-0305

Mountain View
2450 Charleston Rd.
Mountain View, CA 94043
650-969-1938

APPENDIX B
(CONTINUED)

REI (*continued*)

San Carlos
1119 Industrial Rd., Ste. A
San Carlos, CA 94070
650-508-2330

San Francisco
840 Brannan St.
San Francisco, CA 94103
415-934-1938

San Jose
400 El Paseo de Saratoga
San Jose, CA 95130
408-871-8765

Santa Rosa
2715 Santa Rosa Ave.
Santa Rosa, CA 95407
707-540-9025

SONOMA OUTFITTERS
sonomaoutfitters.com
145 3rd St.
Santa Rosa, CA 95401
800-290-1920 or 707-528-1920

TOM HARRISON MAPS
tomharrisonmaps.com

APPENDIX C:
HIKING STORES

ANY MOUNTAIN
anymountain.net
See page 289 for locations.

LOMBARDI SPORTS
lombardisports.com
1600 Jackson St.
San Francisco, CA 94109
888-456-6223 or 415-771-0600

REI
rei.com
See page 289 for locations.

SONOMA OUTFITTERS
sonomaoutfitters.com
145 3rd St.
Santa Rosa, CA 95401
800 290 1920 or 707-528-1920

SPORTS AUTHORITY
sportsauthority.com

Brentwood
5641 Lone Tree Way
Brentwood, CA 94513
925-513-6648

Concord
1235 Concord Ave.
Concord, CA 94520
925-687-6300

185 Sun Valley Mall
Concord, CA 94520
925-685-1022

Corte Madera
435 Corte Madera Town Center
Corte Madera, CA 94925
415-927-1464

Daly City
301 Gellert Blvd.
Daly City, CA 94015
650-301-9000

Dublin
7885 Dublin Blvd.
Dublin, CA 94568
925-556-3504

East Palo Alto
1775 E. Bayshore Rd.
East Palo Alto, CA 94303
650-838-0715

Emeryville
3839 Emery St., Ste. 300
Emeryville, CA 94608
510-450-9400

Fairfield
1451 Gateway Blvd.
Fairfield, CA 94533
707-399-9578

Fremont
43485 Boscell Rd.
Fremont, CA 94538
510-498-8510

Milpitas
GREAT MALL OF THE BAY AREA
1200 Great Mall Dr.
Milpitas, CA 95035
408-934-0280

111 Ranch Dr.
Milpitas, CA 95035
408-934-3000

Mountain View
635 San Antonio Rd.
Mountain View, CA 94040
650-941-8611

APPENDIX C
(CONTINUED)

SPORTS AUTHORITY (*continued*)

Novato
212 Vintage Way, Bldg. L-1
Novato, CA 94945
415-892-2060

San Francisco
233 Winston Dr.
San Francisco, CA 94132
415-682-8605

1690 Folsom St.
San Francisco, CA 94103
415-734-9373

San Jose
680 Blossom Hill Rd.
San Jose, CA 95123
408-229-6200

5170 Stevens Creek Blvd.
San Jose, CA 95129
408-244-4525

San Leandro
1933 Davis St.
San Leandro, CA 94577
510-632-6100

San Mateo
2250 Bridgepointe Pkwy.
San Mateo, CA 94403
650-286-9900

Santa Clara
2855 Stevens Creek Blvd., Ste. 1002
Santa Clara, CA 95050
408-261-1922

Santa Rosa
1970 Santa Rosa Ave.
Santa Rosa, CA 95407
707-523-4700

Sunnyvale
125 E. El Camino Real
Sunnyvale, CA 94086
408-732-6400

Union City
31200 Court House Dr.
Union City, CA 94587
510-491-0473

Vacaville
1071 Helen Power Dr.
Vacaville, CA 95687
707-451-6800

Walnut Creek
Plaza Escuela
1675 Olympic Blvd.
Walnut Creek, CA 94596
925-942-0490

SPORTS BASEMENT
sportsbasement.com

Campbell
THE PRUNEYARD
1875 S. Bascom Ave., Ste. 240
Campbell, CA 95008
408-899-5783

San Francisco
1590 Bryant St.
San Francisco, CA 94103
415-575-3000

THE PRESIDIO OF SAN FRANCISCO
610 Old Mason St.
San Francisco, CA 94129
415-437-0100

Sunnyvale
1177 Kern Ave.
Sunnyvale, CA 94085
408-732-0300

Walnut Creek
1881 Ygnacio Valley Rd.
Walnut Creek, CA 94598
925-941-6100

INDEX

DEAR CUSTOMERS AND FRIENDS,

SUPPORTING YOUR INTEREST IN OUTDOOR ADVENTURE, travel, and an active lifestyle is central to our operations, from the authors we choose to the locations we detail to the way we design our books. Menasha Ridge Press was incorporated in 1982 by a group of veteran outdoorsmen and professional outfitters. For many years now, we've specialized in creating books that benefit the outdoors enthusiast.

Almost immediately, Menasha Ridge Press earned a reputation for revolutionizing outdoors- and travel-guidebook publishing. For such activities as canoeing, kayaking, hiking, backpacking, and mountain biking, we established new standards of quality that transformed the whole genre, resulting in outdoor-recreation guides of great sophistication and solid content. Menasha Ridge continues to be outdoor publishing's greatest innovator.

The folks at Menasha Ridge Press are as at home on a white-water river or mountain trail as they are editing a manuscript. The books we build for you are the best they can be, because we're responding to your needs. Plus, we use and depend on them ourselves.

We look forward to seeing you on the river or the trail. If you'd like to contact us directly, join in at www.trekalong.com or visit us at www.menasharidge.com. We thank you for your interest in our books and the natural world around us all.

SAFE TRAVELS,

Bob Sehlinger

BOB SEHLINGER
PUBLISHER

3 1901 05773 5237